# Drug Hepatotoxicity

*Editor*

NIKOLAOS T. PYRSOPOULOS

# CLINICS IN LIVER DISEASE

www.liver.theclinics.com

*Consulting Editor*
NORMAN GITLIN

November 2013 • Volume 17 • Number 4

**ELSEVIER**

1600 John F. Kennedy Boulevard • Suite 1800 • Philadelphia, Pennsylvania, 19103-2899

http://www.theclinics.com

**CLINICS IN LIVER DISEASE Volume 17, Number 4**
**November 2013 ISSN 1089-3261, ISBN-13: 978-0-323-26106-7**

Editor: Kerry Holland
Developmental Editor: Donald Mumford

*Clinics in Liver Disease* (ISSN 1089-3261) is published quarterly by Elsevier Inc., 360 Park Avenue South, New York, NY 10010-1710. Months of issue are February, May, August, and November. Business and Editorial Offices: 1600 John F. Kennedy Blvd., Ste. 1800, Philadelphia, PA 19103-2899. Customer Service Office: 3251 Riverport Lane, Maryland Heights, MO 63043. Periodicals postage paid at New York, NY and additional mailing offices. Subscription prices are $282.00 per year (U.S. individuals), $139.00 per year (U.S. student/resident), $387.00 per year (U.S. institutions), $374.00 per year (foreign individuals), $192.00 per year (foreign student/ resident), $465.00 per year (foreign instituitions), $326.00 per year (Canadian individuals), $192.00 per year (Canadian student/resident), and $465.00 per year (Canadian institutions). Foreign air speed delivery is included in all *Clinics* subscription prices. All prices are subject to change without notice. **POSTMASTER:** Send address changes to *Clinics in Liver Disease*, Elsevier Health Sciences Division, Subscription Customer Service, 3251 Riverport Lane, Maryland Heights, MO 63043. **Customer Service: Telephone: 1-800-654-2452 (U.S. and Canada); 314-447-8871 (outside U.S. and Canada). Fax: 314-447-8029. E-mail: journalscustomer service-usa@elsevier.com (for print support); journalsonlinesupport-usa@elsevier.com (for online support).**

*Reprints.* For copies of 100 or more of articles in this publication, please contact the Commercial Reprints Department, Elsevier Inc., 360 Park Avenue South, New York, NY 10010-1710. Tel.: 212-633-3874; Fax: 212-633-3820; E-mail: reprints@elsevier.com.

*Clinics in Liver Disease* is covered in *MEDLINE/PubMed (Index Medicus)*, Science Citation Index Expanded, Journal Citation Reports/Science Edition, and Current Contents/Clinical Medicine.

Printed and bound by CPI Group (UK) Ltd, Croydon, CR0 4YY

Transferred to digital print 2012

# Contributors

## CONSULTING EDITOR

**NORMAN GITLIN, MD, FRCP (LONDON), FRCPE (EDINBURGH), FACG, FACP**
Formerly, Professor of Medicine, Chief of Hepatology, Emory University; Currently, Consultant, Atlanta Gastroenterology Associates, Atlanta, Georgia

## EDITOR

**NIKOLAOS T. PYRSOPOULOS, MD, PhD, MBA, FACP, AGAF**
Associate Professor of Medicine, Director of Gastroenterology and Hepatology, Medical Director Liver Transplantation, Rutgers New Jersey Medical School, University Hospital, Newark, New Jersey

## AUTHORS

**RITU AGARWAL, MD**
Assistant Professor of Medicine, Icahn School of Medicine at Mount Sinai, New York, New York

**NICHOLAS AGRESTI, MD**
Department of Medicine, Memorial Health, University Medical Center, Savannah, Georgia

**KAWTAR ALKHALLOUFI, MD**
Howard University College of Medicine, Washington, DC

**JENNIFER S. AU, MD**
Division of Gastroenterology/Hepatology, Scripps Clinic, Scripps Translational Science Institute, La Jolla, California

**KALYAN RAM BHAMIDIMARRI, MD, MPH**
Assistant Professor, Division of Gastroenterology, Department of Medicine, University of Miami Miller School of Medicine, Miami, Florida

**CHALERMRAT BUNCHORNTAVAKUL, MD**
Division of Gastroenterology and Hepatology, Department of Medicine, Hospital of the University of Pennsylvania, University of Pennsylvania, Philadelphia, Pennsylvania; Division of Gastroenterology and Hepatology, Department of Medicine, Assistant Professor of Medicine, Rajavithi Hospital, College of Medicine, Rangsit University, Ratchathewi, Bangkok, Thailand

**MICHAEL DEMYEN, MD**
Assistant Professor, Department of Medicine, Rutgers New Jersey Medical School, Newark, New Jersey

**DOUGLAS T. DIETERICH, MD**
Professor of Medicine, Icahn School of Medicine at Mount Sinai, New York, New York

**CHRISTIN M. GIORDANO, MPAS, PA-C**
University of Central Florida College of Medicine, Orlando, Florida

**HYOSUN HAN, MD**
Icahn School of Medicine at Mount Sinai, New York, New York

**NEIL KAPLOWITZ, MD**
USC Research Center for Liver Disease, Department of Medicine, Keck School of
Medicine, University of Southern California, Los Angeles, CA

**WILLIAM M. LEE, MD**
Professor of Internal Medicine, Division of Digestive and Liver Diseases, University of
Texas Southwestern Medical Center at Dallas, Dallas, Texas

**JOSH LEVITSKY, MD, MS**
Associate Professor, Division of Gastroenterology and Hepatology, Department of
Medicine, Northwestern University Feinberg School of Medicine, Chicago, Illinois

**JAMES H. LEWIS, MD**
Professor of Medicine, Division of Gastroenterology and Hepatology, Department of
Medicine, Georgetown University Medical Center, Washington, DC

**VALERIE MARTEL-LAFERRIERE, MD**
Icahn School of Medicine at Mount Sinai, New York, New York

**VICTOR J. NAVARRO, MD**
Chief, Division of Hepatology, Einstein Healthcare Network, Philadelphia, Pennsylvania

**CHRISTOPHER B. O'BRIEN, MD, AGAF, FRCMI**
Professor of Clinical Medicine, Division of Liver and GI Transplantation, University of
Miami School of Medicine, Miami, Florida

**JIE OUYANG, MD, PhD**
Department of Pathology, Florida Hospital Medical Center and University of
Central Florida, Orlando, Florida

**NEEHAR D. PARIKH, MD, MS**
Transplant Hepatology Fellow, Division of Gastroenterology and Hepatology, Department
of Medicine, Northwestern University Feinberg School of Medicine, Chicago, Illinois

**VAISHALI PATEL, MBBS, MD**
Division of Gastroenterology, Hepatology, and Nutrition, Virginia Commonwealth
University Medical Center, Virginia Commonwealth University, Richmond, Virginia

**PAUL J. POCKROS, MD**
Division of Gastroenterology/Hepatology, Director, Liver Disease Center, Scripps
Clinic, Clinical Director of Research, Scripps Translational Science Institute, La Jolla,
California

**NIKOLAOS T. PYRSOPOULOS, MD, PhD, MBA, FACP, AGAF**
Associate Professor of Medicine, Director of Gastroenterology and Hepatology, Medical
Director Liver Transplantation, Rutgers New Jersey Medical School, University Hospital,
Newark, New Jersey

**K. RAJENDER REDDY, MD**
Division of Gastroenterology and Hepatology, Department of Medicine, Professor of Medicine, Hospital of the University of Pennsylvania, University of Pennsylvania, Philadelphia, Pennsylvania

**ARIE REGEV, MD**
Head, Safety Advisory Hub, Chairman, Liver and GI Safety Committee, Global Patient Safety, Eli Lilly and Company, Lilly Corporate Center; Adjunct Associate Professor of Medicine, Division of Gastroenterology and Hepatology, Indiana University School of Medicine, Indianapolis, Indiana

**ARUN J. SANYAL, MBBS, MD**
Chair, Division of Gastroenterology, Hepatology, and Nutrition, Virginia Commonwealth University Medical Center, Virginia Commonwealth University, Richmond, Virginia

**EUGENE SCHIFF, MD**
Chair, Division of Hepatology and the University of Miami Center for Liver Diseases, University of Miami, Miami, Florida

**LEONARD B. SEEFF, MD**
Consultant in Hepatology, Formerly The Hill Group and the U.S. Food and Drug Administration, Bethesda, Maryland

**JONATHAN G. STINE, MD**
Clinical Instructor of Medicine, Division of Gastroenterology and Hepatology, Department of Medicine, Georgetown University Medical Center, Washington, DC

**AMEET V. THATISHETTY, MD**
Department of Medicine, Memorial Health, University Medical Center, Savannah, Georgia

**SWAN N. THUNG, MD**
Department of Pathology, Icahn School of Medicine at Mount Sinai, New York, New York

**ALBERTO UNZUETA, MD**
Instructor in Medicine, Division of Hospital Internal Medicine, College of Medicine, Mayo Clinic, Phoenix, Arizona

**HUGO E. VARGAS, MD**
Professor of Medicine, Chair, Division of Hepatology, College of Medicine, Mayo Clinic, Phoenix, Arizona

**LIYUN YUAN, MD, PhD**
USC Research Center for Liver Disease, Department of Medicine, Keck School of Medicine, University of Southern California, Los Angeles, CA

**XARALAMBOS B. ZERVOS, DO**
Medical Director Liver Transplant, Staff Physician, Department of Gastroenterology, Digestive Disease Center, Cleveland Clinic Florida, Weston, Florida

**XUCHEN ZHANG, MD, PhD**
Department of Pathology, VA Connecticut Health System and Yale University School of Medicine, New Haven, Connecticut

# Contents

> Drug-induced liver injury (DILI) represents a broad spectrum of liver manifestations. However, the most common manifestation is hepatocyte death following drug intake. DILI can be predictable and dose dependent with a notable example of acetaminophen toxicity. Idiosyncratic DILI occurs in an unpredictable fashion at low frequencies, implying that environmental and genetic factors alter the susceptibility of individuals to the insult (drugs).

> Drug-induced cholestasis manifests as an acute self-limiting injury or as a chronic perpetuating injury, resulting in duct loss and cirrhosis. The number of drugs implicated in drug-induced cholestasis grows every year as new drugs are developed and approved. Other agents such as herbals, nutritional supplements, and complementary and alternative medicines are also reported to cause cholestatic liver injury. Recent literature on molecular transporters involved in bile transport has improved our understanding of patterns of drug-induced liver injury and the mechanisms of cholestasis. This article summarizes the probable offending drugs and the diagnosis and management of drug-induced cholestasis.

> Nonalcoholic fatty liver disease (NAFLD) is currently the most common cause of chronic liver disease in the United States. The term *NALFD* was first used by Ludwig in 1980 to describe the presence of hepatic steatosis and steatohepatitis in a series of patients with no identifiable cause. Since then, our insight into the pathogenesis of NAFLD has expanded significantly. We now know that NAFLD is closely related to metabolic syndrome and chronic low-grade inflammation. In the following review, the authors summarize the current evidence about drugs that lead to hepatic steatosis and steatohepatitis and pathogenic mechanisms thereof.

> Drug-induced hepatotoxicity is underrecognized but increasingly identified as causing acute and chronic liver disease. Several prescription drugs,

over-the-counter medications, dietary and/or supplementary agents, and herbal products are hepatotoxic. Drug-induced liver injury mimics other primary acute and chronic liver diseases and it should be considered in patients with hepatobiliary disease. Certain drugs result in specific histopathologic patterns of liver injury, which may help in sorting out the responsible drug. The diagnosis of drug-induced hepatotoxicity is challenging. It involves excluding other possible causes, careful medication history, the latent period between drug exposure and symptom onset and/or abnormal liver tests, and histopathologic findings.

Collectively, the various classes of antibiotics are a leading cause of drug-induced liver injury (DILI). However, acute antibiotic-associated DILI can be difficult to diagnose, as the course of therapy is usually brief, and other confounding factors are often present. In addition to the broad clinicopathologic spectrum of hepatotoxicity associated with the antimicrobials, the underlying infectious disease being treated may itself be associated with hepatic dysfunction and jaundice. This review provides summarized information on several classes of antimicrobial agents, highlighting new agents causing DILI and updating information on older agents.

Nonsteroidal anti-inflammatory drugs are among the most prescribed medications worldwide. After antibiotics and anticonvulsants they are considered the most common medications associated with drug-induced liver injury mainly through an idiosyncratic form of hepatotoxicity. In rare cases severe hepatotoxicity has been described with significant morbidity and mortality. Genetic risk factors have been reported with diclofenac and lumiracoxib. Postmarketing surveillance and monitoring is crucial to identify severe cases of hepatotoxicity.

Antiretroviral-related hepatotoxicity occurs commonly in patients with human immunodeficiency virus (HIV). Liver injury ranges from unconjugated hyperbilirubinemia and nodular regenerative hyperplasia to lactic acidosis and toxic hepatitis. Effective antiretroviral therapy has changed coinfected patients' primary morbidities and mortality to chronic liver disease rather than complications from HIV. Treatment for hepatitis C virus (HCV) is strongly encouraged early in all coinfected patients. However, drug–drug interactions must be considered to ensure safe and tolerable use alone or in combination with antiretroviral therapies. The first-generation and newer HCV direct-acting antivirals are promising in coinfected patients, with minimal side effects and hepatotoxicity.

Most hepatotoxicity secondary to chemotherapy is idiosyncratic and, therefore, neither dose dependent nor predictable. Some chemotherapy is cleared by the liver and requires dose adjustment in the face of significant liver dysfunction. In addition, preexisting abnormal liver function has been shown to increase the risk of hepatotoxicity. In addition to typical hepatocellular injury, other presentations, including cholestasis and hepatic sinusoidal obstruction syndrome, also commonly occur. The outcomes can range from asymptomatic liver function test abnormalities,

human immunodeficiency virus infection. However, with careful monitoring, even significant interactions can be effectively managed.

Arie Regev

Drugs that caused severe drug-induced liver injury (DILI) in humans have typically not shown clear hepatotoxic signals in preclinical assessment. However, clinical trial databases may show evidence of a drug's potential for severe DILI if clinical and laboratory data are evaluated for evidence of milder liver injury. The most specific indicator during a clinical trial for a drug's potential to cause severe DILI is occurrence of cases of drug induced hepatocellular injury accompanied by altered liver function (eg, elevated direct bilirubin). Meticulous causality assessment of hepatic cases and strict adherence to hepatic discontinuation rules are critical components of this approach.

# CLINICS IN LIVER DISEASE

---

**RELATED INTEREST**

*Infectious Disease Clinics of North America*, June 2013, (Vol. 27, No. 2)
**Infectious Disease Challenges in Solid Organ Transplant Recipients**
Princy N. Kumar, MD, and Joseph Timpone, MD, *Editors*

---

**DOWNLOAD
Free App!**

*Review Articles*
THE CLINICS

**NOW AVAILABLE FOR YOUR iPhone and iPad**

# Preface

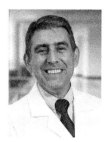

Nikolaos T. Pyrsopoulos, MD, PhD, MBA, FACP, AGAF
*Editor*

The art and science of medicine is evolving along with technology. This has led to the discovery of a vast amount of new therapies. Unequivocally, an immense amount of research should ideally be performed prior to the approval of these new therapies to ensure safety and tolerability along with the efficacy of these compounds. Unfortunately there have been several cases in which liver toxicity is identified sooner or later. These observations lead to the conclusion that drugs, herbal, and alternative treatment–induced liver toxicity is one of the major public health issues around the world. This is an important cause of morbidity and mortality following the aforementioned agents taken even in therapeutic doses. This has led to the withdrawal of a substantial number of medications not only prior to their approval but even after the approval of the compound, or with an inclusion of a "black box warning." It is of great concern that patients with evidence of drug, herbal, and alternative compound–induced hepatotoxicity may present a wide spectrum of symptomatology. Findings range from an asymptomatic increase of the liver enzymes up to and including fulminant hepatic failure requiring liver transplantation.

In this issue of *Clinics in Liver Disease*, distinguished scientists and experts in this field share their findings and experiences of their scientific work, formulating a thorough comprehensive review on the most important and timely topics in drug hepatotoxicity. A full span of very basic articles that discusses drug metabolism, drug-induced cholestasis, and pathological manifestations of drug-induced hepatotoxicity as well as other important articles devoted to clinical, epidemiologic, and therapeutic interventions such as drug-induced acute liver failure are included. Herbal, complementary, and alternative medicine-induced liver injury is a worldwide issue as the potential misconception that this kind of treatment is "benign as it comes from mother earth."

I would like to express my appreciation to the authors of these articles who devoted much of their time to review the literature and publish their own experience on this very

Clin Liver Dis 17 (2013) xiii–xiv
http://dx.doi.org/10.1016/j.cld.2013.09.013
1089-3261/13/$ – see front matter © 2013 Elsevier Inc. All rights reserved.

**liver.theclinics.com**

important topic. I would also like to express my gratitude to Dr Norman Gitlin and Ms Kerry Holland for giving me the opportunity to edit this issue.

Nikolaos T. Pyrsopoulos, MD, PhD, MBA, FACP, AGAF
Rutgers New Jersey Medical School
University Hospital
MSB H level Rm - 536
185 S. Orange Avenue Rm H-536
Newark, NJ 07101-1709, USA

E-mail address:
pyrsopni@njms.rutgers.edu

# Mechanisms of Drug-induced Liver Injury

Liyun Yuan, MD, PhD, Neil Kaplowitz, MD*

## KEYWORDS

- Idiosyncratic drug-induced liver injury • Cell death • Reactive metabolites
- Oxidative stress • Stress signaling • Mitochondria • Adaptive immunity
- HLA associations

## KEY POINTS

- Idiosyncratic drug-induced liver injury (DILI) is the result of the interplay between the environment, drugs, and host (genetic, age, sex, immune factors, pre-existing diseases).
- Idiosyncratic DILI is often mediated by the adaptive immune response. Meanwhile, some drugs and metabolites can directly damage mitochondria, produce reactive oxygen species, and alter signaling pathway.
- To defend against the hazards induced by drugs, hepatocytes exhibit adaptive mechanisms, including upregulation of Nrf2 signaling, mitophagy, and autophagy to cope with stress.
- The innate and adaptive immune systems can adapt to dampen the response.
- The battle between hazardous and adaptive responses determines the development of severe injury, restoration of the liver after mild injury (so-called adaptation), or no injury at all.

Drug-induced liver injury (DILI) occurs in an incidence of 10 to 15 in 10, 000 to 100,000 in the United States,[1,2] yet it has caused remarkable fatalities from acute liver failure yearly. Acetaminophen (APAP) alone accounts for half of the overall cases of acute liver failure in the United States.[3,4] DILI can also mimic all forms of acute or chronic liver diseases (hepatitis, cholestasis, or a mixed),[5] which is often underrecognized because of the complexity of clinical scenarios. Most DILI cases are idiosyncratic. A threshold dose (50–100 mg) may be required for DILI to occur.[6,7] When the dose threshold is exceeded, injury occurs in a very small number of individuals. Although APAP hepatotoxicity is dose dependent, idiosyncratic injury has been observed with a lower dose (less than 4 g per day) depending on individual susceptibility (ie, alcohol intake, fasting).

Over the past decades, much effort has been put into research to understand the mechanisms of hepatotoxicity and explore biomarkers for DILI surveillance. The

USC Research Center for Liver Disease, Department of Medicine, Keck School of Medicine, University of Southern California, 2011 Zonal Avenue (HMR101), Los Angeles, CA 90033, USA
* Corresponding author.
*E-mail address:* kaplowit@usc.edu

Clin Liver Dis 17 (2013) 507–518
http://dx.doi.org/10.1016/j.cld.2013.07.002
1089-3261/13/$ – see front matter © 2013 Elsevier Inc. All rights reserved.
liver.theclinics.com

central question of pathogenesis is how a drug or its metabolites initiate and propagate cell death within the liver with the assistance of surrounding immune cells.

## NECROSIS, APOPTOSIS, AND NECROPTOSIS

The fundamental process in DILI is the death of hepatocytes (in some circumstances, cholangiocytes or endothelial cells) in the background or recruitment of inflammation. DILI manifests clinically with hepatocellular injury, cholestasis, or a mixture of both.

Necrosis and apoptosis, theoretically, are 2 distinct modes of cell death. The fundamental differences between necrosis and apoptosis are the integrity of the plasma membrane, and involvement of caspase activation. Apoptosis is a sterile, "clean" programmed cell death characterized by cell shrinkage and chromatin fragmentation. The rapid removal of apoptotic cells by phagocytes or other cells minimizes the surrounding inflammation. Mechanistically, apoptosis is mediated by adenosine triphosphate (ATP) -dependent intracellular proteolytic cascades involving caspases which is triggered by the extrinsic pathway related to death ligand/receptors binding at the plasma membrane, or intrinsic pathways triggered by oxidative stress, radiation, DNA damage, or toxins leading to increasing permeability of mitochondrial outer membrane. Idiosyncratic DILI is mainly mediated by the innate or adaptive immune response involving death ligands such as tumor necrosis factor-$\alpha$ (TNF-$\alpha$) and FasL. TNF-$\alpha$ and FasL bind to death receptors of hepatocytes, triggering their demise of apoptosis.

Necrosis involves cell swelling, membrane bleb formation, and eventually the rupture of plasma membrane. The release of cellular components from necrotic cells elicits an inflammatory response. Necrosis is considered an oncotic lysis caused by loss of ion homeostasis as a result of severe mitochondria dysfunction and profound ATP depletion.

Necrosis was conventionally considered an incidental, "unwanted" cell death in a nonregulated manner. Increasing evidence has shown that necrosis can be tightly regulated. One of the remarkable observations is that when an apoptotic pathway was initiated on TNF-$\alpha$/TNF receptor binding in L929 cells,[8] inhibition of apoptosis with caspase inhibitors or ATP depletion leads to the shifting of cell demise to necrosis. Many terms have been used to categorize this type of cell death, such as necroptosis, programmed necrosis, regulated necrosis. It involves activation of receptor-interacting protein kinases[9,10] 1 and 3 (RIP1 and RIP3), and participation of mitochondria. This cell death has been implicated in pathophysiology of many diseases, such as acute pancreatitis,[11] brain injury,[12] and viral infection.[13,14]

APAP-induced cell death of hepatocytes has characteristic morphologic changes of necrosis. Mechanistically, the reactive metabolite, N-acetyl-p-benzo-quinoneimine (NAPQI), leads to profound mitochondrial glutathione (GSH) depletion, covalent binding, severe impairment of mitochondrial function, and cessation of ATP production, which lead to disruption of ion homeostasis and consequently oncotic necrosis. Interestingly, many stress kinases, such as c-Jun N-terminal kinase (JNK),[15] glycogen synthase kinase-3$\beta$,[16] apoptosis signal-regulating kinase-1 (ASK1),[17] mixed-lineage kinase-3 (MLK3),[18] Protein Kinase C (PKC),[19] and RIP1(unpublished, Dara L and Kaplowitz N), have been found to regulate the process actively, suggesting that APAP-induced necrosis might be a programmed necrosis.

### THE INVOLVEMENT OF REACTIVE METABOLITES

The fact that liver is the central organ for drug metabolism places it as a prime target for reactive metabolites of drugs. In most cases, drugs or their reactive metabolites are detoxified via phase II conjugation (glucuronidation, acetylation, sulphation, glutathione conjugation) and excreted out of cells through multi-drug-resistance-associated protein transporters (phase III). Reactive metabolites are often produced through oxidation and reduction by cytochrome P450 (phase I). A balance between production and detoxification/transport are critical in determining the most upstream aspects of DILI, namely, exposure of hepatocytes to some threshold level of reactive chemicals. Dose and lipophilicity (favoring hepatic distribution) are key additional factors in determining achievement of a threshold exposure to initiate hepatocellular stress or injury. DILI is often primed by reactive metabolites and their covalent binding to cellular proteins. Inhibition of bile salt export pump may aggravate hepatotoxicity[20,21] not only by causing cholestasis in some cases, but more importantly by bile acid retention causing mitochondrial and endoplasmic reticulum stress, which may amplify injury or sensitize hepatocytes to other injury mechanisms.

APAP metabolism has been well characterized. APAP is predominantly metabolized through sulphation and glucuronidation. A small proportion of APAP is oxidized by cytochrome P450 isoform 2E1 (to lesser extent 1A2 and 3A4) to a reactive form, NAPQI. NAPQI readily attacks free thiols, leading to rapid and selective GSH depletion in cytosol and mitochondria. When GSH is depleted, NAPQI covalently binds to thiol groups of cellular and mitochondrial proteins, causing mitochondria dysfunction, and the production of mitochondrial reactive oxygen species (mROS), MAP kinase activation, and downstream events leading to necrosis (see Involvement of Stress Signaling).

Oxidative stress and covalent binding activate not only toxic signaling but also protective and adaptive pathways. One such pathway is nuclear factor erythroid 2-related factor 2 (Nrf2)/Keap1 signaling.[22,23] Nrf2 is usually maintained at a very low level in the cytosol as newly synthesized Nrf2 is rapidly bound to Kelch-like ECH-associated protein 1 (Keap1), an adaptor of Culin E3 ligase, which shuttles Nrf2 to Culin E3 ligase complex for ubiquitin proteasomal degradation.[24] Keap 1 has 25 cysteine residues and acts as a redox and electrophilic sensor. The Keap-1 homodimer binds to a single Nrf2 molecule at DLG motif with a low affinity and ETGE motif with a high affinity.[25,26] According to the "hinge and latch" model,[25,26] when thiols of Keap1 are oxidized or covalently bound to electrophiles such as NAPQI, the conformation of Keap1 changes and Nrf2 dissociates from DLG binding site, while the remaining bound to Keap1 at ETGE motif. Keap1 is thus occupied by Nrf2 that is not further ubiquitinated, which allows de novo newly synthesized Nrf2 to translocate to the nucleus where it binds to the antioxidant response element promoters and activate the transcription of many antioxidant genes, including glutamate-cysteine ligase, thioredoxin reductase, peroxiredoxin, and glutathione S-transferase,[27,28] increasing glutathione synthesis and ROS detoxification. Meanwhile, increased expression of multi-drug-resistance-associated proteins by Nrf2 activation enhances the export of drugs/metabolites out of cells.

## INVOLVEMENT OF STRESS SIGNALING

JNK activation in response to TNF-$\alpha$ is usually rapidly dampened by NF-$\kappa$B transcription of survival genes. Thus the activation is transient and often nontoxic. Sustained JNK activation, however, leads to lethal consequences. This sustained JNK activation has been extensively studied in the APAP mouse model. Inhibition of JNKs with a small synthetic molecule (SP600125) or silencing of JNK expression with siRNA protects against APAP hepatotoxicity.[15,29] JNK is a family of serine/threonine kinases belonging to the MAPK family. Upstream is MAP3K (eg, ASK1 or MLK3) that phosphorylates and activates MAP2K (eg, MKK4/7), which in turn phosphorylates JNK. Knockout of ASK1 blunts JNK activation and attenuates APAP toxicity.[17] Silencing glycogen synthase kinase-3β or MLK3 blunts early-phase JNK activation and also exhibits a similar protective effect.[16,18]

JNK can be activated by many stressors, such as ROS, UV light, and cytokines. In APAP models, mitochondrial ROS seems to play a crucial role in prolonged JNK activation. The authors observed that sustained JNK activation occurred on profound GSH depletion and covalent binding in mitochondria in the APAP model, which might at least be achieved by modifying several redox-sensitive regulators of JNKs, such as thioredoxin (Trx), GSH S-transferase Pi (GST-Pi), and JNK phosphatases. ASK1 is held inactive by Trx at physiologic conditions and Trx oxidation allows the dissociation of ASK1 for activation.[30] GSH S-transferase Pi (GST-Pi) interacts directly with JNK as an inhibitor in nonstressed cells. ROS induces polymerization of GST-Pi via intermolecular disulfides, causing dissociation of GSTρ polymer from JNK.[31]

A crucial downstream target of JNK is mitochondria. Sustained, activated JNK was found to translocate to mitochondria, further impairing mitochondrial function, and amplifying oxidative stress. This self-amplifying process eventually leads to collapse of mitochondrial function and cell death. The authors' laboratory has identified an important mitochondrial outer membrane protein Sab (SH3 domain-binding protein that preferentially associates with Btk), which binds JNK and mediates its effect on mitochondria.[32] Silencing Sab expression abolished sustained JNK activation, blocked JNK translocation, and attenuated APAP toxicity. The details of how Sab, once phosphorylated by JNK and mediated inhibition of the electron transport (↑ROS), is currently not known.

## THE INVOLVEMENT OF MITOCHONDRIAL DYSFUNCTION

The mechanisms of hepatocyte apoptosis and necrosis converge on mitochondria. The release of cytochrome C, apoptosis-inducing factor, and Smac from the mitochondrial intermembrane space are crucial to activate caspases and execute apoptosis in the presence of adequate ATP,[33] which requires permeabilization of the outer mitochondrial membrane (OMM). Necrosis occurs via mitochondrial permeability transition (MPT). MPT is composed of voltage-dependent anion channel from OMM, adenine nucleotide translocase from the inner mitochondrial membrane (IMM), and cyclophilin D from the matrix. This putative pore spans the mitochondrial outer and inner membranes. Its opening dissipates the proton gradient, resulting in the collapse of mitochondrial membrane potential and cessation of ATP production. As a consequence, mitochondria swell and OMM ruptures, releasing pro-apoptotic factors.[34] However, necrosis is more likely the outcome in the setting of MPT opening, because MPT causes profound ATP depletion and MPT usually occurs in the context of oxidative stress, which inactivates caspases.

Selectively permeabilizing OMM allows the release of the pro-apoptotic factors from the intermembrane space without disrupting IMM. Mitochondrial outer membrane permeability (MOMP) is primarily governed by Bax and Bak, which oligomerize and insert into the outer mitochondrial membrane to create pores for the release of cytochrome c and Smac/Diablo. Bax/Bak is regulated by pro-survival Bcl-2 members (Bcl-2, Bcl-XL, and Mcl1) and pro-apoptotic BH3-only members (Bim, Bid, Puma, Bad, and Noxa).[35,36] The pro-survival factors, such as Bcl-2 and Bcl-XL, directly inhibit Bax/Bak, whereas pro-apoptotic factors, such as tBid and Bim, directly activate Bak/Bax, or de-repress Bak/Bax through binding and inhibiting Bcl-2 and Bcl-XL.

Programmed necrosis is considered an "aborted" apoptosis. When an innate immune response is activated by lipopolysaccharide, TNF-α is released and binds to the membrane receptors, promoting cell death cascades, particularly JNK signaling.

Necrosis occurs when the cell death signaling propagates on ligand binding (TNF-α/ TNF receptor) at the cytoplasmic membrane, but fails to execute apoptosis while the executioner caspases are suppressed with inhibitors, such as Z-VAD-FMK. The caspases destroy RIP1 and RIP3. Recent studies[37,38] showed that when caspases are inhibited under these conditions, RIP1/RIP3 form a complex that translocates to mitochondria, where it activates mitochondrial fission necessary for cell death.

ROS/RNS generated by mitochondria are crucial in the mitochondrial death pathway in the APAP model and has been clearly demonstrated with a regioisomer of APAP, 3'-hydroxyacetanilide (AMAP).[39] AMAP has a comparative metabolic profile to APAP, but the attack of its reactive metabolite spares mitochondria. With AMAP treatment, mitochondrial GSH is preserved and no hepatotoxicity occurs.[40,41] The unsaturated lipid at mitochondrial membrane, such as cardiolipin, is particularly vulnerable to mROS attack. Cardiolipin collaborates with Bax polymer to promote OMM opening.[42] Some researchers[43] also showed that cardiolipin retains cytochrome c at IMM through electrostatic interaction. Cardiolipin peroxidation abrogates this association and frees cytochrome c, a necessary step for the release of cytochrome c to execute apoptosis. Release of mROS is able to activate JNK signaling in the cytoplasm, as noted above. JNK translocates to mitochondria and leads to a self-amplifying cycle of JNK activation. Sustained JNK activation can alter the balance of the Bcl-2 family by activating pro-apoptotic members and inactivating anti-apoptotic members or lead to sufficient ROS generation to cause MPT opening (**Fig. 1**).

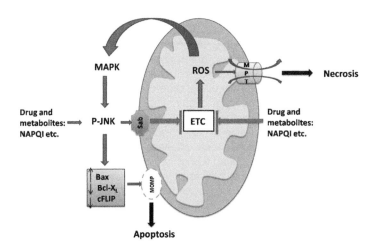

**Fig. 1.** JNK signaling and mitochondrial involvement in the death of hepatocytes. Sustained JNK activation and mitochondrial reactive oxygen species (ROS) generation are critical to induce cell death, particularly in the APAP model. In the APAP model, profound GSH depletion and covalent binding of NAPQI lead to generation of mitochondrial ROS, which activates mitogen-activated protein kinases (MAPK), including apoptosis signal-regulating kinase-1 (ASK1) and mixed-lineage kinase-3 (MLK3). Both ASK1 and MLK3 activate MKK4/ 7, which in turn phosphorylates and activates JNK. Phosphorylated JNK translocates to mitochondria, where it binds to and phosphorylates Sab, a mitochondrial outer membrane scaffold protein and this somehow leads to further impairment of electron transport chain (ETC) and enhancement of mitochondrial ROS generation. This self-amplifying process leads to sustained JNK activation and overwhelming production of mitochondrial ROS in the APAP model. As a result, MPT collapses ATP production and necrosis occurs. In the model of TNF-α-TNF/D-galactosamine, sustained JNK activation leads to MOMP and apoptosis by modulating the Bcl2 family.

Unfit mitochondria may influence the susceptibility to DILI, which is exemplified by heterozygous mouse knockout of superoxide dismutase 2 (Sod2+/−), which exhibits greater vulnerability to liver injury from drugs such as troglitzone[44] and flutamide[45] as well as APAP.[46] SOD2(MnSOD) resides solely in mitochondrial matrix and regulates mitochondrial redox by scavenging superoxide. Null knockout (Sod2−/−) is not viable. The heterozygous knockout has preserved GSH/GSSG level, glutathione peroxidase, and catalase at birth, but exhibits cumulative mitochondrial oxidative stress over time. With extrinsic insults (such as a drug) to mitochondria, the threshold of mitochondrial damage and/or mROS is lowered to elicit apoptosis or necrosis.

## THE INVOLVEMENT OF MITOCHONDRIAL ADAPTATION

Mitochondria provide a primary energy source for the cell to function and cope with stress. Cyclical fusion and fission coupled with mitophagy are key in maintaining quality control and mitochondrial fitness.[47] Mitochondrial fission is mediated by Drp1, a large GTPase in the dynamin family. Drp1 is recruited from cytosol by a group of adaptor proteins, including Mff, Mid49, and Mid51, and constricts both OMM and IMM at the site where mitochondria make contact with endoplasmic reticulum. Mitochondrial fusion involves OMM fusion and IMM fusion. OMM fusion is mediated by Mfn1 and Mfn2. IMM fusion is mediated by Opa1.

Many environmental insults or drugs (tetracycline, amiodarone, valproate, and various antiviral nucleoside analogs) can directly damage mitochondria and deplete mitochondrial DNA. Inhibition of the electron transport chain leads to an accumulation of reducing equivalents, which generate ROS. Damage from ROS, such as oxidation of mitochondrial proteins, lipids, and DNA, builds up within mitochondria. DILI related to mitochondrial toxicity is generally characterized by microvesicular steatosis, focal necrosis, and cholestasis. The number of mitochondria in these cases is decreased, which represents a special case when the drug or metabolite directly targets mitochondria and selective mitochondrial dysfunction is the cause of the phenotype. This selective mitochondrial dysfunction should be distinguished from examples where the immune system is playing a major role in inducing the injury and the effects of the drug/metabolite on mitochondria influence the susceptibility or severity of immune (innate or adaptive)-mediated killing.

Mitochondrial fusion-fission is a self-repair mechanism by which the damage to mtDNA/proteins/lipids is dissipated by fusion with healthy mitochondria and cumulative damage is contained for elimination. Fusion allows component exchange/sharing of healthy mitochondria with damaged ones, thus rescuing stress and mitigating damage. The cumulative damage would eventually pose harm to the cells. Elimination of the damaged cells is necessary to maintain quality control further. Two major enzymes: PINK1 and PARKIN, coordinate and flag the damaged cells for autophagic degradation.[48] The hypothesis is that the damaged components aggregate at the tip of mitochondria. On mitochondrial depolarization, PINK1, a membrane kinase, concentrates on the outer membrane of dysfunctional mitochondria. PINK1 recruits PARKIN, an E3 ligase, which ubiquitinates outer membrane proteins for proteosomal and autophagic degradation.[49–51] Mitochondrial fission then allows the segregation of damaged parts, which are subsequently engulfed by the autophagosome for elimination.

When the damage is overwhelming and/or the repair system is severely impaired, stressed cells commit suicide. There is a close link between mitochondrial fission and cell death (both apoptosis and necrosis). Bax is found to colocalize with Drp1 and Mffs.[52] Oligermerization of Bax (to promote MOMP) is accompanied by

Drp1-dependent fission. Lack of Drp1 delays cell death by decreasing cytochrome c release.[53] However, inhibition of Drp1 (sequestered in cytoplasm) also protects against necrosis (eg, APAP and necroptosis models). The link between JNK, ROS, MOMP, MPT with Drp1 is not completely understood. There have even been suggestions that partial membrane remodeling without full fission is implicated in cell death.

## THE ROLE OF ADAPTIVE IMMUNITY AND INNATE IMMUNITY IN DILI

Some DILI cases (for example, sulindac, phenytoin, and amoxicillin-clavulanic acid) have classic features of an allergic reaction, such as a rash, fever, and eosinophilia. The hypothesis is the drug or its metabolites act as haptens and covalently bind to a liver protein such as cytochrome p450. The drug-protein adducts are further processed in the macrophage/dendritic cell and presented as an antigen in complex with major histocompatibility complex class II molecules, triggering the adaptive immune response by binding to T-cell receptors of CD4 cells, leading to CD8 cytotoxic T-cell activation. The sensitized CD8 T cells express FasL, TNF-$\alpha$, and perforin that mediate cell death of hepatocytes. Although most idiosyncratic DILI cases lack features of the systemic allergic reaction, adaptive immunity is believed to play a pivotal role in the initiation and propagation of liver injury.[54] Several genome-wide association studies have revealed striking HLA haplotype associations with DILI. HLA-DRB1*1501 allele has a strong association with Augmentin-induced cholestatic liver injury.[55–57] The same allele is also associated with an increased risk of lumiracoxib-related hepatitis.[58] In the case of flucloxacillin, there is a strong link between HLA-B*5701 and DILI.[59] The carriers of this specific allele have an 80-fold increased risk of developing liver injury. Striking HLA haplotype associations suggest that DILI occurs as a consequence of a genetic predisposition targeted at adaptive immune response and antigen presentation/recognition. However haptenization alone is not sufficient to trigger the injury. Intrahepatic or extrahepatic stress caused by inflammation, infection, or oxidative stress is believed to costimulate the adaptive immune response as well as to predispose hepatocytes for immune-mediated cell death.

Following some extent of initial cell death, the released cellular content of dead cells may activate innate immune cells including Kupffer cells, infiltrating monocytes and neutrophils in a paracrine fashion. High mobility group box 1 as well as heat shock proteins and DNAs are released from necrotic hepatocytes.[60,61] These molecules have been termed damage-associated molecular patterns. Damage-associated molecular patterns are able to bind to toll-like receptors of innate immune cells and promote the production of the cytokines, such as TNF-$\alpha$, IFN$\gamma$, and IL-1, which could further modulate the intracellular events. Hepatic inflammation is frequently observed in DILI. It is conceivable these pro-inflammatory cytokines sensitize hepatocytes to biochemical stress, or regulate the adaptive immune-mediated cell injury. Trovafloxacin causes idiosyncratic liver injury in human, but is nontoxic to mice. Co-administration of lipopolysaccharide and trovafloxacin renders mice susceptible to severe hepatic necrosis,[62,63] suggesting that an innate immune response could mediate DILI. However, clinical relevance of this model is unclear because the injury caused by this drug in humans seems to involve the adaptive immune system. The role of innate immune response in APAP-induced hepatic necrosis is quite controversial. It is thought that innate immunity is more likely beneficial in the clearance of necrotic cells and promoting tissue repair.

Some drugs, especially biologic immune modulators, can activate underlying autoimmune hepatitis. In addition, a few other drugs (eg, minocycline, nitrofurantoin) seem

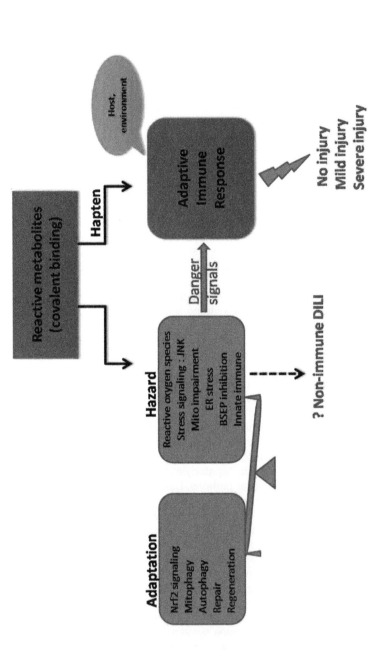

**Fig. 2.** Hypothetical mechanisms of idiosyncratic drug-induced liver injury (IDILI). Adaptive immune response plays a major role in IDILI and this may be to some extent regulated by cellular events induced by drug and reactive metabolites. Specifically, drug or reactive metabolites may generate hazards in hepatocytes by inducing endoplasmic reticulum (ER) stress, generating ROS, activating stress signaling, impairing mitochondrial function, and so on. To defend against these hazards, hepatocytes respond through adaptive mechanisms including nuclear factor erythroid 2-related factor 2 (Nrf-2) signaling, mitophagy, and autophagy to cope with stress. The innate and adaptive immune systems can adapt to dampen the response. The ultimate outcome of liver is no injury, mild injury, or severe injury. Although nonimmune IDILI remains a theoretical possibility as a consequence of the hazards of reactive metabolites, aside from a small number of drugs that directly damage mitochondria, there are very few, if any, proven examples of this possibility. BSEP, bile salt export pump.

to cause a rare form of idiosyncratic drug-induced liver injury indistinguishable from autoimmune hepatitis, but responsive to drug withdrawal.[64] These cases represent an interesting liver manifestation as a result of interaction between drugs and the host immune system.

## SUMMARY

Idiosyncratic DILI is the result of the interplay between the environment, drugs, and host (genetic, age, sex, immune factors, pre-existing diseases) (**Fig. 2**). Idiosyncratic DILI is often mediated by the adaptive immune response. Meanwhile, some drugs and metabolites can directly damage mitochondria, produce ROS, and alter signaling pathway. To defend against the hazards induced by drugs, hepatocytes exhibit adaptive mechanisms including upregulation of Nrf2 signaling, mitophagy, and autophagy to cope with stress. Furthermore, the innate and adaptive immune systems can adapt to dampen the response. Ultimately, the battle between hazardous and adaptive responses determines the development of severe injury, restoration of the liver after mild injury (so-called adaptation), or no injury at all.

## REFERENCES

1. Kaplowitz N. Idiosyncratic drug hepatotoxicity. Nat Rev Drug Discov 2005;4(6): 489–99.
2. Holt M, Ju C. Drug-induced liver injury. Handb Exp Pharmacol 2010;(196):3–27.
3. Khandelwal N, James LP, Sanders C, et al. Unrecognized acetaminophen toxicity as a cause of indeterminate acute liver failure. Hepatology 2011;53(2): 567–76.
4. Larson AM, Polson J, Fontana RJ, et al. Acetaminophen-induced acute liver failure: results of a United States multicenter, prospective study. Hepatology 2005; 42(6):1364–72.
5. Abboud G, Kaplowitz N. Drug-induced liver injury. Drug Saf 2007;30(4):277–94.
6. Lammert C, Einarsson S, Saha C, et al. Relationship between daily dose of oral medications and idiosyncratic drug-induced liver injury: search for signals. Hepatology 2008;47(6):2003–9.
7. Lammert C, Bjornsson E, Niklasson A, et al. Oral medications with significant hepatic metabolism at higher risk for hepatic adverse events. Hepatology 2010; 51(2):615–20.
8. Vercammen D, Beyaert R, Denecker G, et al. Inhibition of caspases increases the sensitivity of L929 cells to necrosis mediated by tumor necrosis factor. J Exp Med 1998;187(9):1477–85.
9. Declercq W, Vanden Berghe T, Vandenabeele P. RIP kinases at the crossroads of cell death and survival. Cell 2009;138(2):229–32.
10. Vandenabeele P, Declercq W, Van Herreweghe F, et al. The role of the kinases RIP1 and RIP3 in TNF-induced necrosis. Sci Signal 2010;3(115):re4.
11. He S, Wang L, Miao L, et al. Receptor interacting protein kinase-3 determines cellular necrotic response to TNF-alpha. Cell 2009;137(6):1100–11.
12. Chavez-Valdez R, Martin LJ, Flock DL, et al. Necrostatin-1 attenuates mitochondrial dysfunction in neurons and astrocytes following neonatal hypoxia-ischemia. Neuroscience 2012;219:192–203.
13. Cho YS, Challa S, Moquin D, et al. Phosphorylation-driven assembly of the RIP1-RIP3 complex regulates programmed necrosis and virus-induced inflammation. Cell 2009;137(6):1112–23.

14. Upton JW, Kaiser WJ, Mocarski ES. Virus inhibition of RIP3-dependent necrosis. Cell Host Microbe 2010;7(4):302–13.
15. Gunawan BK, Liu ZX, Han D, et al. c-Jun N-terminal kinase plays a major role in murine acetaminophen hepatotoxicity. Gastroenterology 2006;131(1):165–78.
16. Shinohara M, Ybanez MD, Win S, et al. Silencing glycogen synthase kinase-3beta inhibits acetaminophen hepatotoxicity and attenuates JNK activation and loss of glutamate cysteine ligase and myeloid cell leukemia sequence 1. J Biol Chem 2010;285(11):8244–55.
17. Nakagawa H, Maeda S, Hikiba Y, et al. Deletion of apoptosis signal-regulating kinase 1 attenuates acetaminophen-induced liver injury by inhibiting c-Jun N-terminal kinase activation. Gastroenterology 2008;135(4):1311–21.
18. Sharma M, Gadang V, Jaeschke A. Critical role for mixed-lineage kinase 3 in acetaminophen-induced hepatotoxicity. Mol Pharmacol 2012;82(5):1001–7.
19. Saberi B, Shinohara M, Ybanez MD, et al. Regulation of H(2)O(2)-induced necrosis by PKC and AMP-activated kinase signaling in primary cultured hepatocytes. Am J Physiol Cell Physiol 2008;295(1):C50–63.
20. Dawson S, Stahl S, Paul N, et al. In vitro inhibition of the bile salt export pump correlates with risk of cholestatic drug-induced liver injury in humans. Drug Metab Dispos 2012;40(1):130–8.
21. Morgan RE, Trauner M, van Staden CJ, et al. Interference with bile salt export pump function is a susceptibility factor for human liver injury in drug development. Toxicol Sci 2010;118(2):485–500.
22. Kaspar JW, Niture SK, Jaiswal AK. Nrf2:INrf2 (Keap1) signaling in oxidative stress. Free Radic Biol Med 2009;47(9):1304–9.
23. Niture SK, Kaspar JW, Shen J, et al. Nrf2 signaling and cell survival. Toxicol Appl Pharmacol 2010;244(1):37–42.
24. Kaspar JW, Niture SK, Jaiswal AK. Antioxidant-induced INrf2 (Keap1) tyrosine 85 phosphorylation controls the nuclear export and degradation of the INrf2-Cul3-Rbx1 complex to allow normal Nrf2 activation and repression. J Cell Sci 2012;125(Pt 4):1027–38.
25. Tong KI, Kobayashi A, Katsuoka F, et al. Two-site substrate recognition model for the Keap1-Nrf2 system: a hinge and latch mechanism. Biol Chem 2006;387(10–11):1311–20.
26. Tong KI, Padmanabhan B, Kobayashi A, et al. Different electrostatic potentials define ETGE and DLG motifs as hinge and latch in oxidative stress response. Mol Cell Biol 2007;27(21):7511–21.
27. Copple IM, Goldring CE, Jenkins RE, et al. The hepatotoxic metabolite of acetaminophen directly activates the Keap1-Nrf2 cell defense system. Hepatology 2008;48(4):1292–301.
28. Copple IM, Goldring CE, Kitteringham NR, et al. The Nrf2-Keap1 defence pathway: role in protection against drug-induced toxicity. Toxicology 2008;246(1):24–33.
29. Kaplowitz N, Shinohara M, Liu ZX, et al. How to protect against acetaminophen: don't ask for JUNK. Gastroenterology 2008;135(4):1047–51.
30. Saitoh M, Nishitoh H, Fujii M, et al. Mammalian thioredoxin is a direct inhibitor of apoptosis signal-regulating kinase (ASK) 1. EMBO J 1998;17(9):2596–606.
31. Adler V, Yin Z, Fuchs SY, et al. Regulation of JNK signaling by GSTp. EMBO J 1999;18(5):1321–34.
32. Win S, Than TA, Han D, et al. c-Jun N-terminal kinase (JNK)-dependent acute liver injury from acetaminophen or tumor necrosis factor (TNF) requires mitochondrial Sab protein expression in mice. J Biol Chem 2011;286(40):35071–8.

33. Wang C, Youle RJ. The role of mitochondria in apoptosis*. Annu Rev Genet 2009;43:95–118.
34. Honda HM, Korge P, Weiss JN. Mitochondria and ischemia/reperfusion injury. Ann N Y Acad Sci 2005;1047:248–58.
35. Youle RJ, Strasser A. The BCL-2 protein family: opposing activities that mediate cell death. Nat Rev Mol Cell Biol 2008;9(1):47–59.
36. Youle RJ. Cell biology. Cellular demolition and the rules of engagement. Science 2007;315(5813):776–7.
37. Zhang DW, Shao J, Lin J, et al. RIP3, an energy metabolism regulator that switches TNF-induced cell death from apoptosis to necrosis. Science 2009; 325(5938):332–6.
38. Wang Z, Jiang H, Chen S, et al. The mitochondrial phosphatase PGAM5 functions at the convergence point of multiple necrotic death pathways. Cell 2012; 148(1–2):228–43.
39. Rashed MS, Streeter AJ, Nelson SD. Investigations of the N-hydroxylation of 3'-hydroxyacetanilide, a non-hepatotoxic positional isomer of acetaminophen. Drug Metab Dispos 1989;17(4):355–9.
40. Rashed MS, Nelson SD. Characterization of glutathione conjugates of reactive metabolites of 3'-hydroxyacetanilide, a nonhepatotoxic positional isomer of acetaminophen. Chem Res Toxicol 1989;2(1):41–5.
41. Rashed MS, Myers TG, Nelson SD. Hepatic protein arylation, glutathione depletion, and metabolite profiles of acetaminophen and a non-hepatotoxic regioisomer, 3'-hydroxyacetanilide, in the mouse. Drug Metab Dispos 1990; 18(5):765–70.
42. Kuwana T, Mackey MR, Perkins G, et al. Bid, Bax, and lipids cooperate to form supramolecular openings in the outer mitochondrial membrane. Cell 2002; 111(3):331–42.
43. Ott M, Robertson JD, Gogvadze V, et al. Cytochrome c release from mitochondria proceeds by a two-step process. Proc Natl Acad Sci U S A 2002;99(3): 1259–63.
44. Lee YH, Chung MC, Lin Q, et al. Troglitazone-induced hepatic mitochondrial proteome expression dynamics in heterozygous Sod2(+/−) mice: two-stage oxidative injury. Toxicol Appl Pharmacol 2008;231(1):43–51.
45. Kashimshetty R, Desai VG, Kale VM, et al. Underlying mitochondrial dysfunction triggers flutamide-induced oxidative liver injury in a mouse model of idiosyncratic drug toxicity. Toxicol Appl Pharmacol 2009;238(2):150–9.
46. Fujimoto K, Kumagai K, Ito K, et al. Sensitivity of liver injury in heterozygous Sod2 knockout mice treated with troglitazone or acetaminophen. Toxicol Pathol 2009;37(2):193–200.
47. Youle RJ, van der Bliek AM. Mitochondrial fission, fusion, and stress. Science 2012;337(6098):1062–5.
48. Jin SM, Youle RJ. PINK1- and Parkin-mediated mitophagy at a glance. J Cell Sci 2012;125(Pt 4):795–9.
49. Jin SM, Lazarou M, Wang C, et al. Mitochondrial membrane potential regulates PINK1 import and proteolytic destabilization by PARL. J Cell Biol 2010;191(5): 933–42.
50. Lazarou M, Narendra DP, Jin SM, et al. PINK1 drives Parkin self-association and HECT-like E3 activity upstream of mitochondrial binding. J Cell Biol 2013;200(2): 163–72.
51. Narendra DP, Jin SM, Tanaka A, et al. PINK1 is selectively stabilized on impaired mitochondria to activate Parkin. PLoS Biol 2010;8(1):e1000298.

52. Suen DF, Norris KL, Youle RJ. Mitochondrial dynamics and apoptosis. Genes Dev 2008;22(12):1577–90.
53. Montessuit S, Somasekharan SP, Terrones O, et al. Membrane remodeling induced by the dynamin-related protein Drp1 stimulates Bax oligomerization. Cell 2010;142(6):889–901.
54. Kaplowitz N. Dealing with stress. Hepatology 2012;55(1):3–13.
55. Hautekeete ML, Horsmans Y, Van Waeyenberge C, et al. HLA association of amoxicillin-clavulanate–induced hepatitis. Gastroenterology 1999;117(5): 1181–6.
56. Lucena MI, Molokhia M, Shen Y, et al. Susceptibility to amoxicillin-clavulanate-induced liver injury is influenced by multiple HLA class I and II alleles. Gastroenterology 2011;141(1):338–47.
57. O'Donohue J, Oien KA, Donaldson P, et al. Co-amoxiclav jaundice: clinical and histological features and HLA class II association. Gut 2000;47(5):717–20.
58. Singer JB, Lewitzky S, Leroy E, et al. A genome-wide study identifies HLA alleles associated with lumiracoxib-related liver injury. Nat Genet 2010;42(8):711–4.
59. Daly AK, Donaldson PT, Bhatnagar P, et al. HLA-B*5701 genotype is a major determinant of drug-induced liver injury due to flucloxacillin. Nat Genet 2009; 41(7):816–9.
60. Kubes P, Mehal WZ. Sterile inflammation in the liver. Gastroenterology 2012; 143(5):1158–72.
61. Antoine DJ, Williams DP, Kipar A, et al. High-mobility group box-1 protein and keratin-18, circulating serum proteins informative of acetaminophen-induced necrosis and apoptosis in vivo. Toxicol Sci 2009;112(2):521–31.
62. Luyendyk JP, Maddox JF, Cosma GN, et al. Ranitidine treatment during a modest inflammatory response precipitates idiosyncrasy-like liver injury in rats. J Pharmacol Exp Ther 2003;307(1):9–16.
63. Shaw PJ, Hopfensperger MJ, Ganey PE, et al. Lipopolysaccharide and trovafloxacin coexposure in mice causes idiosyncrasy-like liver injury dependent on tumor necrosis factor-alpha. Toxicol Sci 2007;100(1):259–66.
64. Czaja AJ. Drug-induced autoimmune-like hepatitis. Dig Dis Sci 2011;56(4): 958–76.

# Drug-Induced Cholestasis

Kalyan Ram Bhamidimarri, MD, MPH, Eugene Schiff, MD*

## KEYWORDS

- Drugs • Cholestasis • Liver injury • Bile duct injury • Management

## KEY POINTS

- Drug-induced cholestasis can result in acute or chronic liver injury.
- Most cases of cholestatic drug-induced liver injury appear to resolve shortly after the drug's withdrawal, but a subset of cases can progress to chronic cholestasis, cirrhosis, and subsequent hepatic decompensation.
- Early recognition and prompt withdrawal of the offending drug is the mainstay in the initial management.
- This review summarizes the implicated drugs, diagnostic tools, and management of drug-induced cholestasis.
- Proper reporting of the adverse drug reactions and outcomes is important as new drugs are being developed and approved.

## INTRODUCTION

Drug-induced liver injury (DILI) poses a significant health and economic burden in the modern health care system.[1] Despite the advancements in health care, DILI is often a diagnosis of exclusion, and the current data on understanding of the pathogenesis, recognition of risk factors, and tools for diagnosis are limited. Heterogeneity of clinical presentation, lack of standardized diagnostic criteria, delay in diagnosis, and the recognition of culprit drugs, and underreporting of cases and outcomes are some of the important reasons for the paucity of data in this field.[2]

There are 3 clinical patterns of DILI: hepatocellular, cholestatic, and mixed. Hepatocellular injury appears distinct from cholestatic and mixed patterns, with predominant cytolytic injury resulting in elevation of serum transaminases before jaundice. Although cholestatic and mixed patterns of injury are theoretically different, they resemble each other in several aspects. The term cholestasis refers to stagnant bile or the failure of bile to reach the small intestine.[3] Cholestatic injury is defined as an elevation of alkaline phosphatase (ALP) greater than 2 times the upper limit of normal (ULN) and/or the ratio of serum alanine aminotransferase (ALT)/serum activity of ALP of less than 2 (both enzymes are expressed as multiples of the ULN).[4] As there is no gold standard for diagnosis, drug-induced cholestasis is usually a diagnosis of exclusion.[4]

University of Miami, 1500NW 12th Avenue, Suite 1101, Miami, FL 33136, USA
* Corresponding author.
*E-mail address:* ESchiff@med.miami.edu

Clin Liver Dis 17 (2013) 519–531
http://dx.doi.org/10.1016/j.cld.2013.07.015
1089-3261/13/$ – see front matter © 2013 Elsevier Inc. All rights reserved.

Drug-induced cholestasis can be broadly classified into acute and chronic liver injury, the former being more common than the latter.[5]

## EPIDEMIOLOGY

DILI accounts for approximately 13% of cases of acute liver failure in the United States, and is a major reason for drug abandonment by the drug regulatory agencies during the developmental phases of several candidate molecules.[5,6] The true incidence of drug-induced cholestasis cannot be estimated with accuracy because of the limited number of population-based studies, heterogeneity in geographic distribution, and underreporting of the cases. A French population-based study showed an annual crude incidence rate of DILI to be around 13.9 cases per 100,000 inhabitants, of which 47% were due to cholestatic or mixed injury.[7] A recent review of major DILI case series reported a rate of 20% to 40% for a cholestatic pattern of DILI and 12% to 20% for a mixed pattern of DILI.[8] Drugs can cause cholestatic liver injury in a dose-dependent or idiosyncratic manner, the latter being more common. Idiosyncratic DILI from a single drug is rare and unpredictable, and its frequency is less than 1 per 10,000 to 100,000 subjects.[9]

## RISK FACTORS

The risk factors for drug-induced cholestasis are poorly understood. Age, gender, ethnicity, comorbidities, drug composition, and use of concomitant drugs or interplay of 1 or more factors can predispose the risk for DILI.[10] Cholestatic and mixed pattern of DILI is predominantly reported in older males, whereas hepatocellular injury is commonly reported in younger females.[9–11] Age older than 60 years is conferred as an independent risk factor for cholestatic DILI, irrespective of the drug involved.[10] Older age is also implicated as a risk factor for drug-induced cholestasis from amoxicillin-clavulanate.[10] Although the age and gender associations are ill conceived, it is speculated that age-related physiologic changes in receptor/transporter expression, body-fat content, volumes of distribution, and hormone status are responsible for such observations.[10]

Genome-wide association studies have enabled the identification of certain genetic determinants that can influence a disease state. One such breakthrough is in the identification of human leukocyte antigen (HLA) B*5701, which is strongly associated with flucloxacillin-induced cholestatic DILI.[12] Similar genetic associations for amoxicillin-clavulanate–induced DILI are HLA haplotypes -DRB and -DQB which were described in a few earlier studies but were not corroborated in later studies.[13] Women with intrahepatic cholestasis of pregnancy appear to be susceptible to drug-induced cholestasis from steroids (oral contraceptives or hormone replacement therapy), which again illustrates a common genetic determinant, the MDR3/BSEP polymorphism.[14] Evidence from such data appears promising, but genome-wide testing in epidemiologic proportions for numerous implicated drugs is impractical.

Drugs can cause liver injury in a dose-dependent or idiosyncratic manner. The mechanism of idiosyncratic drug injury is unpredictable and uncertain, but a component of dose dependency has been postulated in recent studies.[10,15] Individuals taking drug doses of more than 50 mg per day had increased propensity to sustain serious liver injury than those who were taking lower daily doses. Cholestatic or mixed DILI was observed in 30% to 50% of patients who were taking medications at doses greater than 50 mg per day.[10,15]

Apart from drug dosage, chemical composition of the drugs plays an important role in the causation of DILI. Estrogens and its metabolites have been known for a long time to modulate cholangiocyte functions, thereby playing a pathogenic role in intrahepatic cholestasis.[16] Oral contraceptives especially high in estrogen content have been implicated in various studies as a cause of drug-induced cholestasis. The estimated prevalence rates in Europe and North America in the past were reported to be approximately 1 in 10,000 but current reported rates have declined to less than 1%, which parallels the use of contraceptives with lower estrogen doses.[9,11] Anabolic steroids with 17α carbon substitutions (particularly alkyl or methyl substitution) are well known to induce a bland type of cholestatic injury. Other anabolic steroids and dietary supplements predominantly used for body building have also been implicated in the causation of drug-induced cholestasis.[5] Drugs that have greater than 50% hepatic metabolism have a greater propensity to cause DILI, and those that are highly lipophilic are prone to cause cholestatic DILI.[10,15]

## PATHOGENESIS

Drugs and toxins that are absorbed into the portal circulation are taken up by the transporters at the basolateral membrane of the hepatocytes. Detoxification of the drugs involve phase I and II reactions in the hepatocytes, and the metabolites are then effluxed into the canaliculi to be excreted in the bile. The efflux of bile is facilitated by the canalicular transporters of the multidrug-resistance protein (MRP) family, which includes other glycoproteins, MRP2 (ABCC2), MDR1 (ABCB1), MDR3 (ABCB4), and BSEP (ABCB11).[17] Drugs and metabolites that affect these canalicular efflux transporters are particularly involved in cholestatic DILI. The bile salt export pump (BSEP), discovered in 1998, plays a critical role in the secretion of bile into the canaliculi and in the physiologic maintenance of the bile acids by modulating the enterohepatic circulation. Several variant mutations of BSEP are now identified, of which the V444A polymorphism is particularly associated with drug-induced cholestasis. Most drugs implicated in cholestatic injury are reported to inhibit BSEP and, conversely, most patients with mutations in MDR3 or BSEP are reported to have a 3-fold increase in their risk for cholestatic DILI.[18] Other transporter molecules are also involved in the pathogenesis of cholestatic DILI, but more data are awaited.

## ASSOCIATION OF CAUSALITY

There are no standard diagnostic criteria for DILI. Therefore, several scores or scales like, the Naranjo Adverse Drug Reactions Probability Scale, the DILIN Causality Score, the Roussel Uclaf Causality Assessment Method (RUCAM) scale, the Maria and Victorino scale, and the Digestive Disease Week Japan (DDW-J) have been proposed to evaluate the causality.[4,9] The RUCAM, published in 1990 by the Council for International Organizations of Medical Sciences, is an objective and consistent assessment by means of a semiquantitative evaluation of causality, which assigns a score to 6 important domains.[9,19]

The 3 chronologic criteria are:

- Time to onset of the reaction from drug intake and from drug withdrawal
- Course of the reaction
- Rechallenge: response to readministration of the drug

The 3 clinical criteria are:

- Signs and symptoms suggestive of causal role of the drug (fever, rash, or any other hypersensitivity reaction)

- Result of specific tests suggestive of DILI (not usually present, and so previous information on hepatotoxicity of the drug can be used)
- Exclusion of non–drug-related causes[20,21]

Rechallenge can confirm the diagnosis, but should not be used because a recurrent injury may be more severe, especially if the mechanism of injury is immunologic.[5] The final score can range from −5 to +14; based on this, a causal relationship is established as highly probable (>8), probable (6–8), possible (3–5), unlikely (1–2), or excluded (<0). The rest of the scoring systems have been used in a varied manner, and although complex the RUCAM score is well tested, validated, and widely used. Therefore, the diagnosis of DILI should be based on the physician's clinical judgment and discretion.[4]

## CLASSIFICATION OF DRUG-INDUCED CHOLESTASIS

Drug-induced cholestasis can be broadly classified into (1) acute (<6 months), which occurs primarily as a result of alteration in the secretion of bile into the canaliculus: (a) inflammatory (with hepatocellular injury) or (b) bland (without hepatocellular injury); (2) chronic (>6 months), which occurs as a result of injury to the bile ducts or ductules: (a) vanishing bile duct syndrome (ductopenic cholestasis) or (b) sclerosing cholangitis.[3] Acute cholestatic injury is more common than chronic drug-induced cholestasis.

## ACUTE CHOLESTATIC DILI

Acute cholestatic DILI is the most frequent form of drug-induced cholestasis, which can be divided into hepatocellular or bland cholestasis (**Fig. 1**). Although more than 1 drug can be involved in the causation of DILI, single-prescription medication was implicated in 73% of the cases.[9] Drug classes mostly associated with this type of injury are anti-infectious agents, anti-diabetics, anti-inflammatory agents, psychotropic agents, cardiovascular agents, steroids, and other miscellaneous drugs.[7,9,10]

Antimicrobials are the most common drug class associated with cholestatic DILI, with a reported association of 32% to 45.5% of DILI cases.[9,11] The risk of liver injury from amoxicillin-clavulanate was first described in 1988, and it was subsequently noted that the risk is higher with the combination than with amoxicillin alone.[22] Amoxicillin-clavulanate is the single most common agent implicated in cholestatic injury, accounting to 59 of 461 (12.8%) and 23 of 300 (7.6%) of all cases of DILI in 2 large series,[9,11] and an estimated 9.9 cases of jaundice per 100,000 prescriptions.[23] Development of liver injury is usually seen within 4 weeks and can occur in the early phase, late phase, or, more commonly, after the discontinuation of the drug. Most cases resolve within a few weeks of self-limited course but there are rare instances of prolonged severe DILI, liver transplantation, and death.[24,25] Female sex, age older than 65 years, and repeated courses of treatment (2 or more) have all been associated with an increased risk of acute liver injury from amoxicillin-clavulanate.[22,24] Other penicillins such as flucloxacillin, dicloxacillin, cloxacillin, oxacillin, amoxicillin, benzyl penicillin, carbenicillin, and ticarcillin have all been reported to cause cholestatic DILI.[3,9,26] The incidence of amoxicillin-associated DILI is reported to be around 0.1 to 3 per 100,000 prescriptions, with that of flucloxacillin-associated DILI being around 1.8 to 3.6 per 100,000 prescriptions.[22,27] Flucloxacillin is not available in the United States but is commonly used in other parts of the world. Risk factors and the range of spectrum of liver injury from other penicillins are similar to those of amoxicillin-clavulanate. Chronic cholestatic injury and cirrhosis have been reported with flucloxacillin and benzyl penicillin.[26,28–30] Most cephalosporins induce a mild cholestatic DILI in up to

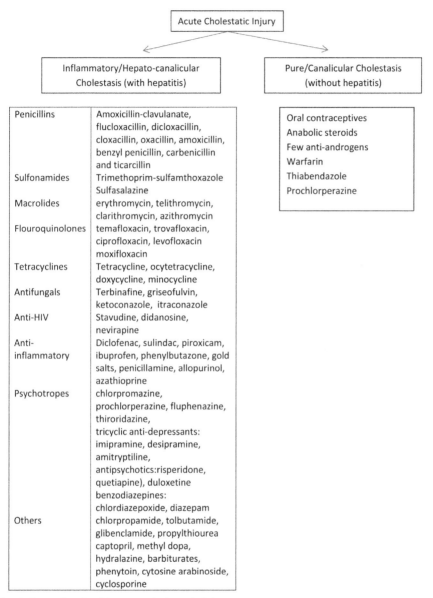

**Fig. 1.** Drugs involved in acute cholestatic injury.

25% of adult and 40% of pediatric populations, which occurs within a few days of treatment initiation.[31] Ceftriaxone has the propensity to form sludge/cholelithiasis and mirrors clinical features of acute cholecystitis, whereas other drugs in the class induce an immune-mediated injury.[31]

Sulfonamides are the oldest class of antimicrobials and are among the top few drugs associated with cholestatic DILI. Sulfa drugs accounted for 1 per 1000 users[27] and around 4.3% of DILI cases in recent studies.[9] Most cases are mild and occur within the first 4 weeks of treatment initiation, but severe cases resulting in death and liver transplantation have also been reported.[9,27,31]

Macrolide antibiotics, erythromycin, telithromycin, clarithromycin, and azithromycin are all reported to cause DILI. Erythromycin-associated cholestatic injury is reported to be around 3.6 per 100,000 users, and most cases have a good outcome with prompt recovery.[32,33] Clarithromycin-associated cholestatic DILI can be mild to severe, and a few cases of death and liver transplantation have been reported.[31] Mild cholestatic injury was observed in the premarketing phase of telithromycin, but occurrence of hepatocellular DILI is seen more common than cholestatic DILI in the postmarketing phase, which has greatly limited the use of this medication.[34]

Flouroquinolones can vary in their propensity to cause DILI, based on their individual molecular structure. Unlike other quinolones, temafloxacin and trovafloxacin have a highly lipophilic difluorophenyl side chain and thus have more potential to cause cholestatic DILI. There are several reported cases of acute liver failure, death, and liver transplantation with the use of temafloxacin and trovafloxacin.[35] Although mild elevation in liver enzymes is noted in 1% to 5% of cases using ciprofloxacin, levofloxacin, and moxifloxacin, cholestatic DILI is rare and occurs in approximately 1 case per 5 million prescriptions.[31]

Tetracycline-related hepatotoxicity was first reported in 1964, and earlier cases were associated larger intravenous doses and pregnancy. The hepatotoxicity seems to be predictable owing to the dose dependency, and with the current use of low-dose oral tetracyclines the incidence of liver injury is rare, accounting for 1.3 to 3.7 cases per 100,000 prescriptions.[27] Hepatotoxicity from doxycycline, minocycline, and tigecycline is very rare and generally has a good prognosis.[31]

Terbinafine is an oral antifungal agent commonly used to treat dermatomycosis or onychomycosis. Symptomatic cholestatic DILI is reported in 1 case per 45,000 to 54,000 exposed subjects[36] and in 1.3% of DILI cases in the United States.[9] Severe cholestatic DILI and liver transplantation has been reported in association with terbinafine.[37] Other antifungals such as griseofulvin, ketoconazole, and itraconazole have also been associated with cholestatic DILI, of which itraconazole toxicity occurs via inhibition of MDR3/ABCB4.[3,38]

Antiretroviral medications are commonly involved in DILI; however, the presence of underlying liver disease or other intrahepatic processes in human immunodeficiency virus (HIV)-positive patients may contribute to the severity of liver injury. Antiretroviral medications accounted for approximately 29% of all AIDS cases with jaundice in a cohort of African Americans and Hispanics.[39] Stavudine, didanosine, nevirapine, and lamivudine were reported to the World Health Organization as suspect drugs associated with liver injury.[40] Didanosine is frequently associated with cholestatic DILI and noncirrhotic portal hypertension, which is a frequent cause of liver-related mortality (26%) in exposed persons.[41,42]

Anti-inflammatory drugs such as nonsteroidal anti-inflammatory drugs (NSAIDs), immunomodulators, and other antirheumatic drugs, such as diclofenac, sulindac, piroxicam, ibuprofen, phenylbutazone, gold salts, penicillamine, allopurinol, and azathioprine, are reported to cause drug-induced cholestasis.[3,43] Azathioprine-associated cholestatic DILI appears to be an idiosyncratic reaction that occurs within the first 3 months of treatment initiation, and the incidence rates are generally between 1.4% and 10%.[44–46] Discontinuation of azathioprine leads to prompt recovery in a majority of cases, whereas continued use can lead to a nodular regenerative hyperplasia that can result in portal hypertension and life-threatening complications.[44]

Psychotropes such as phenothiazines (chlorpromazine, prochlorperazine, fluphenazine, thioridazine), tricyclic antidepressants (imipramine, desipramine, amitriptyline), antipsychotics (risperidone, quetiapine), duloxetine, and some benzodiazepines (chlordiazepoxide, diazepam) are all associated with cholestatic hepatitis.[3]

Chlorpromazine-induced jaundice occurs in about 0.1% of cases, usually as a result of hypersensitivity reaction. It is estimated that one-third of the cases from acute cholestatic injury recover within 4 weeks after the cessation of the drug, one-third recover in a few months, and one-third develop chronic cholestatic injury resulting in ductopenia and cirrhosis.[3,47] Duloxetine-associated liver injury appears to be dose dependent.[48,49]

Antidiabetic or oral hypoglycemic agents (eg, chlorpropamide, tolbutamide, glibenclamide), antithyroid drugs (eg, propylthiourea), antihypertensives (eg, captopril, methyldopa, hydralazine), anticonvulsants (eg, barbiturates, phenytoin), and some chemotherapy agents (eg, cytosine arabinoside, cyclosporine) are also associated with drug-induced cholestasis.[3]

Oral contraceptives are well known to cause acute canalicular or bland cholestasis. The incidence reports from earlier studies were higher, accounting for 1 in 4000 to 10,000 exposed individuals when higher-dose estrogens were used, but the current incidence rates are as low as 1% probably because of lower estrogen content in the tablets.[3,9,11] Androgens, anabolic steroids, body-building supplements, and some antiestrogens are also linked to drug-induced cholestasis.

### Clinical Features and Management

The clinical presentations of drug-induced cholestasis from various drugs are nonspecific and variable, and depend on the mechanism of injury.[50] Idiosyncratic reactions are unpredictable, and occur earlier than those that are dose dependent or immunologically mediated. In general, most cases remain asymptomatic, but vague symptoms such as fatigue, malaise, anorexia, and nausea occur after the onset of liver injury. Fever and rash may follow those that induce hypersensitivity reactions. Painless jaundice with or without pruritus can be seen, which can resolve shortly after drug withdrawal or persist in those who sustain chronic cholestatic injury. Pain is usually not associated with intrahepatic cholestasis from DILI, but a few cases may present with right upper quadrant pain that mimics acute cholecystitis, cholangitis, or choledocholithiasis. Acute liver injury can potentially lead to fulminant or subfulminant liver failure, at which time changes in mental status and bleeding diathesis prevail. Alcohol, sepsis, autoimmune cholangiopathic disorders, infectious hepatitis (especially hepatitis A and E), and certain viruses can all mimic drug-induced cholestasis. DILI is frequently a diagnosis of exclusion, so a detailed history of presenting illness, travel, medications, and drug abuse would help rule out other possible causes of liver injury.

There is no hallmark test or marker for the diagnosis of DILI. Routine biochemical tests, international normalized ratio (INR), serologic markers, and biliary imaging are usually the initial battery of tests that need to be conducted to exclude the common causes. An R value can be calculated as the ratio of ALT to ALP (both accounted for as multiples of their respective ULN). An R value of less than or equal to 2 characterizes cholestatic DILI, an R value ranging from 2 to 5 characterizes mixed DILI, and an R value greater than or equal to 5 characterizes hepatocellular DILI. INR should be closely monitored in those with severe DILI, and early referral to a transplant center is strongly recommended. Serologic testing for autoimmune and infectious panels in addition to biliary imaging with ultrasonography or magnetic resonance imaging can further help to narrow down the differential diagnoses. Although not mandatory in every case, a liver biopsy may become essential in cases of acute on chronic liver failure, to estimate the underlying fibrosis and to prognosticate recovery versus the need for liver transplant.[4]

## Pathology

Findings on liver biopsies of patients with DILI are nonspecific and nondiagnostic of any particular drug. Cholestatic DILI is the most common type of injury seen on histology, approximating two-thirds of all DILI cases, and can be divided into acute and chronic injury.[51] Acute cholestatic DILI is the commonest pattern and, as discussed earlier, can be divided into inflammatory or bland cholestasis. The former, also known as cholestatic hepatitis or hypersensitivity cholestasis, is accompanied by inflammatory cells (mononuclear cells) mediating hepatocellular injury and hepatocellular cholestasis in the centrilobular area.[52] Eosinophils can be present, usually in patients who incite a hypersensitivity reaction, and their presence is associated with a favorable prognosis.[8]

In pure cholestasis as seen with contraceptives, anabolic steroids, warfarin, thiabendazole, and prochlorperazine, the bile pigment accumulates in the dilated canaliculi, hepatocyte cytoplasm, and Kupffer cells, and there is remarkable paucity of inflammatory cells. Hepatocyte necrosis occurs predominantly in the centrilobular area, and bile duct injury is usually absent. Electron microscopy also suggests canalicular cholestasis and injury.[3]

Acute ductular cholangitis or cholangiolitis is infrequent and is seen with psychotropic agents such as barbiturates and phenytoin. Portal triaditis and inflammatory infiltrate (lymphocytes, neutrophils, eosinophils) are found around the bile ducts/ductules. Feathery degeneration of hepatocytes, hepatocyte necrosis, and granulomas can also be seen.[3]

## CHRONIC CHOLESTATIC DILI

Chronic drug-induced cholestasis is infrequent, and typically occurs as a result of protracted liver injury more than 6 months after the initial cholestatic insult (**Fig. 2**). Such chronic cholestasis has been reported with about 40 drugs.[3] It can present in 2 forms: vanishing bile duct syndrome (ductopenic cholestasis) or sclerosing cholangitis. Such chronic cholestasis mimics primary biliary cirrhosis (PBC) and would eventually lead to fibrosis and cirrhosis, although few reports of resolution are present in the literature.[53]

Vanishing bile duct syndrome is a rare form of drug-induced chronic intrahepatic cholestasis. Chronic cholestasis that is incited primarily continues for longer periods, resulting in chronic bile duct injury, bile duct loss, cirrhosis, and subsequent hepatic decompensation. Drugs that are implicated in the causation of vanishing bile duct syndrome are neuroleptic agents (chlorpromazine, imipramine, carbamazepine, amitriptyline, haloperidol, cyproheptadine, phenytoin), antibiotics (amoxicillin, flucloxacillin, quinolones, clindamycin, macrolides, tetracyclines), complementary and alternative medicines (ajmaline, glycyrrhizin), NSAIDs (diclofenac, ibuprofen), amiodarone, cimetidine, thiabendazole, zonisamide, and so forth. Of the whole list, chlorpromazine, ajmaline, and flucloxacillin are the commonly reported drugs associated with vanishing bile duct syndrome.[19] Chlorpromazine can result in prolonged cholestasis lasting more than a year in about 7% to 10% of cases after an acute hepatic insult, with several of them progressing to vanishing bile duct syndrome.[3,19]

Drugs can also cause injury to the major ducts or ductules, mimicking sclerosing cholangitis and causing intrahepatic and extrahepatic cholestasis. Floxuridine (FUDR) is the classic prototype drug of the past, which was administered via the hepatic artery as an intra-arterial infusion for the local treatment of liver metastasis and is associated with segmental or multiple bile duct structures. The mechanism of cholestasis works by causing injury to the hepatic arterioles that supply the biliary radicles

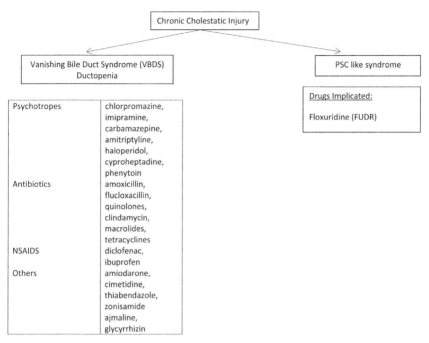

**Fig. 2.** Drugs involved in chronic cholestatic injury. NSAIDS, nonsteroidal anti-inflammatory drugs; PSC, primary sclerosing cholangitis.

and thereby induce ischemic cholangiopathy. Such injury was reported within a few months of initiation of treatment in 5% to 25% of the subjects.[3]

### Clinical Features and Management

The clinical features of the 2 subtypes of chronic cholestasis mimic PBC or primary sclerosing cholangitis. Initial abnormalities include a cholestatic pattern of liver enzymes with jaundice, which remains protracted over several months to years. Pruritus, fatigue, and xanthoma formation are also noted. Resolution of jaundice alone, but with persistence of cholestatic biochemical pattern or complete resolution of cholestasis has been reported in a subset of patients. Patients with unresolved cholestasis can progress to secondary biliary cirrhosis with subsequent development of complications of portal hypertension, resulting in death or liver transplantation. Periodic monitoring of biochemical tests, INR, and biliary imaging are necessary to exclude other possible causes.

### Pathology

Some of the histologic features seen in acute cholestatic injury can overlap in chronic cholestatic DILI, but marked bile duct injury is the hallmark of this condition. Cholestasis, polymorphous inflammatory infiltrate, ductopenia, ductular proliferation, duct fibrosis, copper accumulation, and varying stages of lobular fibrosis are commonly found. Hepatic lobular inflammation and necrosis is usually mild or absent. The biopsy should be carefully reviewed to exclude other causes of cholestasis or to diagnose presence of concomitant liver diseases.[3,8]

## TREATMENT

There is no proven medical therapy for the treatment of chronic cholestatic DILI. The treatment of drug-induced cholestasis is largely supportive, which involves prompt withdrawal of the offending drug and avoiding drug rechallenge.[4,21,52] Patients with mild injury can continue taking the drug with periodic monitoring, especially if the medication is crucial. Cessation of the offending drug is important if the patient is symptomatic or develops severe cholestatic injury as evidenced by jaundice, elevation of serum bilirubin ($>3 \times$ ULN), or prolongation of INR ($>1.5 \times$ ULN).[4] Ursodiol (UDCA) is frequently prescribed, but the data on its efficacy are variable and inconsistent. The major benefit from UDCA is protection against cytotoxicity caused by toxic bile salts, stimulation of hepatobiliary secretion, antioxidant activity, enhancement in glutathione levels, and the inhibition of liver cell apoptosis.[54] Management of pruritus can be challenging and crucial. Topical emollients, cholestyramine, colestipol, antihistamines, rifampin, phenobarbital, and opioid analogues can be used to ameliorate pruritus. Ultraviolet B phototherapy appears to be a promising and well-tolerated treatment in patients who have failed conventional therapy for pruritus.[55] Biliary stenting and drainage appears to be beneficial in managing symptoms and in patients with bile duct strictures.[53] Although corticosteroids do not have a proven benefit, they may be used in severe cholestatic injury caused by hypersensitivity, as in the case of amoxicillin-clavulanate.[4,21,56] Steroid-sparing agents such as azathioprine and mycophenolate mofetil have also been tried, with some benefit. Liver transplantation is the only definitive therapy for patients who develop severe acute liver injury resulting in fulminant hepatic failure, and those who develop secondary biliary cirrhosis and decompensation.[57]

## PROGNOSIS

Drug-induced liver injury leading to jaundice is well known to be associated with poor prognosis and a mortality rate of around 10% without liver transplantation.[58] Previously, cholestatic DILI was thought to have a better prognosis than hepatocellular DILI, but evidence from recent literature suggests that the mortality rate for cholestatic DILI is around 5% to 14.3%, with the rate for mixed DILI at around 2.1% to 5%.[8,9,11] Biochemical abnormalities in cholestatic DILI take a longer time to normalize compared with hepatocellular DILI. Approximately 5% to 13.6% of patients developed chronic liver injury after an acute drug-induced cholestatic insult.[59] Drugs implicated in the development of chronic cholestasis can lead to chronic bile duct injury and cirrhosis. More long-term studies are needed to further prognosticate on the severity of liver disease and outcomes.

## SUMMARY

Drug-induced cholestasis can result in acute or chronic liver injury. Most cases of cholestatic DILI appear to resolve shortly after drug withdrawal, but a subset of cases can progress to chronic cholestasis, cirrhosis, and subsequent hepatic decompensation. Early recognition and prompt withdrawal of the offending drug is the mainstay of the initial management. This review summarizes the implicated drugs, diagnostic tools, and the management of drug-induced cholestasis. Proper reporting of the adverse drug reactions and outcomes are important as new drugs are being developed and approved.

## REFERENCES

1. Siddique A, Kowdley KV. Approach to a patient with elevated serum alkaline phosphatase. Clin Liver Dis 2012;16(2):199–229.
2. Ghabril M, Chalasani N, Bjornsson E. Drug-induced liver injury: a clinical update. Curr Opin Gastroenterol 2010;26(3):222–6.
3. Degott C. Drug-induced liver injury. Cholestatic injury, acute and chronic. Pathol Oncol Res 1997;3(4):260–3.
4. Tajiri K, Shimizu Y. Practical guidelines for diagnosis and early management of drug-induced liver injury. World J Gastroenterol 2008;14(44):6774–85.
5. Navarro VJ, Senior JR. Drug-related hepatotoxicity. N Engl J Med 2006;354(7): 731–9.
6. Ostapowicz G, Fontana RJ, Schiodt FV, et al. Results of a prospective study of acute liver failure at 17 tertiary care centers in the United States. Ann Intern Med 2002;137(12):947–54.
7. Sgro C, Clinard F, Ouazir K, et al. Incidence of drug-induced hepatic injuries: a French population-based study. Hepatology 2002;36(2):451–5.
8. Bjornsson ES, Jonasson JG. Drug-induced cholestasis. Clin Liver Dis 2013; 17(2):191–209.
9. Chalasani N, Fontana RJ, Bonkovsky HL, et al. Causes, clinical features, and outcomes from a prospective study of drug-induced liver injury in the United States. Gastroenterology 2008;135(6):1924–34, 1934.e1–4.
10. Lucena MI, Andrade RJ, Kaplowitz N, et al. Phenotypic characterization of idiosyncratic drug-induced liver injury: the influence of age and sex. Hepatology 2009;49(6):2001–9.
11. Andrade RJ, Lucena MI, Fernández MC, et al. Drug-induced liver injury: an analysis of 461 incidences submitted to the Spanish registry over a 10-year period. Gastroenterology 2005;129(2):512–21.
12. Daly AK, Donaldson PT, Bhatnagar P, et al. HLA-B*5701 genotype is a major determinant of drug-induced liver injury due to flucloxacillin. Nat Genet 2009; 41(7):816–9.
13. Andrade RJ, Lucena MI, Alonso A, et al. HLA class II genotype influences the type of liver injury in drug-induced idiosyncratic liver disease. Hepatology 2004;39(6):1603–12.
14. Meier Y, Zodan T, Lang C, et al. Increased susceptibility for intrahepatic cholestasis of pregnancy and contraceptive-induced cholestasis in carriers of the 1331T>C polymorphism in the bile salt export pump. World J Gastroenterol 2008;14(1):38–45.
15. Lammert C, Bjornsson E, Niklasson A, et al. Oral medications with significant hepatic metabolism at higher risk for hepatic adverse events. Hepatology 2010; 51(2):615–20.
16. Mancinelli R, Onori P, Demorrow S, et al. Role of sex hormones in the modulation of cholangiocyte function. World J Gastrointest Pathophysiol 2010;1(2): 50–62.
17. Pauli-Magnus C, Meier PJ. Hepatobiliary transporters and drug-induced cholestasis. Hepatology 2006;44(4):778–87.
18. Lang C, Meier Y, Stieger B, et al. Mutations and polymorphisms in the bile salt export pump and the multidrug resistance protein 3 associated with drug-induced liver injury. Pharmacogenet Genomics 2007;17(1):47–60.
19. Velayudham LS, Farrell GC. Drug-induced cholestasis. Expert Opin Drug Saf 2003;2(3):287–304.

20. Teschke R, Schwarzenboeck A, Hennermann KH. Causality assessment in hepatotoxicity by drugs and dietary supplements. Br J Clin Pharmacol 2008;66(6): 758–66.

21. Suk KT, Kim DJ. Drug-induced liver injury: present and future. Clin Mol Hepatol 2012;18(3):249–57.

22. Garcia Rodriguez LA, Stricker BH, Zimmerman HJ. Risk of acute liver injury associated with the combination of amoxicillin and clavulanic acid. Arch Intern Med 1996;156(12):1327–32.

23. Hussaini SH, O'Brien CS, Despott EJ, et al. Antibiotic therapy: a major cause of drug-induced jaundice in southwest England. Eur J Gastroenterol Hepatol 2007; 19(1):15–20.

24. Lucena MI, Andrade RJ, Fernández MC, et al. Determinants of the clinical expression of amoxicillin-clavulanate hepatotoxicity: a prospective series from Spain. Hepatology 2006;44(4):850–6.

25. Fontana RJ, Shakil AO, Greenson JK, et al. Acute liver failure due to amoxicillin and amoxicillin/clavulanate. Dig Dis Sci 2005;50(10):1785–90.

26. Olsson R, Wiholm BE, Sand C, et al. Liver damage from flucloxacillin, cloxacillin and dicloxacillin. J Hepatol 1992;15(1–2):154–61.

27. de Abajo FJ, Montero D, Madurga M, et al. Acute and clinically relevant drug-induced liver injury: a population based case-control study. Br J Clin Pharmacol 2004;58(1):71–80.

28. Turner IB, Eckstein RP, Riley JW, et al. Prolonged hepatic cholestasis after flucloxacillin therapy. Med J Aust 1989;151(11–12):701–5.

29. Davies MH, Harrison RF, Elias E, et al. Antibiotic-associated acute vanishing bile duct syndrome: a pattern associated with severe, prolonged, intrahepatic cholestasis. J Hepatol 1994;20(1):112–6.

30. Andrade RJ, Guilarte J, Salmerón FJ, et al. Benzylpenicillin-induced prolonged cholestasis. Ann Pharmacother 2001;35(6):783–4.

31. Andrade RJ, Tulkens PM. Hepatic safety of antibiotics used in primary care. J Antimicrob Chemother 2011;66(7):1431–46.

32. Derby LE, Jick H, Henry DA, et al. Erythromycin-associated cholestatic hepatitis. Med J Aust 1993;158(9):600–2.

33. Lockwood AM, Cole S, Rabinovich M. Azithromycin-induced liver injury. Am J Health Syst Pharm 2010;67(10):810–4.

34. Brinker AD, Wassel RT, Lyndly J, et al. Telithromycin-associated hepatotoxicity: clinical spectrum and causality assessment of 42 cases. Hepatology 2009; 49(1):250–7.

35. Lucena MI, Andrade RJ, Rodrigo L, et al. Trovafloxacin-induced acute hepatitis. Clin Infect Dis 2000;30(2):400–1.

36. Gupta AK, del Rosso JQ, Lynde CW, et al. Hepatitis associated with terbinafine therapy: three case reports and a review of the literature. Clin Exp Dermatol 1998;23(2):64–7.

37. Agarwal K, Manas DM, Hudson M. Terbinafine and fulminant hepatic failure. N Engl J Med 1999;340(16):1292–3.

38. Yoshikado T, Takada T, Yamamoto T, et al. Itraconazole-induced cholestasis: involvement of the inhibition of bile canalicular phospholipid translocator MDR3/ABCB4. Mol Pharmacol 2011;79(2):241–50.

39. Akhtar AJ, Shaheen M. Jaundice in African-American and Hispanic patients with AIDS. J Natl Med Assoc 2007;99(12):1381–5.

40. Bjornsson E, Olsson R. Suspected drug-induced liver fatalities reported to the WHO database. Dig Liver Dis 2006;38(1):33–8.

41. Cachay ER, Peterson MR, Goicoechea M, et al. Didanosine exposure and noncirrhotic portal hypertension in an HIV clinic in North America: a follow-up study. Br J Med Med Res 2011;1(4):346–55.
42. Kovari H, Ledergerber B, Peter U, et al. Association of noncirrhotic portal hypertension in HIV-infected persons and antiretroviral therapy with didanosine: a nested case-control study. Clin Infect Dis 2009;49(4):626–35.
43. Levy C, Lindor KD. Drug-induced cholestasis. Clin Liver Dis 2003;7(2):311–30.
44. Bastida G, Nos P, Aguas M, et al. Incidence, risk factors and clinical course of thiopurine-induced liver injury in patients with inflammatory bowel disease. Aliment Pharmacol Ther 2005;22(9):775–82.
45. Gisbert JP, Gonzalez-Lama Y, Mate J. Thiopurine-induced liver injury in patients with inflammatory bowel disease: a systematic review. Am J Gastroenterol 2007; 102(7):1518–27.
46. Roda G, Caponi A, Belluzzi A, et al. Severe cholestatic acute hepatitis following azathioprine therapy in a patient with ulcerative pancolitis. Dig Liver Dis 2009; 41(12):914–5.
47. Moradpour D, Altorfer J, Flury R, et al. Chlorpromazine-induced vanishing bile duct syndrome leading to biliary cirrhosis. Hepatology 1994;20(6):1437–41.
48. Lammert C, Einarsson S, Saha C, et al. Relationship between daily dose of oral medications and idiosyncratic drug-induced liver injury: search for signals. Hepatology 2008;47(6):2003–9.
49. Vuppalanchi R, Hayashi PH, Chalasani N, et al. Duloxetine hepatotoxicity: a case-series from the drug-induced liver injury network. Aliment Pharmacol Ther 2010;32(9):1174–83.
50. Clarke JD, Cherrington NJ. Genetics or environment in drug transport: the case of organic anion transporting polypeptides and adverse drug reactions. Expert Opin Drug Metab Toxicol 2012;8(3):349–60.
51. Kleiner DE. The pathology of drug-induced liver injury. Semin Liver Dis 2009; 29(4):364–72.
52. Ramachandran R, Kakar S. Histological patterns in drug-induced liver disease. J Clin Pathol 2009;62(6):481–92.
53. Vuppalanchi R, Chalasani N, Saxena R. Restoration of bile ducts in drug-induced vanishing bile duct syndrome due to zonisamide. Am J Surg Pathol 2006;30(12):1619–23.
54. Perez MJ, Briz O. Bile-acid-induced cell injury and protection. World J Gastroenterol 2009;15(14):1677–89.
55. Decock S, Roelandts R, Steenbergen WV, et al. Cholestasis-induced pruritus treated with ultraviolet B phototherapy: an observational case series study. J Hepatol 2012;57(3):637–41.
56. Herrero-Herrero JI, Garcia-Aparicio J. Corticosteroid therapy in a case of severe cholestatic hepatitis associated with amoxicillin-clavulanate. J Med Toxicol 2010;6(4):420–3.
57. Geubel AP, Sempoux CL. Drug and toxin-induced bile duct disorders. J Gastroenterol Hepatol 2000;15(11):1232–8.
58. Lewis JH, Zimmerman HJ. Drug- and chemical-induced cholestasis. Clin Liver Dis 1999;3(3):433–64, vii.
59. Andrade RJ, Lucena MI, Kaplowitz N, et al. Outcome of acute idiosyncratic drug-induced liver injury: long-term follow-up in a hepatotoxicity registry. Hepatology 2006;44(6):1581–8.

# Drug-Induced Steatohepatitis

Vaishali Patel, MBBS, MD, Arun J. Sanyal, MBBS, MD*

KEYWORDS

- Nonalcoholic fatty liver disease • Nonalcoholic steatohepatitis
- Microvesicular and macrovesicular steatosis • Drug-induced steatohepatitis

KEY POINTS

- Hepatic steatosis and steatohepatitis can arise from the interplay of several inciting factors, including alcohol, drugs, and metabolic syndrome as nonalcoholic fatty liver disease (NAFLD).
- Drugs induce fat deposition in the liver in microvesicular or macrovesicular distribution.
- Most drugs implicated in steatosis and steatohepatitis can induce both to a variable extent.
- It is difficult to ascertain whether an implicated drug leads to de novo steatosis and/or steatohepatitis versus worsening of underlying NAFLD.
- The pathogenesis of drug-induced steatohepatitis often involves mitochondrial dysfunction.

## DEFINITION OF NAFLD

Hepatic steatosis is defined as fat deposition within hepatocytes (**Fig. 1**). It is seen microscopically as vacuoles in a microvesicular or macrovesicular distribution. Microvesicular steatosis is characterized by multiple small, fat vesicles distributed throughout the hepatocyte, whereas macrovesicular steatosis is characterized by a large droplet of fat within the cytoplasm, which pushes the nucleus to the edge of the cell. Although microvesicular steatosis is more commonly seen in Reye syndrome and other forms of mitochondrial injury, nonalcoholic fatty liver disease (NAFLD) typically has macrovesicular distribution of fat deposits. Several drugs can lead to both forms of hepatic steatosis. Although the triggering events differ, each of these insults can lead to excessive hepatic fat deposition, increased reactive oxygen species (ROS) formation, mitochondrial dysfunction, and Endoplasmic Reticulum (ER) stress that induces inflammation, cell death and eventually leads to fibrosis.

Disclosure: This work has been supported by the NIH T32 Training Grant.
Division of Gastroenterology, Hepatology, and Nutrition, Virginia Commonwealth University Medical Center, Virginia Commonwealth University, MCV Box 980341, Richmond, VA 23298-0341, USA
* Corresponding author.
E-mail address: asanyal@mcvh-vcu.edu

Clin Liver Dis 17 (2013) 533–546
http://dx.doi.org/10.1016/j.cld.2013.07.012
1089-3261/13/$ – see front matter © 2013 Elsevier Inc. All rights reserved.

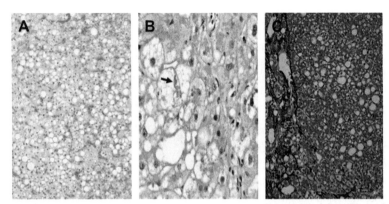

**Fig. 1.** Histologic appearance of hepatic steatosis and steatohepatitis. (*A*) Simple steatosis. Vacuoles represent areas of fat accumulation (hematoxylin-eosin). (*B*) Steatohepatitis demonstrating ballooning degeneration (*arrow*) and fat deposition (hematoxylin-eosin). (*C*) Steatohepatitis with hepatic perisinusoidal fibrosis (Prussian blue staining). Original magnification 200x.

Traditionally, NAFLD is defined as fat infiltration in the liver parenchyma in people who do not consume alcohol in quantities that are considered to be hepatotoxic. NAFLD is a manifestation of the metabolic syndrome and it is often associated with obesity, dyslipidemia, and type 2 diabetes mellitus.[1,2] With the spread of the obesity epidemic, the disease burden of NAFLD is increasing, both in terms of geography and the age of presentation. It is now the most common cause of chronic liver disease in the United States, affecting about a third of the population.[3,4]

There are 2 principal phenotypes of NAFLD: (1) nonalcoholic fatty liver (NAFL) and (2) nonalcoholic steatohepatitis (NASH). NAFL is defined by the presence of steatosis without inflammation. NASH is defined by the presence of steatosis, inflammation and hepatocyte ballooning injury.[2] NASH progresses to cirrhosis in up to a fifth of patients. Apart from this, several cases of cryptogenic cirrhosis are attributed to NAFLD.[2–6]

## DIAGNOSING DRUG-INDUCED STEATOHEPATITIS

Drug-induced liver injury (DILI) is diagnosed in a person when worsening of the baseline liver function is caused by prescription or nonprescription drugs. The diagnosis of DILI requires consideration of the following:

1. The biochemical and histologic pattern of liver injury
2. Lead time between the initiation of the suspected drug and the onset of liver disease
3. Evidence of improvement of liver function after discontinuation of the drug

The diagnosis of DILI is challenging in many cases because there is no specific maker for DILI. The literature is sparse for newer agents and herbal products. Moreover, the clinical presentation and microscopic appearance of liver injury may be nonspecific and rechallenge is not safe. Hence, several scoring systems have been developed to objectively diagnose DILI, such as the Roussel-Uclaf Causality Assessment Method (RUCAM), the Maria and Victorino method, and the Naranjo scale.[7] RUCAM is the most commonly used instrument for the diagnosis of DILI. According to RUCAM, DILI is most likely when it develops within 90 days of the initiation of the drug and improves within 15 to 30 days of discontinuation in cases of hepatocellular and cholestatic patterns of injury, respectively. Drug-induced steatohepatitis may occur after many months of use and may not resolve within 15 days.[8,9] RUCAM is, thus, suboptimal for the diagnosis of drug-induced steatohepatitis. The situation is further complicated by a high prevalence of NAFLD in the general population. Hence, even if the disease is previously undiagnosed, several patients have risk factors associated with NAFLD, making it difficult to differentiate drug-induced steatohepatitis from de novo NAFLD. It is possible that drugs may exacerbate preexisting NAFLD.[10,11]

## PATHOGENESIS OF DRUG-INDUCED STEATOHEPATITIS
### Mitochondrial Structure: Link Between β-oxidation of Fatty Acids and Fuel Synthesis

Mitochondria are double-membrane bound organelles involved in several biochemical reactions, including lipid metabolism and ATP synthesis **Fig. 2**. The outer mitochondrial membrane surrounds the intermembrane space, and the inner mitochondrial membrane (IMM) encloses the mitochondrial matrix. The mitochondrial DNA (mtDNA) is located within the mitochondrial matrix. Respiratory chain complexes I, II, III, and IV and ATP synthase are partially embedded in the IMM. Mitochondrial pyruvate dehydrogenase transforms the pyruvate coming from glucose into acetyl coenzyme A (CoA). Long-chain fatty acids (LCFA) are transported inside the mitochondrial matrix via the carnitine shuttle as long-chain fatty acyl-CoA (LCFA-CoA). Each cycle of β-oxidation yields one molecule of acetyl-CoA. β-oxidation, conversion of pyruvate

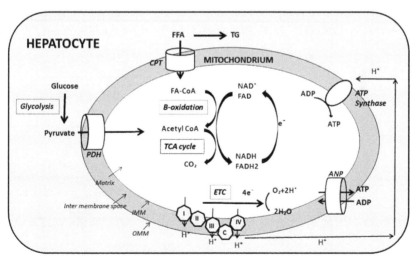

**Fig. 2.** Normal mitochondrial function: long-chain fatty acids (FFA) enter mitochondria via the carnitine palmitoyl shuttle (CPT) and form a complex with coenzyme A (CoA). They undergo β-oxidation, which yields one molecule of acetyl CoA per cycle. Acetyl CoA is also formed from pyruvate via the pyruvate dehydrogenase complex (PDH). Acetyl CoA is finally metabolized to carbon dioxide and water in the tricarboxylic Acid (TCA) cycle. β-oxidation, synthesis of acetyl CoA, and TCA cycle lead to the formation of reduced NAD⁺ and FAD, which are oxidized by releasing electrons. Electrons low through the electron transport chain (ETC) release protons and result in production of water. In energy-depleted state, ADP enters the mitochondrial matrix by the adenine nucleotide transporter (ANP). Protons are used in synthesis of ATP from ADP by ATP synthase. ATP can then leave the mitochondrium via the ANP. IMM, inner mitochondrial membrane; OMM, outer mitochondrial membrane.

to acetyl CoA by the pyruvate dehydrogenase complex, and metabolism of acetyl-CoA by the tricarboxylic acid cycle produce NADH and FADH2. These molecules are, in turn, oxidized by transferring their electrons to the mitochondrial respiratory chain. As electrons flow through the electron transport chain (ETC), 3 protons from the mitochondrial matrix are pushed into the intermembrane space at the level of complexes I, III, and IV. This process increases the electrochemical gradient across the IMM. In an energy-depleted state, ADP enters the mitochondrial matrix via the adenine nucleotide translocator (ANT). The increased transmembrane potential allows ADP to drag along protons, which results in the generation of ATP via ATP synthase. ATP can then leave the mitochondrion via the ANT. These processes are well coordinated and ultimately result in the production of oxygen, water, and ATP. However, at the level of complexes I and III, electrons can interact directly with protons and result in the production of ROS.[10,12]

### Mechanisms of Hepatic Steatosis

Hepatic steatosis in NAFLD results predominantly from a combination of increased dietary intake, peripheral lipolysis, and de novo fatty acid synthesis **Fig. 3**.[13] Drugs that lead to steatosis and steatohepatitis primarily interfere with mitochondrial respiration, β-oxidation, or both.[14] It is important to understand that the ETC and β-oxidation of fatty acids are metabolically inter-connected. Hence, drugs affecting one pathway invariably inhibit the other.[15] When hepatic mitochondrial β-oxidation is severely inhibited, the impairment of fatty acyl-CoA β-oxidation increases fatty acyl-CoA and nonesterified fatty acids, which are converted into triglycerides resulting in hepatic steatosis.[12] Besides inducing steatosis, the inhibition of β-oxidation and ETC results in increased ROS formation and, in more severe cases, hepatic necrosis.[14,16–19]

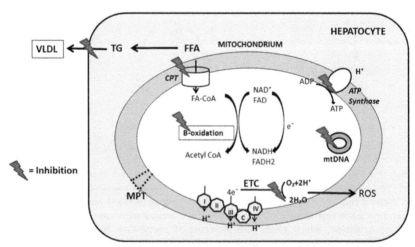

**Fig. 3.** Mechanisms of hepatic steatosis and injury in drug-induced steatohepatitis. Inhibition of entry of long-chain fatty acids (FFA) via the carnitine palmitoyl shuttle (CPT) and inhibition of β-oxidation lead to increased free fatty acids, which are esterified into triglycerides. Transport of triglycerides (TG) as very low-density lipoprotein (VLDL) can be blocked by some drugs. Blocking the flow of electrons through the ETC leads to accumulation of electrons. These electrons can directly interact with oxygen to produce ROS. Certain drugs directly damage mtDNA and can induce mitochondrial permeability transition (MPT) pore formation.

Drugs that inhibit mitochondrial β-oxidation do so by several mechanisms:

- Inhibition of entry of LCFA into the mitochondrial matrix, which is seen with the antidiabetic drug troglitazone, which inhibits mitochondrial acyl-CoA synthase[20]
- Sequestration of CoA in the form of a drug-CoA thioester as seen in valproate toxicity[21]
- Inhibition of enzymes catalyzing β-oxidation, for example, glucocorticoids inhibit acyl-CoA dehydrogenases[10,22]

Rarely, other mechanisms that result in increased hepatic fat are involved. Some drugs can lead to increased synthesis or decreased secretion of hepatic triglycerides as seen with protease inhibitors and dexamethasone, respectively.[23,24] De novo fatty acid synthesis is transiently increased by some antipsychotic medications by an increase in the active form of sterol regulatory element binding protein-1c (SREBP-1c).[25]

### Mechanisms of Steatohepatitis

The causes of the progression of steatosis to steatohepatitis in DILI are not well understood and mostly extrapolated from NASH literature.[10–12] One of the most-studied hypothesis is that mitochondrial dysfunction leads to and worsens drug-induced uncoupling of β-oxidation and phosphorylation, which results in the production of ROS. Reduced energy availability and direct damage form ROS, in turn, induce hepatocyte necrosis.[12] ROS cause additional damage by interaction with nonesterified polyunsaturated fatty acids to produce lipid peroxidation products, which have a longer half-life than ROS and cause damage by diffusing to surrounding cells. ROS also lead to nuclear translocation of the transcription factor, nuclear factor-κβ (NF-κβ). NF-κβ upregulates genes that promote insulin resistance[26] and several inflammatory cytokines, including tumor necrosis factor (TNF)–α[25]; interleukin (IL)-8, which promotes polymorphonuclear (PMN) infiltration[26]; and transforming growth factor (TGF)-β. TGF-β, in turn, stimulates hepatic stellate cell proliferation and fibrosis.[16,26] NF-κβ also promotes apoptotic cell death by inducing transcriptional expression of the normally repressed fatty acid synthetase (FAS)-ligand. FAS ligand binds to FAS on adjacent hepatocytes, leading to caspase-9 activation. Caspase-9 then activates other caspases to promote apoptotic hepatocyte cell death.[16]

## PATHOLOGIC SPECTRUM OF DRUG-INDUCED STEATOSIS AND STEATOHEPATITIS

Drugs implicated in hepatic steatosis can be divided on basis of hepatic microscopy into those that cause microvesicular steatosis and those that predominantly lead to macrovesicular steatosis (**Table 1**). Characteristics and mechanism of injury by individual drugs are described later.

### Drugs Causing Microvesicular Steatosis

#### Aspirin
Aspirin is metabolized to salicylic acid and then salicyl-CoA. In aspirin poisoning, this process leads to excessive utilization of CoA, thus blocking the entry of LCFA entry into mitochondria and arresting β-oxidation.[27] Aspirin can also directly uncouple respiration. It promotes mitochondrial permeability transition pore formation that leads to mitochondrial death, which triggers cell death by apoptosis and necrosis.[28] Aspirin use in children with viral infections has been associated with Reye syndrome. The pathogenesis of Reye syndrome involves widespread arrest of β-oxidation, increased ureagenesis and ketogenesis, and severe hypoglycemia caused by the inability to convert lactate to glucose. Diffuse hepatic microvesicular steatosis is seen in this

**Table 1**
**Drugs causing steatosis and steatohepatitis**

| Drug | Common Liver Pathology | Mechanism of Liver Injury |
|---|---|---|
| Aspirin | Microvesicular steatosis | Arrest B oxidation by consuming CoA; increase mitochondrial permeability by MPT pore formation |
| Valproate | Microvesicular steatosis | Inhibit CPT-1 activity, sequestering CoA; arresting ETC and ATP synthesis; promotes weight gain |
| Cocaine | Microvesicular steatosis | Undergoes n-oxidation to produce hepatotoxic products and inhibition of β-oxidation |
| NRITs (zidovudine and didanosine) | Microvesicular steatosis | Mitochondrial dysfunction by mtDNA depletion and stimulation of autophagy |
| Tetracycline | Microvesicular steatosis | Inhibit β-oxidation of fatty acids and VLDL secretion |
| NSAIDs (ibuprofen and naproxen) | Microvesicular steatosis | Inhibit β-oxidation of short- and medium-chain fatty acids |
| Glucocorticoids | Macrovesicular steatosis | Promote weight gain and glucose intolerance; inhibit mitochondrial β-oxidation, decrease hepatic triglyceride secretion, and induce lipid peroxidation |
| Amiodarone | Macrovesicular steatosis, steatohepatitis, and phospholipidosis | Decreases β-oxidation of fatty acids; increases lipid peroxidation, ROS generation, and lipogenesis |
| 5-fluorouracil | Macrovesicular steatosis | Unknown |
| Irinotecan | Steatohepatitis | Unknown |
| Methotrexate | Macrovesicular steatosis and steatohepatitis | Inhibits mitochondrial electron transport chain |
| Tamoxifen | Macrovesicular steatosis and steatohepatitis | Promotes de novo fatty acid synthesis and inhibits fatty acid β-oxidation |
| Petrochemicals (eg vinyl chloride) | Microvesicular steatosis and steatohepatitis | Unknown |

*Abbreviations:* CPT, carnitine palmitoyl shuttle; MPT, mitochondrial permeability transition; NRITs, nucleoside reverse transcriptase inhibitors; NSAIDs, nonsteroidal antiinflammatory drugs; VLDL, very low-density lipoprotein.

rapidly fatal disease.[19] Since the 1980s, the incidence of Reye syndrome in developed countries has significantly declined.

### Cocaine

Cocaine-induced hepatotoxicity ranges from hepatic steatosis (both microvesicular and macrovesicular) in milder cases to centrilobular necrosis in more severe ones. Inflammation is characteristically sparse.[29] Hepatic n-oxidation of cocaine and its metabolites leads to progressively more hepatotoxic products.[30] A recent lipidomic analysis of mice livers has revealed that cocaine use leads to the inhibition of hepatic β-oxidation of fatty acids, which contributes to the accumulation of hepatic triglycerides, long-chain acylcarnitines, and phospholipids.[31]

### Valproate

Valproate is a branched-chain fatty acid that causes microvesicular steatosis and cirrhosis. In one report, up to 60% of patients treated with valproate had ultrasound evidence of hepatic steatosis.[32] Valproate is initially metabolized by cytochrome P-450 enzymes to 4-ene-valproate. Both valproate and 4-ene-valproate then form complexes with CoA, sequestering CoA as well as competitively inhibiting carnitine palmitoyl shuttle I activity. Valproate can release protons and, thus, arrest the ETC and ATP synthesis.[21] Besides mitochondrial dysfunction, with prolonged use, valproate promotes weight gain and systemic insulin resistance, which may lead to worsening of the underlying NAFLD.[32]

### Nucleoside reverse transcriptase inhibitors, thymidine analogues

Although hepatotoxicity can be seen with all groups of HIV antiretroviral therapy, nucleoside reverse transcriptase inhibitors (NRTIs) have been associated with hepatic steatosis. With prolonged use, thymidine analogues, zidovudine and didanosine (but not the cytidine analogue lamivudine) can lead to hepatic microvesicular steatosis and steatohepatitis. A few cases of acute liver failure have been reported.[33,34] These drugs deplete mtDNA and stimulate autophagy, which leads to ROS formation and further worsening of mitochondrial function.[33–35] NRTI-related hepatic steatosis is more common in obese patients and women.[36] Hence, it is plausible that by inhibition of autophagy, these drugs may worsen and/or unmask underlying NAFLD.[35,37]

### Tetracycline

Intravenous tetracyclines were discontinued in 1991 because of reports of rapid, fulminant, and often fatal hepatotoxicity. Histopathology of tetracycline injury is characterized by generalized microvesicular injury. Tetracyclines inhibit the secretion of hepatic fat as very low-density lipoprotein by inhibiting microsomal triglyceride transfer protein. They also inhibit the mitochondrial β-oxidation of fatty acids.[38]

### Nonsteroidal antiinflammatory drugs (ibuprofen, naproxen)

Nonsteroidal antiinflammatory drugs (NSAIDS) are a leading cause of hepatotoxicity. NSAIDs can cause both cholestatic and hepatocellular patterns of liver injury and, in severe cases, lead to acute liver failure. Only a few NSAIDs have been reported to induce hepatic steatosis. Naproxen and ibuprofen are commonly used NSAIDs in the United States that can lead to microvesicular steatosis. The proposed mechanism is inhibition β-oxidation of short- and medium-chain fatty acids.[39,40]

## Drugs Causing Macrovesicular Steatosis and Steatohepatitis

Most drugs leading to macrovesicular steatosis can also cause steatohepatitis to a varying degree. One exception to this is 5-fluorouracil (5-FU) because its use is associated with isolated macrovesicular steatosis. Individual drugs leading to macrovesicular steatosis and steatohepatitis are summarized later.

### Drugs with true cause-effect relationship with steatosis and steatohepatitis

**Amiodarone** Amiodarone is a potent antiarrhythmic agent that, over prolonged use, causes several adverse effects, including liver dysfunction; pulmonary fibrosis; neurotoxicity; ocular complications; and, because it is structurally similar to thyroxin, thyroid dysfunction.[41,42] These adverse effects are seen in up to 80% of patients taking the drug. Twenty percent to 40% of patients need to discontinue its use because of the adverse effects.[42] In some reports, up to 30% of patients taking the drug have an acute elevation of liver enzymes, usually within 24 hours of intravenous infusion. Liver enzymes may be up to 1.5 to 4.0 times the upper limit of normal even in asymptomatic patients.[41] Although liver enzyme abnormalities are benign in about a fourth of the patients, 1% to 2% develop symptomatic disease in the form of steatohepatitis. Other more aggressive patterns of injury, including extensive hepatocellular necrosis, Reye syndrome–like illness, and cholestatic hepatitis, have also been reported.[41,43,44] With chronic use, amiodarone is concentrated in the liver and can be visualized on imaging studies. With prolonged use, its hepatic levels can be 100 to 500 times higher than serum. Chronic liver injury caused by amiodarone is a function of its cumulative dose. Hence, steatohepatitis can be seen with low daily doses.[10,22] The histopathologic appearance of amiodarone-induced hepatotoxicity is similar to classic NASH. Mallory hyaline deposits and neutrophil infiltration with steatosis may be seen. Some patients develop a distinct pattern of lipid deposition inside lysosomes leading to foamy-appearing hepatocytes and Kupffer cells. This condition is referred to as *phospholipidosis*, and it can be seen in the absence of steatohepatitis.[45,46]

Amiodarone promotes several enzymes involved in de novo fatty acid synthesis, including SREBP-1c, FAS, and ATP citrate lyase.[47] It can inhibit β-oxidation of LCFA by blocking their mitochondrial entry via the carnitine shuttle and by inhibiting long-chain acyl-CoA dehydrogenase.[48,49] It arrests mitochondrial respiration by inhibiting enzymes of the ETC as well as by direct inhibition of electron transport by its benzofuran structure.[50] It is important to note that because of hepatic concentration and long half-life, amiodarone hepatotoxicity not only takes time to resolve but can also occasionally manifest after drug discontinuation.[44]

**Diethylamioethoxyhexestrol and perhexiline maleate** Perhexiline maleate (Pexid) and diethylamioethoxyhexestrol (Coralgil) caused steatohepatitis and phospholipidosis.[51–54] Both drugs have been removed from the market in the United States.

**Chemotherapy-associated steatohepatitis** Irinotecan, 5-FU, and oxaliplatin, along with the biologic agents cituximab (Erbitux) and bevacizumab (Avastin), have improved the survival of patients with colorectal cancer with metastasis.[55–57] When used before surgery, they can downsize the tumor and allow resection in carefully selected patients who otherwise have incurable disease.[58,59] However, the use of these agents has proved to be challenging because they cause steatosis, steatohepatitis, and sinusoidal obstruction syndrome, collectively referred to as chemotherapy-induced liver injury (CALI). 5-FU causes isolated hepatic steatosis. Steatohepatitis is seen following treatment with irinotecan and is referred to as chemotherapy-associated steatohepatitis. Oxaliplatin has been shown to cause sinusoidal obstruction syndrome.[60,61] According to one large study, steatosis involving more than 30% of the hepatocytes was seen in more than 46% of patients and steatohepatitis in about 20% of patients who underwent neoadjuvant chemotherapy for colorectal liver metastasis.[62] A recent consensus statement by the International Hepato-Pancreato-Biliary Association noted that hepatic steatosis and steatohepatitis are associated with poor postoperative outcomes, including slower regeneration and increased mortality.[63] CALI interferes with decreases the accuracy of the preoperative assessment of metastasis. It has been associated with poor surgical outcomes, such as longer operating time, longer hospital stay, postoperative infections, and perioperative hemorrhage. Liver failure leading to portal hypertension and ascites is possible because of poor functional reserve. However, there is evidence that shows no change in outcomes in patients with isolated hepatic steatosis. Another study has shown worse outcomes to be a function of the amount of resection and blood loss rather than the degree of steatosis.[64,65] The problem in interpreting these studies is that it is unclear if those patients who got the drug were somehow different from those who did not. A lack of prechemotherapy data biopsy for diagnoses and the higher prevalence of NAFLD add to the difficulty of establishing causality.[63] The mechanism of hepatic fat accumulation and liver injury induced by these drugs remains to be elucidated.

### Drugs leading to worsening of underlying NAFLD

**Methotrexate** Methotrexate is a folate antagonist. It is used as a chemotherapeutic agent and as an immunosuppressant in the treatment of rheumatoid arthritis, psoriasis, and inflammatory bowel disease. Methotrexate toxicity increases with cumulative doses. Liver pathology ranges from simple steatosis, mild portal inflammation, and focal necrosis to more severe forms of injury, including extensive necrosis, fibrosis, and cirrhosis. Methotrexate can independently cause steatohepatitis and lead to worsening of underlying NASH.[66–68] The risk of developing liver disease with methotrexate use is higher in those with underlying liver disease. The American Association of Dermatology's 2009 guidelines on methotrexate use in psoriasis recommend a liver biopsy after cumulative doses of 3.5 to 4.0 g in patients with no underlying liver disease or risk factors.[66] Methotrexate targets mitochondrial respiration to induce steatohepatitis, and scarring may be caused by its effect on the canals of Hering.[69,70]

**Tamoxifen** Tamoxifen is a selective estrogen receptor modulator widely used for the treatment of patients with breast cancer. Several forms of liver injury, both acute and chronic, have been reported with tamoxifen use. Among these, hepatic steatosis and steatohepatitis are the most commonly seen on microscopic examination.[71,72] Hepatic steatosis develops within 2 years of therapy in patients with breast cancer who are treated with tamoxifen. Overall, about a third of patients develop steatosis.[73,74] Rapid improvement in both steatosis and steatohepatitis is seen with drug withdrawal.[73,75] Several of these patients are obese and have other risk factors for metabolic syndrome. Hence, it has been suggested that tamoxifen may accelerate the development of NAFLD.[71–76] The mechanisms reported include the promotion of de novo fatty acid synthesis and impairment of fatty acid β-oxidation.[11,77]

**Corticosteroids** Glucocorticoids are used widely as immunosuppressants in a variety of autoimmune diseases. Their use over the long-term commonly leads to weight gain, dyslipidemia, and glucose intolerance. Hence, as expected, glucocorticoids lead to steatosis and steatohepatitis by the worsening of metabolic syndrome. Glucocorticoids also inhibit mitochondrial β-oxidation, decrease hepatic triglyceride secretion, and induce the peroxidation of lipids, thus independently causing steatohepatitis.[24,78]

## MANAGEMENT OF PATIENTS WITH DRUG-INDUCED STEATOHEPATITIS

There are no guidelines and there is little evidence from controlled clinical trials that can be applied in the management of patients with drug-induced steatohepatitis. As in other forms of DILI, if the implicated drug has already been discontinued at the time of diagnosis, it should not be reintroduced because of the risk of developing more aggressive liver injury. However, if patients are still on the drug, stop the drug whenever possible and consider alternative forms of therapy, if available. If not, the risks and benefits of continuing the drug versus stopping it should be carefully weighed. The patients' background history and risk factors for NAFLD should be reviewed. If no risk factors for NAFLD can be identified, then steatosis/steatohepatitis in those patients can be exclusively attributed to the drug. In such scenarios, stopping the drug should be favored. Current literature supports that steatosis and steatohepatitis both improve after stopping the implicated drug. Liver enzymes and imaging should be used to confirm improvement after stopping the drug. Magnetic resonance imaging (MRI) is more specific than sonography as a marker of hepatic steatosis. The information gained by an MRI may aid in future drug development and to guide therapy in other patients on that particular drug.

## SUMMARY

Steatohepatitis is a complex disease with several possible etiologic factors. The clinicopathological picture varies depending on the genetic makeup of an individual and the contributing environmental factors, including nutrition excess and exposure to toxins, such drugs and alcohol. In the real world, several of these exposures are usually present simultaneously in the same individual. Hence, classifying steatohepatitis by the cause, such as alcoholic liver disease, NAFLD, or drug-induced steatohepatitis, creates false barriers that may not allow for a unifying diagnosis in an individual patient. Nevertheless, an understanding of each contributing factor adds to our knowledge into the pathogenesis of the disease and can help us in developing individualized diagnostic and therapeutic tools.

## REFERENCES

1. Marchesini G, Bugianesi E, Forlani G, et al. Nonalcoholic fatty liver, steatohepatitis, and the metabolic syndrome. Hepatology 2003;37:917–23.
2. Chalasani N, Younossi Z, Lavine JE, et al. The diagnosis and management of non-alcoholic fatty liver disease: practice guideline by the American Association for the Study of Liver Diseases, American College of Gastroenterology, and the American Gastroenterological Association. Hepatology 2012;55:2005–23.
3. Dam-Larsen S, Franzmann M, Andersen IB, et al. Long term prognosis of fatty liver: risk of chronic liver disease and death. Gut 2004;53:750–5.
4. Matteoni CA, Younossi ZM, Gramlich T, et al. Nonalcoholic fatty liver disease: a spectrum of clinical and pathological severity. Gastroenterology 1999;116: 1413–9.
5. Angulo P. Diagnosing steatohepatitis and predicting liver-related mortality in patients with NAFLD: two distinct concepts. Hepatology 2011;53:1792–4.
6. Caldwell SH, Oelsner DH, Iezzoni JC, et al. Cryptogenic cirrhosis: clinical characterization and risk factors for underlying disease. Hepatology 1999;29:664–9.
7. Rockey DC, Seeff LB, Rochon J, et al. Causality assessment in drug-induced liver injury using a structured expert opinion process: comparison to the Roussel-Uclaf causality assessment method. Hepatology 2010;51:2117–26.
8. Benichou C, Danan G, Flahault A. Causality assessment of adverse reactions to drugs–II. An original model for validation of drug causality assessment methods: case reports with positive rechallenge. J Clin Epidemiol 1993;46:1331–6.
9. Danan G, Benichou C. Causality assessment of adverse reactions to drugs–I. A novel method based on the conclusions of international consensus meetings: application to drug-induced liver injuries. J Clin Epidemiol 1993;46:1323–30.
10. Stravitz RT, Sanyal AJ. Drug-induced steatohepatitis. Clin Liver Dis 2003;7: 435–51.
11. Farrell GC. Drugs and steatohepatitis. Semin Liver Dis 2002;22:185–94.
12. Pessayre D, Fromenty B, Berson A, et al. Central role of mitochondria in drug-induced liver injury. Drug Metab Rev 2012;44:34–87.
13. Donnelly KL, Smith CI, Schwarzenberg SJ, et al. Sources of fatty acids stored in liver and secreted via lipoproteins in patients with nonalcoholic fatty liver disease. J Clin Invest 2005;115:1343–51.

14. Fromenty B, Pessayre D. Inhibition of mitochondrial beta-oxidation as a mechanism of hepatotoxicity. Pharmacol Ther 1995;67:101–54.
15. Watmough NJ, Bindoff LA, Birch-Machin MA, et al. Impaired mitochondrial beta-oxidation in a patient with an abnormality of the respiratory chain. Studies in skeletal muscle mitochondria. J Clin Invest 1990;85:177–84.
16. Koek GH, Liedorp PR, Bast A. The role of oxidative stress in non-alcoholic steatohepatitis. Clin Chim Acta 2011;412:1297–305.
17. Saudubray JM, Martin D, de Lonlay P, et al. Recognition and management of fatty acid oxidation defects: a series of 107 patients. J Inherit Metab Dis 1999;22:488–502.
18. Fromenty B, Grimbert S, Mansouri A, et al. Hepatic mitochondrial DNA deletion in alcoholics: association with microvesicular steatosis. Gastroenterology 1995; 108:193–200.
19. Kimura S, Kobayashi T, Tanaka Y, et al. Liver histopathology in clinical Reye syndrome. Brain Dev 1991;13:95–100.
20. Fulgencio JP, Kohl C, Girard J, et al. Troglitazone inhibits fatty acid oxidation and esterification, and gluconeogenesis in isolated hepatocytes from starved rats. Diabetes 1996;45:1556–62.
21. Eadie MJ, Hooper WD, Dickinson RG. Valproate-associated hepatotoxicity and its biochemical mechanisms. Med Toxicol Adverse Drug Exp 1988;3:85–106.
22. Goldman IS, Winkler ML, Raper SE, et al. Increased hepatic density and phospholipidosis due to amiodarone. AJR Am J Roentgenol 1985;144:541–6.
23. Lenhard JM, Croom DK, Weiel JE, et al. HIV protease inhibitors stimulate hepatic triglyceride synthesis. Arterioscler Thromb Vasc Biol 2000;20:2625–9.
24. Letteron P, Brahimi-Bourouina N, Robin MA, et al. Glucocorticoids inhibit mitochondrial matrix acyl-CoA dehydrogenases and fatty acid beta-oxidation. Am J Physiol 1997;272:G1141–50.
25. Lauressergues E, Staels B, Valeille K, et al. Antipsychotic drug action on SREBPs-related lipogenesis and cholesterogenesis in primary rat hepatocytes. Naunyn Schmiedebergs Arch Pharmacol 2010;381:427–39.
26. Cai D, Yuan M, Frantz DF, et al. Local and systemic insulin resistance resulting from hepatic activation of IKK-beta and NF-kappaB. Nat Med 2005;11: 183–90.
27. Deschamps D, Fisch C, Fromenty B, et al. Inhibition by salicylic acid of the activation and thus oxidation of long chain fatty acids. Possible role in the development of Reye's syndrome. J Pharmacol Exp Ther 1991;259:894–904.
28. Oh KW, Qian T, Brenner DA, et al. Salicylate enhances necrosis and apoptosis mediated by the mitochondrial permeability transition. Toxicol Sci 2003;73: 44–52.
29. Wanless IR, Dore S, Gopinath N, et al. Histopathology of cocaine hepatotoxicity. Report of four patients. Gastroenterology 1990;98:497–501.
30. Roberts SM, Harbison RD, James RC. Human microsomal N-oxidative metabolism of cocaine. Drug Metab Dispos 1991;19:1046–51.
31. Shi X, Yao D, Gosnell BA, et al. Lipidomic profiling reveals protective function of fatty acid oxidation in cocaine-induced hepatotoxicity. J Lipid Res 2012;53: 2318–30.
32. Luef GJ, Waldmann M, Sturm W, et al. Valproate therapy and nonalcoholic fatty liver disease. Ann Neurol 2004;55:729–32.
33. Brivet FG, Nion I, Megarbane B, et al. Fatal lactic acidosis and liver steatosis associated with didanosine and stavudine treatment: a respiratory chain dysfunction? J Hepatol 2000;32:364–5.

34. Chariot P, Drogou I, de Lacroix-Szmania I, et al. Zidovudine-induced mitochondrial disorder with massive liver steatosis, myopathy, lactic acidosis, and mitochondrial DNA depletion. J Hepatol 1999;30:156–60.

35. Stankov MV, Panayotova-Dimitrova D, Leverkus M, et al. Autophagy inhibition due to thymidine analogues as novel mechanism leading to hepatocyte dysfunction and lipid accumulation. AIDS 2012;26:1995–2006.

36. Osler M, Stead D, Rebe K, et al. Risk factors for and clinical characteristics of severe hyperlactataemia in patients receiving antiretroviral therapy: a case-control study. HIV Med 2010;11:121–9.

37. Neuman MG, Schneider M, Nanau RM, et al. HIV-antiretroviral therapy induced liver, gastrointestinal, and pancreatic injury. Int J Hepatol 2012;2012:760706.

38. Letteron P, Sutton A, Mansouri A, et al. Inhibition of microsomal triglyceride transfer protein: another mechanism for drug-induced steatosis in mice. Hepatology 2003;38:133–40.

39. Freneaux E, Fromenty B, Berson A, et al. Stereoselective and nonstereoselective effects of ibuprofen enantiomers on mitochondrial beta-oxidation of fatty acids. J Pharmacol Exp Ther 1990;255:529–35.

40. Victorino RM, Silveira JC, Baptista A, et al. Jaundice associated with naproxen. Postgrad Med J 1980;56:368–70.

41. Lewis JH, Ranard RC, Caruso A, et al. Amiodarone hepatotoxicity: prevalence and clinicopathologic correlations among 104 patients. Hepatology 1989;9:679–85.

42. Podrid PJ. Amiodarone: reevaluation of an old drug. Ann Intern Med 1995;122:689–700.

43. Kalantzis N, Gabriel P, Mouzas J, et al. Acute amiodarone-induced hepatitis. Hepatogastroenterology 1991;38:71–4.

44. Chang CC, Petrelli M, Tomashefski JF Jr, et al. Severe intrahepatic cholestasis caused by amiodarone toxicity after withdrawal of the drug: a case report and review of the literature. Arch Pathol Lab Med 1999;123:251–6.

45. Guigui B, Perrot S, Berry JP, et al. Amiodarone-induced hepatic phospholipidosis: a morphological alteration independent of pseudoalcoholic liver disease. Hepatology 1988;8:1063–8.

46. Lewis JH, Mullick F, Ishak KG, et al. Histopathologic analysis of suspected amiodarone hepatotoxicity. Hum Pathol 1990;21:59–67.

47. Antherieu S, Rogue A, Fromenty B, et al. Induction of vesicular steatosis by amiodarone and tetracycline is associated with up-regulation of lipogenic genes in HepaRG cells. Hepatology 2011;53:1895–905.

48. Fromenty B, Fisch C, Labbe G, et al. Amiodarone inhibits the mitochondrial beta-oxidation of fatty acids and produces microvesicular steatosis of the liver in mice. J Pharmacol Exp Ther 1990;255:1371–6.

49. Kennedy JA, Unger SA, Horowitz JD. Inhibition of carnitine palmitoyltransferase-1 in rat heart and liver by perhexiline and amiodarone. Biochem Pharmacol 1996;52:273–80.

50. Fromenty B, Fisch C, Berson A, et al. Dual effect of amiodarone on mitochondrial respiration. Initial protonophoric uncoupling effect followed by inhibition of the respiratory chain at the levels of complex I and complex II. J Pharmacol Exp Ther 1990;255:1377–84.

51. Pessayre D, Mansouri A, Haouzi D, et al. Hepatotoxicity due to mitochondrial dysfunction. Cell Biol Toxicol 1999;15:367–73.

52. Pessayre D, Bichara M, Degott C, et al. Perhexiline maleate-induced cirrhosis. Gastroenterology 1979;76:170–7.

53. Kubo M, Hostetler KY. Metabolic basis of diethylaminoethoxyhexestrol-induced phospholipid fatty liver. Am J Physiol 1987;252:E375–9.

54. Le Gall JY, Guillouzo A, Glaise D, et al. Perhexiline maleate toxicity on human liver cell lines. Gut 1980;21:977–84.

55. Douillard JY, Cunningham D, Roth AD, et al. Irinotecan combined with fluoro-uracil compared with fluorouracil alone as first-line treatment for metastatic colo-rectal cancer: a multicentre randomised trial. Lancet 2000;355:1041–7.

56. Tournigand C, Andre T, Achille E, et al. FOLFIRI followed by FOLFOX6 or the reverse sequence in advanced colorectal cancer: a randomized GERCOR study. J Clin Oncol 2004;22:229–37.

57. Levi F, Zidani R, Misset JL. Randomised multicentre trial of chronotherapy with oxaliplatin, fluorouracil, and folinic acid in metastatic colorectal cancer. Interna-tional Organization for Cancer Chronotherapy. Lancet 1997;350:681–6.

58. Adam R, Delvart V, Pascal G, et al. Rescue surgery for unresectable colorectal liver metastases downstaged by chemotherapy: a model to predict long-term survival. Ann Surg 2004;240:644–57 [discussion: 657–8].

59. Bismuth H, Adam R, Levi F, et al. Resection of nonresectable liver metastases from colorectal cancer after neoadjuvant chemotherapy. Ann Surg 1996;224: 509–20 [discussion: 520–2].

60. Gentilucci UV, Santini D, Vincenzi B, et al. Chemotherapy-induced steatohepa-titis in colorectal cancer patients. J Clin Oncol 2006;24:5467 [author reply: 5467–8].

61. Rubbia-Brandt L, Audard V, Sartoretti P, et al. Severe hepatic sinusoidal obstruc-tion associated with oxaliplatin-based chemotherapy in patients with metastatic colorectal cancer. Ann Oncol 2004;15:460–6.

62. Brouquet A, Benoist S, Julie C, et al. Risk factors for chemotherapy-associated liver injuries: a multivariate analysis of a group of 146 patients with colorectal metastases. Surgery 2009;145:362–71.

63. Schwarz RE, Berlin JD, Lenz HJ, et al. Systemic cytotoxic and biological thera-pies of colorectal liver metastases: expert consensus statement. HPB (Oxford) 2013;15:106–15.

64. Cho JY, Suh KS, Kwon CH, et al. Mild hepatic steatosis is not a major risk factor for hepatectomy and regenerative power is not impaired. Surgery 2006;139: 508–15.

65. Kooby DA, Fong Y, Suriawinata A, et al. Impact of steatosis on perioperative outcome following hepatic resection. J Gastrointest Surg 2003;7:1034–44.

66. Menter A, Korman NJ, Elmets CA, et al. Guidelines of care for the management of psoriasis and psoriatic arthritis: section 4. Guidelines of care for the manage-ment and treatment of psoriasis with traditional systemic agents. J Am Acad Dermatol 2009;61:451–85.

67. Langman G, Hall PM, Todd G. Role of non-alcoholic steatohepatitis in methotrexate-induced liver injury. J Gastroenterol Hepatol 2001;16:1395–401.

68. Berends MA, van Oijen MG, Snoek J, et al. Reliability of the Roenigk classi-fication of liver damage after methotrexate treatment for psoriasis: a clinico-pathologic study of 160 liver biopsy specimens. Arch Dermatol 2007;143: 1515–9.

69. Hytiroglou P, Tobias H, Saxena R, et al. The canals of Hering might represent a target of methotrexate hepatic toxicity. Am J Clin Pathol 2004;121:324–9.

70. Yamamoto N, Oliveira MB, Campello Ade P, et al. Methotrexate: studies on the cellular metabolism. I. Effect on mitochondrial oxygen uptake and oxidative phosphorylation. Cell Biochem Funct 1988;6:61–6.

71. Ogawa Y, Murata Y, Nishioka A, et al. Tamoxifen-induced fatty liver in patients with breast cancer. Lancet 1998;351:725.
72. Pratt DS, Knox TA, Erban J. Tamoxifen-induced steatohepatitis. Ann Intern Med 1995;123:236.
73. Murata Y, Ogawa Y, Saibara T, et al. Unrecognized hepatic steatosis and non-alcoholic steatohepatitis in adjuvant tamoxifen for breast cancer patients. Oncol Rep 2000;7:1299–304.
74. Bruno S, Maisonneuve P, Castellana P, et al. Incidence and risk factors for non-alcoholic steatohepatitis: prospective study of 5408 women enrolled in Italian tamoxifen chemoprevention trial. BMJ 2005;330:932.
75. Nishino M, Hayakawa K, Nakamura Y, et al. Effects of tamoxifen on hepatic fat content and the development of hepatic steatosis in patients with breast cancer: high frequency of involvement and rapid reversal after completion of tamoxifen therapy. AJR Am J Roentgenol 2003;180:129–34.
76. Saphner T, Triest-Robertson S, Li H, et al. The association of nonalcoholic stea-tohepatitis and tamoxifen in patients with breast cancer. Cancer 2009;115:3189–95.
77. Cole LK, Jacobs RL, Vance DE. Tamoxifen induces triacylglycerol accumulation in the mouse liver by activation of fatty acid synthesis. Hepatology 2010;52:1258–65.
78. Letteron P, Fromenty B, Terris B, et al. Acute and chronic hepatic steatosis lead to in vivo lipid peroxidation in mice. J Hepatol 1996;24:200–8.

# Histopathologic Manifestations of Drug-induced Hepatotoxicity

Xuchen Zhang, MD, PhD[a],*, Jie Ouyang, MD, PhD[b],
Swan N. Thung, MD[c]

## KEYWORDS

- Drugs • Drug-induced hepatotoxicity • Liver injury • Pathology

## KEY POINTS

- The diagnosis of drug toxicity is challenging, both clinically and pathologically.
- The diagnosis often rests on excluding other causes, careful medication history, chronology between drug exposure and findings of abnormal liver tests and/or clinical symptoms, and histopathologic findings.
- Medication history should include prescription drugs, over-the-counter medications, dietary and/or supplementary agents, and herbal products.
- Drug-induced liver injury can mimic any other acute and chronic primary liver diseases.
- Certain agents cause certain types of hepatotoxicity (eg, cholestasis, hepatitis, or cholestatic hepatitis), which helps to identify the responsible drug, especially in polypharmacotherapy.

## INTRODUCTION

Drug-induced hepatotoxicity is also known as drug-induced liver injury (DILI). It is often misdiagnosed because of its clinical and pathologic mimicry of other primary acute and chronic liver diseases. The liver is the main organ in metabolism and detoxification of virtually every foreign substance, including drugs and toxins, which places it as a higher risk for toxic damage by drugs and/or their metabolites compared with other organs.[1,2] DILI has become the leading reason for discontinuation of previously approved drugs.[3] At least two major mechanisms are involved in drug-induced hepatotoxicity: intrinsic and idiosyncratic hepatotoxicity.[4] Intrinsic hepatotoxins, such as acetaminophen, cause hepatocellular damage in a predictable dose-dependent manner. In contrast, most of the other drugs cause hepatotoxicity in an unpredictable

There are no direct or indirect financial conflicts of interest with this article.
[a] Department of Pathology, VA Connecticut Health System and Yale University School of Medicine, 310 Cedar Street, LH 108, New Haven, CT 06516, USA; [b] Department of Pathology, Florida Hospital Medical Center and University of Central Florida, 2855 N Orange Avenue, Orlando, FL 32814, USA; [c] Department of Pathology, Icahn School of Medicine at Mount Sinai, 1468 Madison Avenue, New York, NY 10029, USA
* Corresponding author.
*E-mail address:* xuchen.zhang@yale.edu

Clin Liver Dis 17 (2013) 547–564
http://dx.doi.org/10.1016/j.cld.2013.07.004
1089-3261/13/$ – see front matter Published by Elsevier Inc.

or so-called idiosyncratic fashion. Generally, intrinsic hepatotoxicity demonstrates acute hepatocellular injury with little inflammation, whereas idiosyncratic hepatotoxicity frequently shows inflammation-dominant acute or chronic hepatic injury.

The diagnosis of DILI often relies on exclusion of other primary liver diseases, careful medication history, latent period between drug-exposure and findings of abnormal biochemical liver tests and/or clinical symptoms, and/or histopathologic manifestations. Although liver biopsy is considered the gold standard in the diagnosis of drug-induced hepatotoxicity, it is not a routine procedure in DILI. Liver biopsy is performed when the clinical situations and laboratory findings are not typical of DILI, or when assessing the degree of liver damage and/or repair. In addition, DILI might not have been considered in the clinical differential diagnosis, thus the liver biopsy result would suggest the possibility of DILI.[5] DILI can be classified into two main categories according to the pattern of liver injury (ie, hepatocellular or cholestatic). A combination of the two is mixed hepatocellular-cholestatic injury. Others, such as steatosis and/or steatohepatitis, granulomatous hepatitis, hepatic vascular injuries, cytoplasmic inclusions, lipidosis, pigment deposition, and tumor formation, can also be seen. The pattern of injury can help the pathologist narrow down the differential diagnoses and suggest the most probable drug according to its previously known type of injury. For example, centrilobular (zone 3) necrosis with little or no inflammation would suggest acetaminophen, halothane and other halogenated anesthetics, or toxins such as carbon tetrachloride or *Amanita phalloides* from mushroom poisoning. Extensive microvesicular steatosis may suggest the use of tetracycline and nucleoside analogs such as zidovudine. The histopathologic pattern may also reflect the pathogenesis of the liver injury in a specific agent and, therefore, can be helpful in diagnosis and treatment. For example, zidovudine or didanosine treatment-induced microvesicular steatosis is associated with mitochondrial toxicity, whereas barbiturate-induced ground-glass hepatocytic change is associated with adaptive proliferation of smooth endoplasmic reticulum.

## HEPATOCELLULAR INJURY PATTERN
### Acute Hepatocellular Injury

Acute hepatitis accounts for approximately 90% of drug-induced hepatotoxicity. This liver injury pattern resembles acute viral hepatitis ranging from mild hepatitis with spotty cell death to submassive or massive necrosis leading to fulminant liver failure. Numerous drugs can cause this pattern of liver injury.

### Spotty Cell Death

Spotty cell death is death of isolated hepatocytes in the lobule with inflammatory activity. Hepatocytes undergo two types of cell death: necrosis and apoptosis. Apoptosis is a process of programmed cell death that involves a series of biochemical events that lead to a variety of morphologic changes, including blebbing, cell shrinkage, nuclear fragmentation, chromatin condensation, and chromosomal DNA fragmentation. The condensed cells and fragments in the liver are called apoptotic bodies (previously known as acidophilic bodies) (**Fig. 1**A). Spotty cell death is also seen in acute viral hepatitis. Besides the spotty cell death, lobular lymphocytic infiltrate, portal inflammation, and interface hepatitis are also present. The presence of eosinophils favors drug-induced over viral hepatitis and suggests a better short-term prognosis.[6] However, unlike viral hepatitis, portal inflammation and interface hepatitis in DILI are not the dominant features. Viral serology tests for hepatitis A, B, and C are usually part of the standard evaluation of possible DILI. Testing for hepatitis E virus

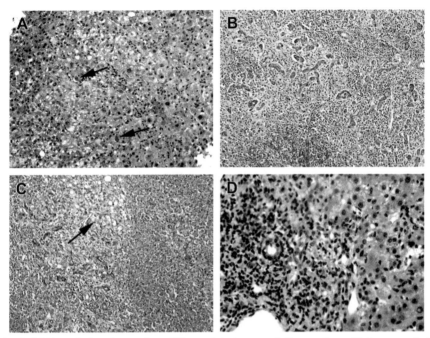

**Fig. 1.** (*A*) Drug-induced acute hepatitis: panlobular necroinflammation with two apoptotic bodies (*arrows*). (*B*) Massive hepatic necrosis due to accidental rechallenge with amoxicillin: ductular hepatocytes and lymphocytic infiltration in the collapsed parenchyma without remaining hepatocytes. (*C*) Confluent necrosis involving zones 2 and 3 (*right side*) with no significant inflammation, and preservation of periportal hepatocytes (*arrow*) containing fat droplets from acetaminophen toxicity. (*D*) Autoimmune-like drug induced hepatitis caused by isoniazid toxicity showing portal tract infiltrated by lymphocytes, plasma cells, and eosinophils with moderate interface hepatitis.

(HEV), however, is rarely included because HEV infection is considered rare in developed countries. An increasing number of cases of HEV infection in developed countries, including the United States, are being recognized.[4] A survey showed that in some areas in the United States, up to 20% of blood donors are immunoglobulin G seropositive for HEV, indicating prior exposure and immunity to the virus.[7] The genotypes 3 and 4 of HEV are swine viruses that are common in domestic and wild pigs. Zoonotic transmission of HEV from both domesticated and wild animals to humans has been described.[8] Because drug-induced hepatotoxicity is a diagnosis of exclusion, and hepatitis E is rarely considered in the evaluation of acute liver injury in the United States, some cases diagnosed as DILI may actually be HEV infection as has also been reported in the United Kingdom.[9,10] Drug-induced hepatotoxicity may also resemble Epstein-Barr virus hepatitis. In this mononucleosis-like hepatitis, sinusoidal beading of lymphocytes is prominent. This type of hepatotoxicity is typically caused by phenytoin; however, it is also seen in dapsone, para-aminosalicylate, and sulphonamides.[1,7,11]

## Confluent and Zonal Necrosis

Death of larger groups of hepatocytes (confluent necrosis) occurs in severe hepatitis. Confluent necrosis can be zonal or nonzonal. Generally, the necrosis produced by intrinsic hepatotoxins is zonal, whereas that produced by idiosyncratic injury is nonzonal. Liver parenchyma is divided into three zones: zone 1 is closest to the vascular supply (periportal), zone 3 abuts the terminal hepatic venule and is most remote from the afferent blood supply (centrilobular), and zone 2 is intermediate (mid-zone). Centrilobular necrosis is the most common type of zonal necrosis and is characteristic of injuries caused by acetaminophen, halothane, and other halogenated anesthetics; and toxins, such as carbon tetrachloride and *Amanita phalloides* from mushroom poisoning. Isolated necrosis affecting zone 1 or 2 only is uncommon. Agents, such as cocaine and ferrous sulfate, typically affect zone 1. Extreme degrees of both zonal and nonzonal necrosis can result in bridging, submassive, or massive necrosis leading to liver failure. Drug-induced confluent, either submassive or massive, necrosis shows collapsed parenchyma intermingled with ductular reaction (ductular hepatocytes) accompanied by mild or no inflammatory infiltrate (see **Fig. 1**B). Massive necrosis of the zonal type tends to retain its zonal territory with preservation of a rim of hepatocytes with or without steatosis in the periportal region (see **Fig. 1**C).

### Chronic Hepatocellular Injury

Many drugs known to cause acute hepatocellular injury are also capable of causing chronic hepatocellular injury. Chronic hepatocellular injury has morphologic features similar to those of chronic viral hepatitis or autoimmune hepatitis (AIH) with variable degrees of necroinflammation and even fibrosis or cirrhosis. Similar to drug-induced acute hepatocellular injury, clinical and serologic studies are also part of the workup to rule out viral or AIH. Most drug-induced acute hepatocellular injuries are followed by recovery without leaving significant fibrosis.[12] However, progression to chronicity has been reported in 5% to 10% of adverse drug reactions.[13] At initial diagnosis, many liver injuries are already in chronic phase owing to unrecognized prolonged exposure to offending drugs. A British study based on histopathologic findings showed that drugs were considered initially in only 39% of cases, chronic hepatitis was present in 45% of patients at presentation, and unrecognized exposure to the drug continued for at least 6 months in 16% of cases.[13] The agents commonly associated with chronic liver disease are amoxicillin-clavulanic acid, bentazepam, and atorvastatin. Herbal medications and dietary and/or supplementary agents causing chronic liver injury are increasingly recognized.[14,15] Drugs, such as methotrexate, hypervitaminosis A, vinyl chloride, thorotrast, and heroin, may lead to fibrosis with only minimal or absent necrosis or inflammation. Persistent exposure to methotrexate, isoniazid, ticrynafen, amiodarone, enalapril, and valproic acid may lead to cirrhosis. Drug-induced submassive or massive necrosis may be followed by fibrosis of the collapsed areas, nodular regeneration, and cirrhosis.

Several drugs, such as clometacin, methyldopa, minocycline, nitrofurantoin, infliximab, and other tumor necrosis factor (TNF)-α blocking agents, can cause autoimmune-like chronic hepatitis that maybe clinically, serologically, and morphologically indistinguishable from AIH.[16,17] Clinical and pathologic diagnoses of drug-induced autoimmune-like hepatitis are challenging. It is often difficult to differentiate drug-induced chronic hepatitis from AIH (see **Fig. 1**D). Furthermore, drugs may trigger the onset of AIH. Careful clinical and pathologic correlation is advised to sort out the correct diagnosis so that proper management can be administered. Early immunosuppression is the treatment of AIH, which can lead to disease remission. Prompt identification and discontinuation of the drug is essential to avoid disease progression and/or chronicity in drug-induced autoimmune-like hepatitis. Failure to properly diagnose and treat AIH and drug-induced autoimmune-like hepatitis could result in clinically devastating acute or chronic outcomes.[17–19] Suzuki and colleagues[18] explored potential hallmarks to differentiate AIH versus drug-induced autoimmune-like hepatitis in liver biopsies and found that interface hepatitis, focal necrosis, and portal inflammation were present in all evaluated cases. Prominent eosinophil infiltration, regarded as one of the histologic findings suggesting drug-induced hepatotoxicity,[5,20] was also not useful in its differential diagnosis from AIH. No single indicative histologic feature could be assigned to either AIH or drug-induced autoimmune-like hepatitis. Then, the investigators established a model combining portal inflammation, portal plasma cells, intra-acinar lymphocytes and eosinophils, rosette formation, and canalicular cholestasis. They concluded that four features (ie, severe portal inflammation, rosette formation, prominent portal plasma infiltrates, and prominent intra-acinar eosinophils) were consistently more prevalent in AIH, whereas portal neutrophils and cholestasis were more prevalent in drug-induced autoimmune-like hepatitis (see **Fig. 1**D). Further investigation is warranted to validate these findings and to incorporate the knowledge into current clinicopathologic diagnosis.

## CHOLESTATIC INJURY PATTERN
### Acute Cholestatic Injury

Cholestatic injury pattern is recognized when cholestasis is present, either in the form of visible bile accumulation in hepatocytes and/or bile canaliculi, or in the form of bile duct loss and/or cholate stasis seen in chronic cholestasis.[5] Bile stasis may be subtle and difficult to identify without the use of special stains. Iron and copper stains are useful in identifying other brown pigments and highlight bile deposition. Drug-induced acute cholestatic injury pattern can be classified into two subtypes: bland (pure) cholestasis and acute cholestatic hepatitis (mixed hepatocellular-cholestatic injury). Bland cholestasis is characterized by the presence of prominent hepatocellular and/or canalicular cholestasis with little or no inflammation and hepatocellular injury. Bile duct injury may be seen (**Fig. 2**A) but does not imply progression to ductopenic chronic cholestasis. Typical examples of drugs that cause the bland cholestasis pattern are anabolic and oral contraceptive steroids (see **Fig. 2**B). The histopathologic differential diagnoses include cholestasis in sepsis, cardiac failure, shock, acute large bile duct obstruction, benign recurrent intrahepatic cholestasis, postoperative cholestasis, and intrahepatic cholestasis of pregnancy. These conditions should be considered within the appropriate clinical settings.[20] Acute cholestatic hepatitis or mixed hepatocellular-cholestatic injury is characterized by cholestasis, which is accompanied by inflammation and hepatocellular injury (see **Fig. 2**C). It can result from a wide variety of drugs, such as antibiotics, including erythromycin and amoxicillin-clavulanate; angiotensin-converting enzyme (ACE) inhibitors; phenothiazine neuroleptics; and many others.[1,21–30] Almost all drugs that produce cholestatic injury are also capable of inducing a mixed injury pattern. Generally, cholestasis, especially mixed injury pattern, is not a feature of viral hepatitis. When cholestasis is present histologically, especially in a mixed injury pattern, DILI should be kept in mind because this type of injury is far more characteristic of drug-induced hepatotoxicity than viral hepatitis.[6]

### Chronic Cholestatic Injury

Most cases of drug-induced acute cholestatic injury are followed by rapid clinical and biochemical recovery on withdrawal of the drug but, in some cases, it may persist. Drug-induced chronic cholestatic injury may take a variety of forms, but the main features are significant bile duct loss and/or the presence of cholate stasis, which may mimic primary biliary cirrhosis, primary sclerosing cholangitis, or vanishing bile duct syndrome. Cholate-stasis is recognized as a rim of pallor hepatocytes adjacent to the portal areas or fibrous septa (see **Fig. 2**D). Special stains for copper or

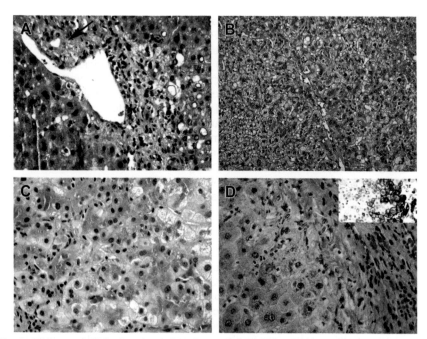

**Fig. 2.** (*A*) Damaged bile duct (*arrow*) in chemotherapy-induced pure cholestatic liver injury. (*B*) Bile plugs in dilated bile canaliculi in androgen-induced cholestasis. (*C*) Drug-induced cholestatic hepatitis, in which there is significant necroinflammation accompanying the cholestasis. (*D*) Cholate-stasis (rim of pallor hepatocytes containing Mallory-Denk hyalines adjacent to the portal areas or fibrous septa) in drug-induced vanishing bile duct syndrome. (*Inset*) Cytokeratin 7 (CK7) immunostain highlights the cholestatic hepatocyte formation.

copper-binding proteins are useful because copper accumulates in cytoplasm of hepatocytes with cholate-stasis. Primary sclerosing cholangitis-like injury is a relatively uncommon pattern that is mainly seen with infusion of chemotherapy agents into the hepatic artery, such as floxuridine and fluorouracil to treat liver metastatic colon cancer, and hepatic arterial chemoembolization in hepatocellular carcinoma.[31,32] The injury has been attributed to indirect bile duct damage secondary to drug-caused vascular injury.[33,34] Primary biliary cirrhosis-like injury is rare and has resulted from the use of herbal drugs or statins.[35,36] Many drugs, including antibiotics such as amoxicillin-clavulanate and flucloxacillin; ACE inhibitors, such as enalapril; antifungals, such as terbinafine; and, rarely, oral contraceptives, can cause bile duct paucity (ductopenia), in which more than 50% of portal tracts have interlobular bile duct loss, to vanishing bile duct syndrome, in which there is near complete absence of bile ducts.[20,37] Cytokeratin 7 immunohistochemistry highlights bile ducts, ductular reaction, and cholestatic hepatocyte formation in chronic cholestasis. Therefore, it aids in the diagnosis of ductopenia, vanishing bile duct syndrome, and chronic cholestasis (see **Fig. 2**D inset). Regeneration and restoration of bile ducts have been reported in some patients with drug-induced ductopenia and vanishing bile duct syndrome.[38,39]

## STEATOSIS AND STEATOHEPATITIS PATTERN

Many drugs can cause steatosis and steatohepatitis, which may resemble alcoholic fatty liver disease or nonalcoholic fatty liver disease. Nonalcoholic fatty liver disease can be seen in individuals with obesity, diabetes, hypertriglyceridemia, or insulin resistance. The presence of mild-to-moderate degree of steatosis in liver biopsy is common and is not a feature of a specific liver disease. It can be identified in various liver biopsies performed for elevated liver enzyme activities.[40] However, drug-induced injury should always be considered a potential cause of steatosis and steatohepatitis.

### Macrovesicular Steatosis

Macrovesicular steatosis is characterized by the presence of medium or large-sized intracytoplasmic fat droplet that displaces the hepatocellular nucleus to the periphery. It is worth mentioning that multiple fat droplets of varying sizes are frequently observed in a single hepatocyte; this should still be considered as macrovesicular steatosis instead of microvesicular steatosis.[5] In drug-induced hepatotoxicity, macrovesicular steatosis may be the only histologic abnormality (**Fig. 3**A) or it may be accompanied by steatohepatitis showing necroinflammation, ballooning degeneration of hepatocytes with or without Mallory-Denk hyalines, or perisinusoidal fibrosis, which resemble alcohol or non–alcohol-induced steatohepatitis. Mallory-Denk hyalines may be seen but are not necessary for the diagnosis of steatohepatitis. Typically, macrovesicular steatosis is seen in glucocorticoids and methotrexate-induced hepatotoxicity, and in association with variety of other drugs. These include NSAIDs; amiodarone; antihypertensives, such as metoprolol; chlorinated hydrocarbons, such as carbon tetrachloride and chloroform; and total parenteral nutrition. Chemotherapeutic agents, such as 5-fluorouracil, cisplatin, irinotecan and tamoxifen-induced steatosis and/or steatohepatitis, are increasingly recognized. This is also called chemotherapy-associated steatosis or steatohepatitis (CASH).[41,42] Glucocorticoids-associated steatosis is frequently bland, whereas methotrexate-related steatosis can lead to steatohepatitis, fibrosis, and even cirrhosis.

### Microvesicular Steatosis

Microvesicular steatosis is a more serious form of fat deposition in hepatocytes. It is mainly due to mitochondrial injury, which may lead to lactic acidosis. It appears as numerous small fat droplets that fill the cytoplasm of hepatocytes without peripheral displacement of the nucleus. Special stains with oil red O or Sudan black are helpful in differentiating microvesicular steatosis from other foamy cytoplasmic changes but they must be done on frozen sections. Mild necroinflammation and intrahepatic cholestasis may coexist but usually are minimal. Several drugs have been linked with microvesicular steatosis and its associated hepatic failure. Most notable are acetylsalicylic acid (Reye syndrome), valproic acid, tetracycline, and some nucleoside-nucleotide analogs.[5,20] The injury may continue to progress even after the patient has stopped taking the drugs.

### GRANULOMA AND GRANULOMATOUS HEPATITIS

Granulomas are seen in 2.4% to 15% of all liver biopsy specimens.[43] The common causes of granulomas in the liver are infections, sarcoidosis, primary biliary cirrhosis, lymphomas, systemic diseases, and drugs.[44,45] Special stains for microorganisms should always be performed whenever large epithelioid granulomas with or without necrosis are present. Granuloma, especially microgranuloma, is a common finding in drug-induced hepatotoxicity; however, when inflammation also dominates, it should be referred to as granulomatous hepatitis.[5] Drug-induced granulomas are usually non-necrotizing and can be seen either in the portal tracts or within the lobule (see **Fig. 3**B). When granulomas are present in portal tracts, bile duct injury mimicking primary biliary

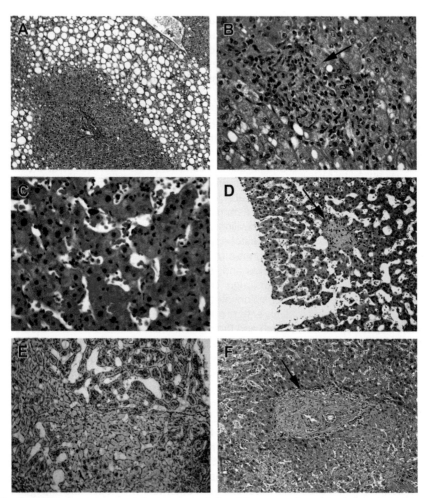

**Fig. 3.** (*A*) Moderate macrovesicular steatosis involving zones 2 and 3 of the acini with no evidence of steatohepatitis. (*B*) Small granulomas with eosinophils in the lobules of liver with lithium-induced toxicity (*arrow*). (*C*) Trapping of red blood cells in spaces of Disse due to damaged endothelial cells in SOS. (*D*) Occlusion of central venule by loose connective tissue in VOD due to medication containing pyrrolizidine alkaloids (*arrow*). (*E*) Oral contraceptive steroid-induced sinusoidal dilatation (reticulin stain). (*F*) Drug-induced OPV. Portal tract contains bile duct and hepatic artery, but without recognizable lumen of the portal vein (*arrow*).

cirrhosis may be seen. Granulomas can also be observed in other patterns of liver injury, such as acute or chronic hepatitis, cholestasis, or steatosis and/or steatohepatitis. Drugs, such as sulfonamide, sulfonylurea, phenytoin, carbamazepine, quinidine, hydralazine, interferon-alfa, etanercept, and many others, have been frequently associated with the development of granuloma or granulomatous hepatitis.[46–51] Uses of mineral oil or paraffin oil have been reported to cause lipogranulomas,[51–54] which are also commonly seen in hepatitis C and fatty liver disease.[45,55] Lipogranulomas generally are located in portal tracts and adjacent to central venules (perivenular) and do not result in significant liver injury. Allopurinol, BCG vaccination, and intravesical therapy for bladder carcinoma are known to cause granuloma formation, sometimes with features of fibrin-ring granuloma,[56–58] which is seen in patients with Q fever or other infections.[59]

## VASCULAR INJURY PATTERNS

Hepatic vasculature has also been targeted in drug-induced hepatotoxicity, which results in a variety of vascular diseases.[34]

### Sinusoidal Obstruction Syndrome

Sinusoidal obstruction syndrome (SOS), also known as hepatic venoocclusive disease (VOD), is caused by toxic injury to sinusoidal endothelial cells. It is characterized by the loss of sinusoidal wall integrity with consequent trapping of red blood cells in Disse spaces (see **Fig. 3**C), sinusoidal congestive obstruction, perisinusoidal fibrosis, hepatic venule fibrotic obstruction (see **Fig. 3**D), nodular regenerative hyperplasia (NRH), or peliosis.[60] SOS/VOD may complicate treatment with different immunosuppressive and chemotherapeutic agents.[34,61–64] It may also result from poisoning with pyrrolizidine alkaloids-containing plants, consumed either as contaminated flour or as traditional and herbal remedies.[15,34,65,66] Recently, studies have shown that defibrotide, a novel polydeoxyribonucleotide with fibrinolytic properties, can be used effectively and safely to treat and prevent SOS/VOD.[67–69]

### Peliosis Hepatis and Sinusoidal Dilatation

Peliosis hepatis is a pathologic entity characterized by the presence of blood-filled lacunar spaces lined by hepatocytes without an endothelial lining. Sinusoidal dilatation is often seen in livers with peliosis hepatis or it occurs independently without peliosis hepatis (see **Fig. 3**E). The most common drugs implicated are androgens and contraceptive steroids.[70,71] Other agents, especially chemotherapeutic drugs, have also been associated with peliosis hepatis and/or sinusoidal dilatation.[72–76]

### NRH and Obliterative Portal Venopathy

NRH and obliterative portal venopathy (OPV), also termed hepatoportal sclerosis (HPS),[77] are underrecognized diseases of uncertain causes that often present as noncirrhotic portal hypertension.[34,78] NRH is characterized by multiple small hyperplastic nodules centered on portal tracts compressing the adjacent, frequently atrophic, liver cells and sinusoids without significant fibrosis. OPV is characterized by portal fibrosis and obliteration of small and medium branches of the portal vein, resulting in portal hypertension (see **Fig. 3**F).[34,79] OPV is frequently associated with nodular regenerative changes (so-called NRH, in the full-blown form) and sinusoidal dilatation.[80,81] The causes of NRH and OPV are unclear. It has been suggested that these lesions are linked by a common pathway of endothelial cell injury. Reported causes for NRH and OPV include chronic exposure to various chemicals (arsenic, copper sulfate, vinyl chloride, thorium dioxide) or drugs (azathioprine, methotrexate, 6-mercaptopurine, oxaliplatin).[34,77,78,82–84] In recent years, cases of OPV and/or NRH are increasingly recognized among patients with HIV receiving highly active antiretroviral therapy (didanosine and stavudine).[85–88]

## CYTOPLASMIC INCLUSIONS, LIPIDOSIS, AND PIGMENTS

Ground-glass inclusion within cytoplasm of hepatocytes is an important histopathologic marker of chronic hepatitis B virus (HBV) infection. Similar ground glass hepatocytes are also recognized in Lafora disease (familial myoclonus epilepsy) (**Fig. 4**A),

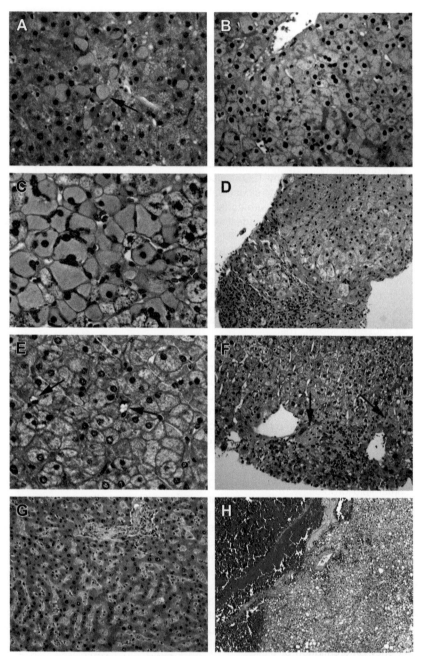

**Fig. 4.** (*A*) Lafora body-like inclusions due to polypharmacotherapy (*arrow*). (*B*) Dilantin toxicity results in formation of induction hepatocytes. (*C*) Hepatic glycogenosis with ground glass hepatocytes. (*D*) Phospholipidosis (*upper*) and steatohepatitis (*lower*) with abundant Mallory-Denk hyalines in amiodarone toxicity. (*E*) Hepatic stellate cells with bubbly cytoplasm and tent shaped nuclei (*arrows*) in hypervitaminosis A (*arrows*). (*F*) Clusters of ceroid (light brown pigment) containing macrophages in centrilobular areas from previous drug-induced injury (*arrows*). (*G*) Increased lipofuscin deposits in pericanalicular region of hepatocytes in chronic drug intake. (*H*) OCPs-induced HCA with fat and glycogenated nuclei within the lesion, and area of hemorrhage.

cyanamide alcohol aversion therapy, type IV glycogenosis (branching enzyme deficiency or Andersen disease), and fibrinogen storage disease. Drugs such as Dilantin and barbiturates are commonly associated with cytoplasmic ground-glass change (induction hepatocytes) due to adaptive proliferation of smooth endoplasmic reticulum (see **Fig. 4**B). Other medications, including immunosuppressive agents, antibiotics, and insulin, have also been reported to cause cytoplasmic ground-glass change, which closely resembles polyglucosan bodies described in humans, animals, and experimental models.[89]

Hepatic glycogenosis (see **Fig. 4**C), characterized by distended cytoplasm filled with pale gray-blue homogeneous material, is seen in adults or children with marked or prolonged hyperglycemia who are treated with insulin, usually in the setting of type I diabetes mellitus.[90,91] It also can be an early manifestation of type 1 diabetes mellitus.[92] Most individuals will have a history of poor glycemic control, elevated liver transaminase activities, and hepatomegaly.[93,94] Hepatic glycogenosis has also been reported in patients following short-term high-dose corticosteroid therapy.[95] Histochemical reactions (periodic acid–Schiff [PAS] or PAS-diastase) on frozen or alcohol-fixed liver specimen confirm the glycogen deposition.

Phospholipidosis, characterized by enlarged, foamy, or granular cytoplasm, is a form of lysosomal lipid accumulation in hepatocytes and/or Kupffer cells. It is well established that a large number of cationic amphiphilic drugs have the potential to induce phospholipidosis. These include agents that are antibiotic, antipsychotic, antidepressant, antianginal, antimalarial, antiarrhythmic, and cholesterol lowering, as well as total parenteral nutrition.[96] Amiodarone, a potent antiarrhythmic agent, is one of the most commonly encountered drugs to cause phospholipidosis.[97] Although drug-induced phospholipidosis often has a background of steatosis and/or steatohepatitis, some drugs may cause phospholipidosis alone (see **Fig. 4**D). Similar to induction hepatocytes, it has been suggested that phospholipidosis represents an adaptive response to cationic amphiphilic drugs rather than a toxic manifestation.[96,98] It is difficult sometimes to distinguish hepatic phospholipidosis from other forms of hepatic lipidosis. Immunohistochemical staining of lysosome-associated protein-2 (LAMP2) and adipophilin (a protein that forms the membrane around non-lysosomal lipid droplets) can be used to differentiate phospholipidosis from other forms of lipidosis.[99]

Hypervitaminosis A refers to the effects of excessive vitamin A intake, for which liver is the most affected organ. Histologically, the hepatic stellate cells (Ito cells) in hypervitaminosis A are typically enlarged and appear increased in numbers. The stellate cell is filled with small lipid droplets, which give rise to its bubbly cytoplasm (see **Fig. 4**E). The small lipid droplets typically cause indentation of the darker nucleus, giving rise to a tent-shaped nucleus. The accumulation of small fat droplets has been described as stellate cell lipidosis.[100,101] Hepatic stellate cells are located in the spaces of Disse. They are modified fibroblasts and, in normal conditions, are capable of storing lipids and vitamin A. The location of the stellate cells and the shape of their nuclei usually permit easy differentiation of stellate cell lipidosis from steatosis. Hypervitaminosis A often results from excess dietary and/or supplementary vitamin A intake or use of oral and/or topical retinoids. Drugs such as methotrexate, valproate, and steroids have also been reported as causative agents. Stellate cell lipidosis can be easily overlooked, in which case hepatic fibrosis and cirrhosis may ensue.[100]

Ceroid-laden macrophages (see **Fig. 4**F) are seen in the resolution phase of hepatocellular injury secondary to drugs, viral hepatitis, or other causes of parenchymal injury.[102] In conjunction with other pathologic changes and clinical information, the presence of ceroid-macrophages is highly suggestive of DILI.

Lipofuscin pigment is produced by lysosomal oxidation of lipids and is often seen in atrophic liver, old age, starvation, chronic wasting diseases, and malignancies (see **Fig. 4**G). Drugs such as 6-mercaptopurine, phenothiazine, aminopyrine, phenacetin, and cascara sagrada have been reported to increase lipofuscin accumulation in cytoplasm of hepatocytes, particularly in the centrilobular zone.[5,102] In cases of excess dietary iron, alcoholism, total parenteral nutrition, or transfusion, hemosiderin can also accumulate in hepatocytes and/or Kupffer cells.

## DRUG-INDUCED HEPATIC NEOPLASMS

Hepatocellular adenoma (HCA) is a benign neoplasm arising from hepatocytes (see **Fig. 4**H) and has risk of malignant transformation. HCA is closely associated with the use of oral contraceptive pills (OCPs), which were first introduced in 1960. However, recent studies showed that cases of HCA associated with OCPs were decreasing since newer formulations with lower hormonal concentrations were introduced.[103] For instance, case series reported before 1985 showed that nearly all HCAs were in women taking OCPs; whereas, in series reported after 1985, fewer cases were associated with OCP use.[103] HCAs associated with OCPs were usually of larger size, had higher risk of rupture and malignant transformation, especially when they were larger than 5 cm.[104] Although rare, long-term use of other drugs such as anabolic and male hormone steroids,[105,106] danazol,[107] oxcarbazepine,[108] carbamazepine,[109] and phenobarbital[110] have also been associated with HCA. Although the association is weak, use of OCPs has also been linked to other hepatic neoplasms, such as focal nodular hyperplasia,[111,112,113] hepatocellular carcinoma,[114] and multifocal epitheloid hemangioendothelioma.[115]

## SUMMARY

DILI is an underrecognized, but increasingly known cause of acute and chronic liver disease. Many new drugs, dietary and/or supplementary agents, and herbal products are increasingly identified as hepatotoxic. DILI can be classified into several pathologic injury patterns. Recognizing these patterns facilitates diagnosis of DILI and identification of possible insulting drugs. Pathologic diagnosis of DILI, however, remains challenging for many reasons. These reasons include (1) different drugs may produce a similar pathologic pattern of injury, whereas one drug may result in different patterns of injury; (2) the pathologic features following a single exposure may be different from those after multiple and/or prolonged exposures; (3) frequently, patients are on multiple medications; and (4) drug-induced liver hepatotoxicity can mimic other primary liver disease. When interpreting a liver biopsy specimen, DILI should always be included in the differential diagnosis, especially when, after excluding other possible causes, the origin of liver injury is still not clear. The diagnosis of drug-induced hepatotoxicity usually rests on careful medical history that includes prescribed and over-the-counter medications, the latent period between drug and/or toxin exposure to clinical symptoms or abnormal liver tests, and results of liver biopsy.

## REFERENCES

1. Lee WM. Drug-induced hepatotoxicity. N Engl J Med 2003;349:474–85.
2. Bleibel W, Kim S, D'Silva K, et al. Drug-induced liver injury: review article. Dig Dis Sci 2007;52:2463–71.
3. Tujios S, Fontana RJ. Mechanisms of drug-induced liver injury: from bedside to bench. Nat Rev Gastroenterol Hepatol 2011;8:202–11.

4. Davern TJ. Drug-induced liver disease. Clin Liver Dis 2012;16:231–45.
5. Kleiner DE. The pathology of drug-induced liver injury. Semin Liver Dis 2009;29: 364–72.
6. Andrade RJ, Robles M, Fernandez-Castaner A, et al. Assessment of drug-induced hepatotoxicity in clinical practice: a challenge for gastroenterologists. World J Gastroenterol 2007;13:329–40.
7. Gan TE, Van der Weyden MB. Dapsone-induced infectious mononucleosis-like syndrome. Med J Aust 1982;1:350–1.
8. Spigset O. Drug-induced hepatic injuries. Tidsskr Nor Laegeforen 1998;118: 2805–8 [in Norwegian].
9. Dalton HR, Fellows HJ, Stableforth W, et al. The role of hepatitis E virus testing in drug-induced liver injury. Aliment Pharmacol Ther 2007;26:1429–35.
10. Davern TJ, Chalasani N, Fontana RJ, et al. Acute hepatitis E infection accounts for some cases of suspected drug-induced liver injury. Gastroenterology 2011; 141:1665–72.e1–9.
11. Lee WM. Drug-induced hepatotoxicity. N Engl J Med 1995;333:1118–27.
12. Bjornsson E, Kalaitzakis E, Av Klinteberg V, et al. Long-term follow-up of patients with mild to moderate drug-induced liver injury. Aliment Pharmacol Ther 2007; 26:79–85.
13. Andrade RJ, Lucena MI, Kaplowitz N, et al. Outcome of acute idiosyncratic drug-induced liver injury: long-term follow-up in a hepatotoxicity registry. Hepatology 2006;44:1581–8.
14. Hou FQ, Zeng Z, Wang GQ. Hospital admissions for drug-induced liver injury: clinical features, therapy, and outcomes. Cell Biochem Biophys 2012;64:77–83.
15. Bunchorntavakul C, Reddy KR. Herbal and dietary supplement hepatotoxicity. Aliment Pharmacol Ther 2013;37:3–17.
16. Efe C. Drug induced autoimmune hepatitis and TNF-alpha blocking agents: is there a real relationship? Autoimmun Rev 2013;12(3):337–9.
17. Czaja AJ. Drug-induced autoimmune-like hepatitis. Dig Dis Sci 2011;56:958–76.
18. Suzuki A, Brunt EM, Kleiner DE, et al. The use of liver biopsy evaluation in discrimination of idiopathic autoimmune hepatitis versus drug-induced liver injury. Hepatology 2011;54:931–9.
19. Lewis JH. Diagnosis: liver biopsy differentiates DILI from autoimmune hepatitis. Nat Rev Gastroenterol Hepatol 2011;8:540–2.
20. Ramachandran R, Kakar S. Histological patterns in drug-induced liver disease. J Clin Pathol 2009;62:481–92.
21. Yoshikado T, Takada T, Yamamoto H, et al. Ticlopidine, a cholestatic liver injury-inducible drug, causes dysfunction of bile formation via diminished biliary secretion of phospholipids: involvement of biliary-excreted glutathione-conjugated ticlopidine metabolites. Mol Pharmacol 2013;83(2):552–62.
22. Vilas-Boas F, Goncalves R, Sobrinho Simoes M, et al. Thalidomide-induced acute cholestatic hepatitis: case report and review of the literature. Gastroenterol Hepatol 2012;35:560–6.
23. Studniarz M, Czubkowski P, Cielecka-Kuszyk J, et al. Amoxicillin/clavulanic acid-induced cholestatic liver injury after pediatric liver transplantation. Ann Transplant 2012;17:128–31.
24. Ruiz Rebollo ML, Aller De La Fuente R, Macho Conesa A, et al. Amoxicillin-induced cholestatic hepatitis. Gastroenterol Hepatol 2011;34:474–7.
25. Stadlmann S, Portmann S, Tschopp S, et al. Venlafaxine-induced cholestatic hepatitis: case report and review of literature. Am J Surg Pathol 2012;36: 1724–8.

26. Nojkov B, Signori C, Konda A, et al. Lenalidomide-associated hepatotoxicity—a case report and literature review. Anticancer Res 2012;32:4117–9.
27. Devarbhavi H. Antituberculous drug-induced liver injury: current perspective. Trop Gastroenterol 2011;32:167–74.
28. Avelar-Escobar G, Mendez-Navarro J, Ortiz-Olvera NX, et al. Hepatotoxicity associated with dietary energy supplements: use and abuse by young athletes. Ann Hepatol 2012;11:564–9.
29. Palta R, Thobani S, Donovan JA, et al. Prolonged cholestasis associated with benazepril therapy. Am J Gastroenterol 2009;104:245–6.
30. Yeung E, Wong FS, Wanless IR, et al. Ramipril-associated hepatotoxicity. Arch Pathol Lab Med 2003;127:1493–7.
31. Alazmi WM, McHenry L, Watkins JL, et al. Chemotherapy-induced sclerosing cholangitis: long-term response to endoscopic therapy. J Clin Gastroenterol 2006;40:353–7.
32. Qu K, Liu C, Wu QF, et al. Sclerosing cholangitis after transcatheter arterial chemoembolization: a case report. Chin Med Sci J 2011;26:190–3.
33. Siddique A, Kowdley KV. Approach to a patient with elevated serum alkaline phosphatase. Clin Liver Dis 2012;16:199–229.
34. Plessier A, Rautou PE, Valla DC. Management of hepatic vascular diseases. J Hepatol 2012;56(Suppl 1):S25–38.
35. Elbl C, Terracciano L, Stallmach TK, et al. Herbal drugs mimicking primary biliary cirrhosis. Praxis (Bern 1994) 2012;101:195–8.
36. Nakayama S, Murashima N. Overlap syndrome of autoimmune hepatitis and primary biliary cirrhosis triggered by fluvastatin. Indian J Gastroenterol 2011; 30:97–9.
37. Macias FM, Campos FR, Salguero TP, et al. Ductopenic hepatitis related to Enalapril. J Hepatol 2003;39:1091–2.
38. Nakanuma Y, Tsuneyama K, Harada K. Pathology and pathogenesis of intrahepatic bile duct loss. J Hepatobiliary Pancreat Surg 2001;8:303–15.
39. Vuppalanchi R, Chalasani N, Saxena R. Restoration of bile ducts in drug-induced vanishing bile duct syndrome due to zonisamide. Am J Surg Pathol 2006;30:1619–23.
40. Kleiner DE, Brunt EM. Nonalcoholic fatty liver disease: pathologic patterns and biopsy evaluation in clinical research. Semin Liver Dis 2012;32:3–13.
41. Khan AZ, Morris-Stiff G, Makuuchi M. Patterns of chemotherapy-induced hepatic injury and their implications for patients undergoing liver resection for colorectal liver metastases. J Hepatobiliary Pancreat Surg 2009;16: 137–44.
42. Tannapfel A, Reinacher-Schick A, Flott-Rahmel B. Steatohepatitis after chemotherapy for colorectal liver metastases (CASH). Pathologe 2011;32:330–5.
43. Coash M, Forouhar F, Wu CH, et al. Granulomatous liver diseases: a review. J Formos Med Assoc 2012;111:3–13.
44. Turhan N, Kurt M, Ozderin YO, et al. Hepatic granulomas: a clinicopathologic analysis of 86 cases. Pathol Res Pract 2011;207:359–65.
45. Gaya DR, Thorburn D, Oien KA, et al. Hepatic granulomas: a 10 year single centre experience. J Clin Pathol 2003;56:850–3.
46. Fiel MI, Shukla D, Saraf N, et al. Development of hepatic granulomas in patients receiving pegylated interferon therapy for recurrent hepatitis C virus post liver transplantation. Transpl Infect Dis 2008;10:184–9.
47. Farah M, Al Rashidi A, Owen DA, et al. Granulomatous hepatitis associated with etanercept therapy. J Rheumatol 2008;35:349–51.

48. Braun M, Fraser GM, Kunin M, et al. Mesalamine-induced granulomatous hepatitis. Am J Gastroenterol 1999;94:1973–4.
49. Ruiz-Valverde P, Zafon C, Segarra A, et al. Ticlopidine-induced granulomatous hepatitis. Ann Pharmacother 1995;29:633–4.
50. Vial T, Descotes J. Drug-induced granulomatous hepatitis. Gastroenterol Clin Biol 1993;17:H44–8.
51. Flamm SL. Granulomatous liver disease. Clin Liver Dis 2012;16:387–96.
52. Trivalle C, Profit P, Bonnet B, et al. Liver lipogranulomas with log-term fever caused by paraffin oil. Gastroenterol Clin Biol 1991;15:551–3.
53. Dincsoy HP, Weesner RE, MacGee J. Lipogranulomas in non-fatty human livers. A mineral oil induced environmental disease. Am J Clin Pathol 1982;78:35–41.
54. Fleming KA, Zimmerman H, Shubik P. Granulomas in the livers of humans and Fischer rats associated with the ingestion of mineral hydrocarbons: a comparison. Regul Toxicol Pharmacol 1998;27:75–81.
55. Zhu H, Bodenheimer HC Jr, Clain DJ, et al. Hepatic lipogranulomas in patients with chronic liver disease: association with hepatitis C and fatty liver disease. World J Gastroenterol 2010;16:5065–9.
56. Villamil-Cajoto I, Jove MJ, Serrano M, et al. Granulomatous hepatitis due to *Mycobacterium* complex following *Bacillus* Calmette-Guérin intravesical instillation. Enferm Infecc Microbiol Clin 2010;28:759–61 [author reply: 761–2].
57. Stricker BH, Blok AP, Babany G, et al. Fibrin ring granulomas and allopurinol. Gastroenterology 1989;96:1199–203.
58. Khanlari B, Bodmer M, Terracciano L, et al. Hepatitis with fibrin-ring granulomas. Infection 2008;36:381–3.
59. Tjwa M, De Hertogh G, Neuville B, et al. Hepatic fibrin-ring granulomas in granulomatous hepatitis: report of four cases and review of the literature. Acta Clin Belg 2001;56:341–8.
60. Rubbia-Brandt L. Sinusoidal obstruction syndrome. Clin Liver Dis 2010;14: 651–68.
61. Sebagh M, Azoulay D, Roche B, et al. Significance of isolated hepatic veno-occlusive disease/sinusoidal obstruction syndrome after liver transplantation. Liver Transpl 2011;17:798–808.
62. Robinson SM, White SA. Hepatic sinusoidal obstruction syndrome reduces the effect of oxaliplatin in colorectal liver metastases. Histopathology 2012;61:1247–8.
63. Tuncer HH, Rana N, Milani C, et al. Gastrointestinal and hepatic complications of hematopoietic stem cell transplantation. World J Gastroenterol 2012;18: 1851–60.
64. Pai RK, van Besien K, Hart J, et al. Clinicopathologic features of late-onset veno-occlusive disease/sinusoidal obstruction syndrome after high dose intravenous busulfan and hematopoietic cell transplant. Leuk Lymphoma 2012;53:1552–7.
65. Gao H, Li N, Wang JY, et al. Definitive diagnosis of hepatic sinusoidal obstruction syndrome induced by pyrrolizidine alkaloids. J Dig Dis 2012;13:33–9.
66. Larrey D, Faure S. Herbal medicine hepatotoxicity: a new step with development of specific biomarkers. J Hepatol 2011;54:599–601.
67. Corbacioglu S, Kernan N, Lehmann L, et al. Defibrotide for the treatment of hepatic veno-occlusive disease in children after hematopoietic stem cell transplantation. Expert Rev Hematol 2012;5:291–302.
68. Platzbecker U, Bornhauser M. SOS for veno-occlusive disease: defibrotide prophylaxis. Lancet 2012;379:1277–8.
69. Richardson PG, Corbacioglu S, Ho VT, et al. Drug safety evaluation of defibrotide. Expert Opin Drug Saf 2013;12:123–36.

70. van Erpecum KJ, Janssens AR, Kreuning J, et al. Generalized peliosis hepatis and cirrhosis after long-term use of oral contraceptives. Am J Gastroenterol 1988;83:572–5.
71. Neri M, Bello S, Bonsignore A, et al. Anabolic androgenic steroids abuse and liver toxicity. Mini Rev Med Chem 2011;11:430–7.
72. Komori H, Beppu T, Baba Y, et al. Histological liver injury and surgical outcome after FOLFOX followed by a hepatectomy for colorectal liver metastases in Japanese patients. Int J Clin Oncol 2010;15:263–70.
73. Gisbert JP, Gonzalez-Lama Y, Mate J. Thiopurine-induced liver injury in patients with inflammatory bowel disease: a systematic review. Am J Gastroenterol 2007; 102:1518–27.
74. Nam SJ, Cho JY, Lee HS, et al. Chemotherapy-associated hepatopathy in Korean colorectal cancer liver metastasis patients: oxaliplatin-based chemotherapy and sinusoidal injury. Korean J Pathol 2012;46:22–9.
75. Ryan P, Nanji S, Pollett A, et al. Chemotherapy-induced liver injury in metastatic colorectal cancer: semiquantitative histologic analysis of 334 resected liver specimens shows that vascular injury but not steatohepatitis is associated with preoperative chemotherapy. Am J Surg Pathol 2010;34:784–91.
76. Agostini J, Benoist S, Seman M, et al. Identification of molecular pathways involved in oxaliplatin-associated sinusoidal dilatation. J Hepatol 2012;56: 869–76.
77. Cazals-Hatem D, Hillaire S, Rudler M, et al. Obliterative portal venopathy: portal hypertension is not always present at diagnosis. J Hepatol 2011;54:455–61.
78. Schouten JN, Garcia-Pagan JC, Valla DC, et al. Idiopathic noncirrhotic portal hypertension. Hepatology 2011;54:1071–81.
79. Krishnan P, Fiel MI, Rosenkrantz AB, et al. Hepatoportal sclerosis: CT and MRI appearance with histopathologic correlation. AJR Am J Roentgenol 2012;198: 370–6.
80. Mendizabal M, Craviotto S, Chen T, et al. Noncirrhotic portal hypertension: another cause of liver disease in HIV patients. Ann Hepatol 2009;8:390–5.
81. Schiano TD, Kotler DP, Ferran E, et al. Hepatoportal sclerosis as a cause of noncirrhotic portal hypertension in patients with HIV. Am J Gastroenterol 2007;102: 2536–40.
82. Lawal TO, Farris AB, El-Rayes BF, et al. Oxaliplatin-induced hepatoportal sclerosis, portal hypertension, and variceal bleeding successfully treated with transjugular intrahepatic portosystemic shunt. Clin Colorectal Cancer 2012;11:224–7.
83. Lopez-Martin C, de la Fuente-Fernandez E, Corbaton P, et al. Nodular regenerative hyperplasia: azathioprine-induced hepatotoxicity in a patient with Crohn's disease. Gastroenterol Hepatol 2011;34:16–9.
84. Calabrese E, Hanauer SB. Assessment of non-cirrhotic portal hypertension associated with thiopurine therapy in inflammatory bowel disease. J Crohns Colitis 2011;5:48–53.
85. Vispo E, Moreno A, Maida I, et al. Noncirrhotic portal hypertension in HIV-infected patients: unique clinical and pathological findings. AIDS 2010;24:1171–6.
86. Schiano TD, Uriel A, Dieterich DT, et al. The development of hepatoportal sclerosis and portal hypertension due to didanosine use in HIV. Virchows Arch 2011; 458:231–5.
87. Jones M, Nunez M. Liver toxicity of antiretroviral drugs. Semin Liver Dis 2012;32: 167–76.
88. Jackson BD, Doyle JS, Hoy JF, et al. Non-cirrhotic portal hypertension in HIV mono-infected patients. J Gastroenterol Hepatol 2012;27:1512–9.

89. Lefkowitch JH, Lobritto SJ, Brown RS Jr, et al. Ground-glass, polyglucosan-like hepatocellular inclusions: a "new" diagnostic entity. Gastroenterology 2006;131: 713–8.

90. Bua J, Marchetti F, Faleschini E, et al. Hepatic glycogenosis in an adolescent with diabetes. J Pediatr 2010;157:1042.

91. Torbenson M, Chen YY, Brunt E, et al. Glycogenic hepatopathy: an underrecognized hepatic complication of diabetes mellitus. Am J Surg Pathol 2006;30: 508–13.

92. Carcione L, Lombardo F, Messina MF, et al. Liver glycogenosis as early manifestation in type 1 diabetes mellitus. Diabetes Nutr Metab 2003;16:182–4.

93. Abaci A, Bekem O, Unuvar T, et al. Hepatic glycogenosis: a rare cause of hepatomegaly in Type 1 diabetes mellitus. J Diabetes Complications 2008;22:325–8.

94. Cuthbertson DJ, Brennan G, Walsh S, et al. Hepatic glycogenosis: abnormal liver function tests in Type 1 diabetes. Diabet Med 2007;24:322–3.

95. Iancu TC, Shiloh H, Dembo L. Hepatomegaly following short-term high-dose steroid therapy. J Pediatr Gastroenterol Nutr 1986;5:41–6.

96. Reasor MJ, Hastings KL, Ulrich RG. Drug-induced phospholipidosis: issues and future directions. Expert Opin Drug Saf 2006;5:567–83.

97. Guigui B, Perrot S, Berry JP, et al. Amiodarone-induced hepatic phospholipidosis: a morphological alteration independent of pseudoalcoholic liver disease. Hepatology 1988;8:1063–8.

98. Degott C, Messing B, Moreau D, et al. Liver phospholipidosis induced by parenteral nutrition: histologic, histochemical, and ultrastructural investigations. Gastroenterology 1988;95:183–91.

99. Obert LA, Sobocinski GP, Bobrowski WF, et al. An immunohistochemical approach to differentiate hepatic lipidosis from hepatic phospholipidosis in rats. Toxicol Pathol 2007;35:728–34.

100. Levine PH, Delgado Y, Theise ND, et al. Stellate-cell lipidosis in liver biopsy specimens. Recognition and significance. Am J Clin Pathol 2003;119:254–8.

101. Nollevaux MC, Guiot Y, Horsmans Y, et al. Hypervitaminosis A-induced liver fibrosis: stellate cell activation and daily dose consumption. Liver Int 2006;26: 182–6.

102. Masia R, Pratt DS, Misdraji J. A histopathologic pattern of centrilobular hepatocyte injury suggests 6-mercaptopurine-induced hepatotoxicity in patients with inflammatory bowel disease. Arch Pathol Lab Med 2012;136:618–22.

103. Chang CY, Hernandez-Prera JC, Roayaie S, et al. Changing epidemiology of hepatocellular adenoma in the United States: review of the literature. Int J Hepatol 2013;2013:604860.

104. Deneve JL, Pawlik TM, Cunningham S, et al. Liver cell adenoma: a multicenter analysis of risk factors for rupture and malignancy. Ann Surg Oncol 2009;16: 640–8.

105. Socas L, Zumbado M, Perez-Luzardo O, et al. Hepatocellular adenomas associated with anabolic androgenic steroid abuse in bodybuilders: a report of two cases and a review of the literature. Br J Sports Med 2005;39:e27.

106. Martin NM, Abu Dayyeh BK, Chung RT. Anabolic steroid abuse causing recurrent hepatic adenomas and hemorrhage. World J Gastroenterol 2008;14: 4573–5.

107. Bork K, Schneiders V. Danazol-induced hepatocellular adenoma in patients with hereditary angio-oedema. J Hepatol 2002;36:707–9.

108. Lautz TB, Finegold MJ, Chin AC, et al. Giant hepatic adenoma with atypical features in a patient on oxcarbazepine therapy. J Pediatr Surg 2008;43:751–4.

109. Tazawa K, Yasuda M, Ohtani Y, et al. Multiple hepatocellular adenomas associated with long-term carbamazepine. Histopathology 1999;35:92–4.
110. Cerminara C, Bagnolo V, De Leonardis F, et al. Hepatocellular adenoma associated with long-term exposure to phenobarbital: a paediatric case report. Childs Nerv Syst 2012;28:939–41.
111. Defrance R, Zafrani ES, Hannoun S, et al. Association of hepatocellular adenoma and focal nodular hyperplasia of the liver in a woman on oral contraceptives. Gastroenterol Clin Biol 1982;6:949–50.
112. Hagay ZJ, Leiberman RJ, Katz M, et al. Oral contraceptives and focal nodular hyperplasia of the liver. Arch Gynecol Obstet 1988;243:231–4.
113. Tajada M, Nerin J, Ruiz MM, et al. Liver adenoma and focal nodular hyperplasia associated with oral contraceptives. Eur J Contracept Reprod Health Care 2001;6:227–30.
114. Ikeda N, Oka K, Yonekawa N, et al. Pelioid-type well-differentiated hepatocellular carcinoma in a patient with a history of taking oral contraceptives: report of a case. Surg Today 2011;41:1270–4.
115. Singhal S, Jain S, Singla M, et al. Multifocal epitheloid hemangioendothelioma of liver after long-term oral contraceptive use—a case report and discussion of management difficulties encountered. J Gastrointest Cancer 2009;40:59–63.

# Clinical Manifestations and Treatment of Drug-induced Hepatotoxicity

Christin M. Giordano, MPAS, PA-C[a],*, Xaralambos B. Zervos, DO[b]

## KEYWORDS

- Drug-induced liver injury • Drug-induced cholestasis
- Drug-induced hepatocellular injury • Management of drug-induced liver injury

## KEY POINTS

- Greater than 1000 medications have been implicated in drug-induced liver injury (DILI), most commonly acetaminophen and antibiotics.
- Greater than 1 in 100 hospitalized patients are diagnosed with DILI and DILI is responsible for greater than 50% of cases of fulminant hepatic failure.
- Drug-induced hepatocellular injury carries a worse prognosis than cholestatic injury.
- Assessing risk factors, time course, and exclusion of other causes of liver injury are essential for proper diagnosis.
- Management includes withdrawing the offending drug, administering proven antidotes when appropriate, symptomatic treatment, and monitoring of biochemical tests.
- Early recognition of DILI and subsequent referral and transfer to a transplant center can be life-saving.
- In most cases, biochemical resolution of DILI occurs within 60 days.

## EPIDEMIOLOGY

Greater than 1000 medications on the market have been associated with causing hepatotoxicity.[1] Drug-induced liver injury (DILI) is implicated in most cases of acute liver failure and hepatotoxicity remains an important cause of drugs withdrawn from the market.[2–5] In addition, whereas DILI may not confer long-term morbidity and mortality in most cases, the combined mortality and transplantation rate is approximately 9%.[6] In fact, the United States Liver Failure Study Group found that acetaminophen (Tylenol) and idiosyncratic drug reactions account for nearly 50% of fulminant hepatic

Financial Disclosures: None.
[a] University of Central Florida College of Medicine, 6850 Lake Nona Boulevard, Orlando, FL 32827, USA; [b] Liver Transplant, Department of Gastroenterology, Digestive Disease Center, Cleveland Clinic Florida, 2950 Cleveland Clinic Boulevard, Weston, FL 33331, USA
* Corresponding author.
E-mail address: cgiordano@knights.ucf.edu

failure in the United States.[7] Although the greatest single cause of new-onset jaundice was from ischemic liver injury in a retrospective study of 732 adult inpatients and outpatients in Indiana, DILI was implicated in 4% of cases. Most of the DILI cases were secondary to acetaminophen use and there were no deaths in a 6-week follow-up period.[8] In a study of postliver transplant patients, antibiotics were the most commonly implicated agent, although 14% of reported cases were due to immunosuppressive agents, including tacrolimus and azathioprine.[9] Other studies confirm nonsteroidal anti-inflammatory drugs and antibiotics, specifically amoxicillin-clavulanic acid (Augmentin, Clavamox), as the most common causes of DILI.[5,7,10,11] Although most cases of DILI can be attributed to a single prescription drug, up to 18% have been the result of multiple agents and dietary supplements have been linked to DILI in 7% to 9% of cases.[11,12]

One study performed on patients admitted to a medicine service demonstrated that DILI had an incidence of 1.4%.[13] Furthermore, the incidence of DILI is quite high in the general population with one study of the French population concluding that it occurs in 14 of 100,000 people each year.[14] However, chronic liver enzyme abnormalities or significant histologic changes are rare. Indeed, one study demonstrated that chronic biochemical changes occurred in only 5.8% of the studied patients and the liver ultrasounds performed 6 months after the initial presentation were normal in all but 2.9% of patients who had steatosis.[15] In another study, jaundice resolved in all cases with a median time to biochemical resolution of 60 days.[16]

Many medications undergo hepatic metabolism and, in fact, one study demonstrated that drugs with greater than 50% hepatic metabolism conveyed a significant risk for alanine transferase (ALT) increases (35% vs 11%), liver failure (28% vs 9%), and mortality related to DILI (23% vs 4%).[17] Although the damage in these cases may be attributed to the induction of hepatic enzymes, other mechanisms for DILI include hypersensitivity, autoimmunity, veno-occlusive disease, and idiosyncratic reactions, as seen in **Box 1**.[2,10]

## TERMINOLOGY

DILI is defined as any liver injury that is caused by medication or herbal supplements that has led to biochemical abnormalities or liver dysfunction with the exclusion of other causes.[11] DILI may be dose-dependent, as seen in medications such as aspirin and acetaminophen, or idiosyncratic.[18] However, both require the exclusion of other causes of liver disease before diagnosis.[18] The clinical presentation may range from asymptomatic elevation of aspartate transferase (AST) and ALT to fulminant hepatic failure. Liver injury can be described as cholestatic, hepatocellular, or mixed in nature.

Cholestatic liver injury is defined by isolated elevations of alkaline phosphatase (ALP), which is released by damaged cholangiocytes, thus suggesting injury to the

---

**Box 1**
**Mechanisms of DILI**

- Hepatic metabolism
- Hypersensitivity/allergic reactions
- Autoimmunity
- Veno-occlusive disease
- Idiosyncratic reactions

bile ducts.[19] Acute drug-induced cholestasis is defined as an elevation of ALP at least 2 times the upper limit of normal (ULN) or an ALT/ALP ratio of less than 2 with both ALT and ALP greater than the ULN.[20]

Increases in both AST and ALT suggest damage to hepatocytes.[19] However, ALT is liver-specific and is the current gold standard biochemical marker for liver injury.[21,22] Hepatocellular injury is most recently defined as ALT elevation of at least 5 times ULN in combination with a bilirubin elevation of at least 2 times ULN.[23,24] Hepatocellular injury is the more commonly occurring presentation and, unfortunately, has been correlated with worse outcome.[16,25] A recent study found that both glutamate dehydrogenase and malate dehydrogenase may confer an added value over ALT by better reflecting recovery from injury as return to normal levels is directly associated with normal liver function.[21]

As one would suspect, mixed injury has elements of both cholestatic and hepatocellular injury with increases in ALT, ALP, and bilirubin.[19] Other clinical manifestations include veno-occlusive disease and steatohepatitis. **Table 1** provides a list of commonly implicated medications along with their common clinical presentation and its definition.

## DIAGNOSIS

When making a diagnosis, assessing risk factors for DILI may help to determine the likelihood of DILI as a cause of abnormal liver enzymes or function. The proven risk factors are provided in **Box 2**. Although it is traditionally believed that women are at a higher risk for DILI, studies fail to confirm any differences in the incidence of DILI between sexes.[9] However, one study did find that men were at higher risk for DILI when they were younger, while women were at higher risk when they were older.[26,27] Interestingly, underlying chronic liver disease does not seem to be a risk factor for DILI in the most cases, although this does not hold true for aspirin, methotrexate, isoniazid, or HIV antiretroviral therapy.[2] In posttransplant patients, primary sclerosing cholangitis as the reason for transplant seemed to be a risk factor for DILI and most cases occurred between 31 and 90 days posttransplant or greater than 501 days posttransplant.[9]

When diagnosing DILI, gathering information as the illness progresses is essential for proper diagnosis.[3] There are several criteria in use for diagnosing DILI and, although none are considered a gold standard, they can be used as tools to assist in the clinical diagnosis of DILI. A summary of the criteria along with their limitations is provided in **Table 2**. Hy's law is considered a more specific indication than ALT and consists of AST and ALT measurements along with bilirubin but, because it does not consider temporal relationships or reports in literature of hepatotoxicity, it is not as sensitive as other available criteria.[21,28] The Roussel Uclaf Causality Assessment Method (RUCAM), also known as the Council for International Organizations of Medical Sciences (CIOMS) scale, was developed at an international meeting in response to the diagnostic challenge DILI provides. It considers the temporal relationship of drug administration and symptom development, prior reports of hepatotoxicity in the literature, exclusion of other causes, extrahepatic manifestations, and rechallenge results.[29] Although it can specifically associate liver injury to a particular medication, it is complicated to administer and rechallenging patients is rare.[30] Thus, modifications to this scale have been proposed.

Perhaps the best modification is the Digestive Disease Week-Japan (DDW-J) scale, which changed the criteria for chronology, concomitant drugs, and extrahepatic manifestations and was found to have a higher sensitivity but lower specificity than the

**Table 1**
**Causes of DILI by clinical presentation**

| Presentation | Definition | Implicated Drugs |
|---|---|---|
| Hepatocellular | ALT >5× ULN and Bilirubin >2× ULN | *Antibiotics:* ciprofloxacin, nitrofurantoin, tetracycline, trimethoprim-sulfamethoxazole<br>*Antidepressants:* bupropion fluoxetine, paroxetine<br>*Anti-inflammatory medications:* acetaminophen, bromfenac, diclofenac, ibuprofen, naproxen<br>*Cardiac medications:* amiodarone, lisinopril, statins<br>*Neurologic/psychiatric medications:* methyldopa, nefazodone, risperidone, sertraline, trazodone, valproic acid<br>*Other:* acarbose, amatoxin, allopurinol, cimetidine, ketoconazole, halothane, isoniazid, omeprazole, protease inhibitors, pyrazinamide, quinidine, rifampin, troglitazone |
| Cholestatic | ALP >2× ULN or ALP/ALT <2 with both ALP and ALT >1× ULN | *Antibiotics:* amoxicilin-clavulanate acid, erythromycin, trimethoprim-sulfamethoxazole<br>*Anti-inflammatory medications:* sulindac<br>*Cardiac medications:* clopidogrel, ACE inhibitors<br>*Neurologic/psychiatric medications:* carbamazepine, chlorpromazine, tricyclic antidepressants<br>*Other:* azathioprine, anabolic steroids, oral contraceptives |
| Mixed | ALT >5× ULN or Bilirubin >2× ULN and ALP >2× ULN or ALP/ALT <2 with both ALP and ALT >1× ULN | *Antibiotics:* clindamycin, sulfonamides<br>*Cardiac medications:* ACE inhibitors, statins<br>*Neurologic/psychiatric medications:* phenytoin, amitriptyline<br>*Other:* azathioprine, protease inhibitors reverse transcriptase inhibitors |
| Veno-occlusive disease leading to portal hypertension | Manifestations include ascites, varices, and hepatic encephalopathy | *Antineoplastic agents:* busulfan, cyclophosphamide<br>*Environmental exposures:* arsenic, vinyl chloride, thorium dioxide<br>*Other:* Vitamin A |
| Steatohepatitis | Fatty infiltration | *Cardiac:* amiodarone<br>*Other:* tamoxifen |

original scale.[31] This scale uses lymphocyte stimulation testing, which involves culturing lymphocytes in the presence of the suspected medication.[32–34] A second modification is known as the Clinical Diagnostic Scale or Maria and Victorino (M&V) scale. Although it is simpler than the RUCAM because it does not consider risk factors or concomitant therapy, it has been shown to be less predictive in cases with long latency periods or with the development of chronic liver injury.[29,35]

## MANAGEMENT

Following the diagnosis of DILI, management is largely supportive except when DILI is the result of acetaminophen toxicity or Amanita mushroom poisoning for which

---

**Box 2**
**Risk factors for DILI**

- Older age
- History of chronic liver disease *if* aspirin, methotrexate, isoniazid, or antiretroviral agents
- Obesity, in particular, central obesity
- Pregnancy
- Regular alcohol concomitant alcohol consumption
- Genetic polymorphisms (ie, HLA-B*5701)
- Male in younger patients, female in older patients
- In postliver transplant patients: history of primary sclerosing cholangitis

---

antitoxins are available (**Table 3**). The only proven treatment of DILI is withdrawal of the causative agent.[2,36] In addition, all patients should have their AST, ALT, ALP, and international normalized ratio (INR) monitored as well as monitoring for changes in mental status consistent with hepatic encephalopathy.[2] Ursodeoxycholic acid

**Table 2**
**Diagnostic criteria in use for DILI**

|  | Criteria | Limitations |
|---|---|---|
| Hy's law | AST and/or ALT >3× ULN *and* Bilirubin >2× ULN without initial ALP >2× ULN *and* No other causes of liver disease | Not specific for a particular drug Does not consider temporal relationship Does not consider literature |
| Roussel Uclaf Causality Assessment Method (RUCAM, also known as CIOMS) | Risk factors Temporal relationship (different for cholestatic and hepatocellular injuries) Exclusion of other causes Concomitant therapy Extrahepatic manifestations Prior reports of hepatotoxicity Rechallenge results | Requires training for administration Weighting of risk factors not significant for most medications Likely not to rechallenge |
| DDW-J | Temporal relationship Eosinophilia Positive lymphocyte stimulation Test | Lower specificity than RUCAM |
| Clinical Diagnostic Scale (also known as the M&V scale) | Temporal relationship Exclusion of other causes Prior reports of hepatotoxicity Rechallenge results | Poor performance with chronic hepatotoxicity and longer time to symptom development Has to be computed for each drug patient is taking Likely not to rechallenge |
| Naranjo Adverse Drug Reaction Probability Scale | Temporal relationship Exclusion of other causes Rechallenge results Prior reports of hepatotoxicity | Not specific for hepatotoxicity Likely not to rechallenge |

| Table 3 Management of DILI | |
|---|---|
| General | • Withdraw offending agent<br>• Monitor biochemical tests, such as ALT, bilirubin, and INR<br>• Monitor for changes in mental status suggesting hepatic encephalopathy<br>• Administer corticosteroids if presentation consistent with drug-induced autoimmune hepatitis<br>• Consider N-acetylcysteine if fulminant presentation<br>• If fulminant hepatic failure develops, consider listing patient for transplant and consider Status 1A listing |
| Cholestatic pattern | • Consider ursodeoxycholic acid<br>• Consider corticosteroids<br>• Treat pruritus: consider emollients, diphenhydramine, bile acid resins, selective norepinephrine reuptake inhibitors |
| Acetaminophen poisoning | • Administer N-acetylcysteine if elevated AST or ALT or detectable serum acetaminophen level, consider IV administration if presentation is >10-h after ingestion or if vomiting precludes oral administration<br>• Continual observation and psychiatry consult if intentional overdose suspected |
| Mushroom poisoning | • Administer silibinin<br>• Administer high-dose penicillin G<br>• Consider administering N-acetylcysteine or cimetidine |

can be considered in cases of cholestatic pattern of injury, although the European Association for the Study of the Liver states that this treatment is experimental.[2,36,37] Other management for cholestasis should include symptomatic treatment of pruritus, such as emollients, hydroxyzine, diphenhydramine, selective norepinephrine reuptake inhibitors, bile acid resins, and rifampicin.[38] Although corticosteroid therapy is experimental in most DILI, it is beneficial and should be administered in cases of drug-induced autoimmune hepatitis.[37,39]

Patients with a detectable serum acetaminophen level or AST or ALT 3 times ULN should be treated with N-acetylcysteine (NAC). One study found that, although oral and intravenous (IV) formulations provided equal efficacy if first administration was within 10 hours of acetaminophen ingestion, IV formulations provided better results if first administration was greater than 10 hours.[40] In addition, providers should consider IV formulations when a patient has intractable vomiting that prevents adequate oral administration. Amanita Paholloides mushroom poisoning has been traditionally treated with silibinin and high-dose penicillin G, with penicillin G being more readily available in the United States.[2,41,42] However, only silibinin has been demonstrated to be effective both in vivo and in vitro and use of penicillin G remains controversial.[42,43] Other therapies that have been used with case reports of success include NAC and cimetidine.[42,43]

Patients who develop fulminant hepatic failure from DILI should be considered for transplant. Patients may be listed as Status 1A if they are 18 or older, have a life expectancy of 7 days or less, have encephalopathy that developed within 8 weeks of the first symptoms of liver disease, do not have a pre-existing liver disease, and are in the intensive care unit with either ventilator dependence, dialysis, or and INR greater than 2.[44] In addition, a recent study suggested that IV NAC may improve transplant-free survival in patients with non-acetaminophen-related fulminant hepatic failure, although NAC administration should not delay referral and workup for transplantation.[45]

## REFERENCES

1. Zimmerman H. Hepatotoxicity: the adverse effects of drugs and other chemicals on the liver. 2nd edition. Philadelphia: Lippincott, Williams &Wilkins; 1999.
2. Dienstag J. Toxic and drug-induced hepatitis. In: Longo D, Fauci A, Kasper DL, et al, editors. Harrison's principles of internal medicine. 18th edition. New York: McGraw-Hill; 2011. Available at. http://accessmedicine.com/content.aspx?aid= 9134024. Accessed March 20, 2013.
3. Lee W, Senior J. Recognizing drug-induced liver injury: current problems, possible solutions. Toxicol Pathol 2005;33:155–64.
4. Kaplowitz N. Drug-induced liver disorders: implications for drug development and regulation. Drug Saf 2001;24:483–90.
5. Chang CY, Schiano TD. Review article: drug hepatoxicity. Aliment Pharmacol Ther 2007;25:1135–51.
6. Bjornsson E, Olsson R. Outcome and prognostic markers in severe-drug induced liver disease. Hepatology 2005;42:481–9.
7. Ostapowicz G, Fontana RJ, Schiodt FV, et al. Results of a prospective study of acute liver failure at 17 tertiary care centers in the United States. Ann Intern Med 2002;137:947–54.
8. Vuppalanchi R, Liangpunsakul S, Chalasani N. Etiology of new-onset jaundice: how often is it caused by idiosyncratic drug-induced liver injury in the United States? Am J Gastroenterol 2007;102:558–62.
9. Sembera S, Lammert C, Talwalkar J, et al. Frequency, clinical presentation and outcomes of drug-induced liver injury after liver transplantation. Liver Transpl 2012;18:803–10.
10. Farrell GC. Liver disease caused by drugs, anesthetics, and toxins. In: Feldman M, Friedman LS, Sleisenger MH, editors. Gastrointenstinal and liver disease. 7th edition. Philadelphia: WB Saunders; 2002. p. 1403–47.
11. Suk KT, Kim DJ. Drug-induced liver injury: present and future. Clin Mol Hepatol 2012;18:249–57.
12. Chalasani N, Fontana RJ, Bonkovsky HL, et al. Causes, clinical features, and outcomes from a prospective study of drug-induced liver injury in the United States. Gastroenterology 2008;135:1924–34.
13. Meier Y, Cavallaro M, Roos M, et al. Incidence of drug-induced liver injury in medical inpatients. Eur J Clin Pharmacol 2005;61:135–43.
14. de Abajo FJ, Montero D, Madurga M, et al. Acute and clinically relevant drug-induced liver injury: a population based case-control study. Br J Clin Pharmacol 2004;58:71–80.
15. Bjornsson E, Kalaitzakis E, Klinteberg V, et al. Long-term follow-up of patients with mild to moderate drug-induced liver injury. Aliment Pharmacol Ther 2007;26: 79–85.
16. De Valle MB, Klinteberg V, Alem N, et al. Drug-induced liver injury in a Swedish university hospital out-patient hepatology clinic. Aliment Pharmacol Ther 2006; 24:1187–95.
17. Lammert C, Bjornsson E, Niklasson A, et al. Oral medications with significant hepatic metabolism at higher risk for hepatic adverse events. Hepatology 2010;51: 615–20.
18. Watkins PB, Seeff LB. Drug-induced liver injury: summary of a single topic clinical research conference. Hepatology 2006;43:618–31.
19. Aragon G, Younossi Z. When and how to evaluate mildly elevated liver enzymes in apparently healthy patients. Cleve Clin J Med 2010;77(3):195–204.

20. Benichou C. Criteria of drug-induced liver disorders. Report of an international consensus meeting. J Hepatol 1990;11:272–6.
21. Schomaker S, Warner R, Bock J, et al. Assessment of emerging biomarkers of liver injury in human subjects. Toxicol Sci 2013;132(2):276–83.
22. Green RM, Flamm S. AGA technical review on the evaluation of liver chemistry tests. Gastroenterology 2002;123(4):1367–84.
23. Aithal GP, Watkins PB, Andrade RJ, et al. Case definition and phenotype standardization in drug-induced liver injury. Clin Pharmacol Ther 2011;89(6):806–15.
24. Temple R. Hy's law: predicting serious hepatotoxicity. Pharmacoepidemiol Drug Saf 2006;15(4):241–3.
25. Andrade RJ, Lucena MI, Fernandez MC, et al. Drug-induced liver injury: an analysis of 461 incidences submitted to the Spanish registry over a 10-year period. Gastroenterology 2005;129:512–21.
26. Bell LN, Chalasani N. Epidemiology of idiosyncratic drug-induced liver injury. Semin Liver Dis 2009;29:337–47.
27. Lucena MI, Andrade RJ, Kaplowitz N, et al. Phenotypic characterization of idiosyncratic drug-induced liver injury: the influence of age and gender. Hepatology 2009;49:2001–9.
28. Food and Drug Administration Website. "Guidance for industry. Drug-induced liver injury: premarketing clinical evaluation." Available at: http://www.fda.gov/downloads/Drugs/GuidanceComplianceRegulatoryInformation/Guidances/UCM174090.pdf. Accessed March 20, 2013.
29. Lucena MI, Camargo R, Andrade R, et al. Comparison of two clinical scales for causality assessment in hepatoxicity. Hepatology 2001;33(1):123–30.
30. Rochon J, Protiva P, Seef L, et al. Reliability of the Roussel Uclaf Causality Assessment Method for assessing causality in drug-induced liver injury. Hepatology 2008;48(4):1175–83.
31. Watanabe M, Shibuya A. Validity study of a new diagnostic scale for drug-induced liver injury in Japan-comparison with two previous scales. Hepatol Res 2004;30:148–54.
32. Takikawa H, Takamori Y, Kumagi T, et al. Assessment of 287 Japanese cases of drug induced liver injury by the diagnostic scale of the International Consensus Meeting. Hepatol Res 2003;27:192–5.
33. Pichler WJ, Tilch J. The lymphocyte transformation test in the diagnosis of drug hypersensitivity. Allergy 2004;59(8):809–20.
34. Merk HF. Diagnosis of drug hypersensitivity: lymphocyte transformation test and cytokines. Toxicology 2005;209(2):217–20.
35. Maria V, Victorino R. Development and validation of a clinical scale for the diagnosis of drug-induced hepatitis. Hepatology 1997;26(3):664–9.
36. Nathwani RA, Kaplowitz N. Drug hepatotoxicity. Clin Liver Dis 2006;10:207–17.
37. European Association for the Study of the Liver. EASL clinical practice guidelines: management of cholestatic liver diseases. J Hepatol 2009;51:237–67.
38. Patel T, Yosipovitch G. Therapy of pruritus. Expert Opin Pharmacother 2010;11(10):1673–82.
39. Czaja A. Drug-induced autoimmune-like hepatitis. Dig Dis Sci 2011;56:958–76.
40. Kanter M. Comparison of oral and IV acetylcysteine in the treatment of acetaminophen poisoning. Am J Health Syst Pharm 2006;63(19):1821–7.
41. Mengs U, Pohl R, Mitchell T. Legalon SIL: the antidote of choice in patients with acute hepatotoxicity from amatoxin poisoning. Curr Pharm Biotechnol 2012;13(10):1964–70.

42. Ward J, Kapadia K, Brush E, et al. Amatoxin poisoning: case reports and review of current therapies. J Emerg Med 2013;44(1):116–21.

43. Magdalan J, Piotrowska A, Gomułkiewicz A, et al. Influence of commonly used clinical antidotes on antioxidant systems in human hepatocyte culture intoxicate with alpha-amanitin. Hum Exp Toxicol 2011;30(1):38–43.

44. Organ Procurement and Transplantation Network. Policy 3.6. Available at: http://optn.transplant.hrsa.gov/PoliciesandBylaws2/policies/pdfs/policy_8.pdf. Accessed March 20, 2013.

45. Lee WM, Hynan LS, Rosaro L, et al. Intravenous N-acetylcysteine improves transplant-free survival in early stage non-acetaminophen acute liver failure. Gastroenterology 2009;137(3):856–64.

# Drug-induced Acute Liver Failure

William M. Lee, MD

## KEYWORDS

- Hepatocyte injury • Encephalopathy • Coagulopathy • Liver transplantation

## KEY POINTS

- Acute liver failure, the most severe form of liver injury, is comprised primarily of instances of drug-induced liver injury (DILI).
- Although acetaminophen overdoses dominate, a significant portion of DILI is related to prescription drugs and complementary and alternative medications.
- Acetaminophen and idiosyncratic cases differ dramatically in clinical and biochemical features and in outcomes.
- Therapy for these conditions has been limited to date, although N-acetylcysteine may be of benefit.
- Survival without transplantation is particularly poor for those with idiosyncratic DILI.
- Efforts to improve outcomes should focus on pathogenesis and improving hepatocyte regeneration.

## BACKGROUND

Acute liver failure (ALF), where loss of hepatocyte function occurs over days or weeks without evidence of cirrhosis, has traditionally been defined by altered mentation accompanied by coagulopathy (prolonged international normalized ratio [INR]). Loss of nearly the entire hepatocyte mass is observed in this setting because of a variety of agents including viruses, toxins, and drugs. Recovery depends on whether the injury is ongoing or self-limited and whether or not hepatocytes are capable of regenerating. It is estimated that approximately 2000 people experience ALF annually in the United States and nearly 60% of these are caused by acetaminophen or idiosyncratic drug reactions, drug-induced liver injury (DILI) in its largest sense. Overall, acetaminophen injury far exceeds idiosyncratic DILI by 4:1 among cases reaching the threshold of ALF. Idiosyncratic reactions to prescription drugs or complementary and alternative medications (CAMS) are referred to as DILI, whereas acetaminophen hepatotoxicity is often referred to separately under the acronym APAP. Over the past 16 years, APAP-related toxicity leading to ALF has comprised 46% of subjects enrolled in the Acute

Division of Digestive and Liver Diseases, University of Texas Southwestern Medical Center at Dallas, 5959 Harry Hines Boulevard, Suite 420, Dallas, TX 75390-8887, USA
*E-mail address:* William.Lee@utsouthwestern.edu

Clin Liver Dis 17 (2013) 575–586
http://dx.doi.org/10.1016/j.cld.2013.07.001
1089-3261/13/$ – see front matter © 2013 Elsevier Inc. All rights reserved.

liver.theclinics.com

Liver Failure Study Group (ALFSG), a network that currently includes 16 transplant centers across the United States.[1] By contrast, DILI-related ALF was observed in 11% of these same subjects. Still, DILI is the largest single group after APAP (**Fig. 1**).

This was not the case before the 1990s when hepatitis B was more prevalent and acetaminophen was not as widely used. Early studies did not mention acetaminophen-related injury; nearly 50% were thought related to acute hepatitis B. Even in the mid-1990s only 20% of cases were determined to be caused by APAP overdoses.[2]

DILI caused by either idiosyncratic reactions or acetaminophen-related hepatic necrosis leads to ALF on very different trajectories. A prescription drug, such as isoniazid, leads to a subacute pattern where injury evolves gradually over several weeks, and encephalopathy occurs generally after a minimum of 2 to 4 weeks from onset of illness. By contrast, acetaminophen-related injury is termed hyperacute rather than subacute and its evolution is measured in hours, with peak injury occurring about 72 hours after a single time point ingestion of a toxic amount (**Table 1**). Although patients with ALF may exhibit these features, patients with APAP more commonly exhibit advanced degrees of hepatic coma on admission to transplant centers, sometimes having signs of cerebral edema that results in uncal herniation and compression of the brainstem that is nearly uniformly fatal. Fortunately, only between 10% and 20% of all patients with ALF show evidence of cerebral edema and its incidence may be declining.[3]

## ACETAMINOPHEN-RELATED ALF

Acetaminophen-related ALF was traditionally recognized as caused by suicidal overdoses, although frequent mention was made in the 1980s of therapeutic misadventures or the "alcohol-Tylenol" syndrome.[4,5] Thus, most cases can be divided into intentional and unintentional cases. Intentional cases represent a single time point ingestion for self-harm, whereas unintentional cases are defined as ingestions in excess of package labeling instructions, occurring over several days (or weeks) with pain (usually chronic back or pancreatic pain, but also postsurgical pain and other

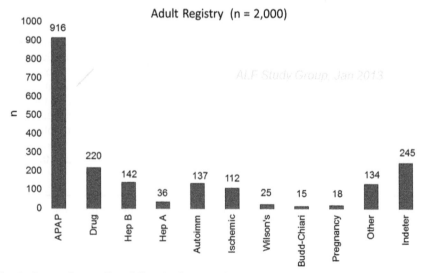

**Fig. 1.** Cause of acute liver failure in the United States.

**Table 1**
**Clinical features of different ALF etiology groups (N = 2000)**

|  | APAP (N = 916) | Drug (N = 220) | Indeterminate (N = 245) | HepA/HepB (N = 36/142) | All Others (N = 441) |
|---|---|---|---|---|---|
| Age (median) | 37 | 46 | 39 | 49/43 | 45 |
| Gender (% female) | 76 | 69 | 59 | 44/44 | 71 |
| Jaundice (days) | 1 | 11.5 | 11 | 4/8 | 7 |
| Coma ≥3 (%) | 53 | 35 | 48 | 56/52 | 38 |
| Alanine aminotransferase | 3773 | 639.5 | 865 | 2275/1649 | 681 |
| Bilirubin (median) | 4.3 | 19.8 | 21.1 | 12.3/18.4 | 13.9 |
| Tx (%) | 9 | 40 | 42 | 33/39 | 32 |
| Spontaneous survival (%) | 63 | 24 | 22 | 50/21 | 31 |
| Overall survival (%) | 70 | 58 | 60 | 72/55 | 58 |

miscellaneous causes).[6] The overall burden of intentional cases greatly exceeds accidental ones in terms of emergency room visits where all patients once recognized should immediately receive the antidote, N-acetylcysteine (NAC; obtained in intravenous form as Acetadote). Among those reaching the threshold of ALF, there are nearly equal numbers of intentional and unintentional cases. Because APAP-related ALF has become commonplace, instances of APAP-related injury should be readily recognized. However, many are already comatose on arrival to the tertiary care facility and the ingestion history may be lacking. Similarly, the use of acetaminophen levels in patients already demonstrating massive hepatocyte injury may create false impressions that the cause is not acetaminophen. Thus, a high index of suspicion is needed to recognize all cases. Recently, it has become apparent that the biochemical profile itself can be a strong indication for acetaminophen hepatotoxicity: the finding of remarkably high aminotransferases (>3500 IU/L) in concert with low bilirubin levels (<5) is the nearly unique signature of APAP injury.[7] Typical aminotransferase levels exceed 10,000 IU/L. Ischemic hepatopathy and rare instances of hepatitis B or herpes simplex hepatitis are the only alternate diagnoses that should be entertained. A point-of-care assay to detect acetaminophen adducts, the by-product of cell injury rather than the parent compound, currently is being developed. Acetaminophen hepatic injury is covered in more detail elsewhere in this issue.

## IDIOSYNCRATIC DRUG-RELATED LIVER INJURY

Most reactions to prescription drugs or CAMs are considered idiosyncratic; they are unpredictable, vary greatly in severity, and occur at varying time intervals after ingestion (anywhere from a few days to 1 year).[8] Their toxicity is usually unrelated to dose, route, or duration of drug administration (although a review of drugs withdrawn from the market in the United States recently found that most were prescribed at daily doses >50 mg per day).[9] Instead, the Greek root of idiosyncrasy emphasizes that it is the unique characteristics of the individual that predispose them to develop a toxic reaction, whereas many others can use the drug safely.[10] It is assumed that the adverse reactions to these xenobiotic compounds have a strong genetic basis.[11] DILI, as a result, has become an important catalyst for pharmacogenomics research.[12] Only a fraction of DILI reactions lead to ALF. Among the first 300 patients enrolled in the National Institutes of Health–supported Drug-Induced Liver Injury Network (DILIN),

33% were hospitalized, 15% were considered severe, and 6% died or underwent transplantation.[13] Thus, only a small fraction of the overall group experienced ALF, although there were 9% fatalities or transplants in the subgroup where hepatocellular injury was present. Thus, the spectrum of types and severity of liver injury caused by DILI overall is broad and expectation for recovery from the average instance of DILI is the rule.

The phenotype associated with ALF is characterized by hepatocellular injury that typically evolves more slowly than acetaminophen and is remarkably rare, with some agents in the range of 1:30,000 to 100,000 prescriptions. A wide variety of medications have been implicated, although not every one can cause these severe forms of liver damage. Antibiotics, anticonvulsants, and nonsteroidal anti-inflammatory agents are among the most commonly implicated medications, with isoniazid continuing its prominent place among those frequently implicated. The ALFSG review of 133 patients enrolled in the registry with ALF determined that antimicrobials were the most common cause for ALF accounting for 46% of cases.[14] **Box 1** lists a current update of commonly seen drugs modified from Reuben and colleagues.[14] Over time the list of agents implicated evolves, because usage changes as new agents come along. For example, phenytoin is used much less currently than it was in an earlier era. Thus, a decline in phenytoin ALF should be seen. Telithromycin (Ketek) was a new antibiotic that gained in popularity as a replacement for macrolide antibiotics because its spectrum of activity included pneumococci resistant to penicillins and even macrolides; however, the identification of several instances of ALF in the 3 years after its approval has led to revised approval with much more limited indications and a black box warning from the Food and Drug Administration.[15,16] It is hoped that isoniazid will lose its primacy as the keystone agent against tuberculosis, but to date that has not happened.

In the paper cited previously that reviewed the experience of 133 ALF DILI cases, spontaneous recovery was limited, although the slower evolution of disease often allowed for transplantation to take place. Transplant-free survival (TFS) was 27%, whereas 42% received a graft, yielding an overall short-term survival of 66%. A recent update of these figures from ALFSG for 220 DILI cases indicated that TFS is even worse, at 23%, with 40% transplanted giving an overall survival of only 58% (William M. Lee, MD, unpublished data, 2013). By comparison, acetaminophen short-term results for 916 individuals admitted with ALF included 63% TFS, 9% transplanted, giving a 70% overall short-term survival. Fewer APAP cases are candidates for liver grafting because of ongoing substance abuse or lack of insurance funding, but they less frequently seem to require rescue. It is postulated that the self-limited duration of injury, despite its severity, allows rapid regeneration and resolution of the hepatic damage. Pathogenesis of the two forms of DILI (APAP and idiosyncratic DILI) remains a black box.[17]

Clinical recognition of DILI ALF is little different from that of APAP except for the slower speed of disease evolution. Any patient in the emergency room showing signs of jaundice and coagulopathy with or without altered mentation should undergo further screening to determine if ALF is present. All patients should receive careful questioning regarding recent medications, CAMs, and any use of acetaminophen-containing compounds and an extensive serologic work-up focusing on determining the cause of the condition. Those with subacute injury of whatever cause may not exhibit significant encephalopathy early on, but linger with modest aminotransferase elevations but elevated INR and bilirubin levels that predict a poor outcome once they persist for more than 10 to 14 days. These patients are more likely to develop ascites, infection, and renal insufficiency. Cause of death in the absence of transplantation is primarily systemic infection or cerebral edema.

| Box 1 |
|---|
| **Drugs implicated in causing acute liver failure** |
| *Antimicrobials* |
| Isoniazid, with or without rifampicin |
| Trimethoprim/sulfamethoxazole |
| Nitrofurantoin |
| Terbinafine |
| Itraconazole |
| Ketoconazole |
| Amoxicillin |
| Ciprofloxacin |
| Azithromycin |
| Telithromycin |
| *Anticonvulsants* |
| Phenytoin |
| Valproic acid |
| Carbamazepine |
| *Complementary and alternative medications* |
| Lipokinetix (usnic acid) |
| Herbalife (unspecified) |
| Ma-huang and other Chinese herbs |
| Hydroxycut (unspecified) |
| *Others* |
| Diclofenac |
| Etodolac |
| Disulfiram |
| Propylthiouracil |
| Methyldopa |
| *Chemotherapeutic agents* |
| Gemtuzumab |
| *Adapted from* Reuben A, Koch DG, Lee WM. Drug-induced acute liver failure: results of a U.S. multicenter, prospective study. Hepatology 2010;52:2068. |

## OVERALL MANAGEMENT

Intensive care management is used for virtually all patients with any degree of enceph-alopathy and can be considered for those with profound coagulopathy where evolu-tion to altered mentation is likely. Extensive guidelines have been established for management, although much is based on expert opinion rather than evidence-based medicine, because large controlled trials are seldom possible, given the orphan status of this syndrome.[18,19] In general, patients are placed with head elevated and receive frequent checks for neurologic function. Most are dehydrated on arrival and require volume resuscitation. Initial serologic testing is used to exclude other causes, even if a putative drug cause has been elicited. In a recent study from the DILIN, 9 out of 318 cases tested for hepatitis E were recategorized as having likely hepatitis E based on the presence of IgM anti–hepatitis E antibody, and in four patients also hepatitis E virus RNA.[20] Only one of these cases manifested signs of ALF. Thus, casting a wide initial testing net for causes and, in particular, repeat questioning of the patient or their family concerning use of antibiotics even remotely or herbal or dietary supplements is remarkably helpful.

There is no certain antidote for ALF at this time. Specific measures are available for acetaminophen (NAC). Although NAC use after onset of encephalopathy theoretically may help prevent worsening, it is being given too late to prevent the unfolding injury. With regard to idiosyncratic DILI, many patients continue to consume the suspect agent after onset of symptoms and this, in general, is harmful, although no study to date has shown with certainty that early withdrawal improves outcomes. In some instances, a drug taken only for 2 to 3 days may lead to a fatal outcome.

### Treatment with NAC

NAC is the recognized antidote for acetaminophen poisoning and long has been claimed to be effective in nonacetaminophen settings, without much supportive evidence. NAC was subjected to a randomized placebo-controlled trial for nonacetaminophen ALF that included DILI as one subgroup. The trial included 173 randomized patients, the largest ever performed in ALF. The group consisted of four causes: (1) DILI; (2) autoimmune hepatitis; (3) hepatitis B; and (4) indeterminate, those where a cause could not be discerned. The primary outcome (improvement in overall survival) was not achieved but significant improvement was observed within early coma grade patients (I to II): spontaneous survival (SS) 52% with NAC versus 30% with placebo.[21] All ALF trials in the modern era are compromised by transplantation that rescues approximately 40% of those with non-APAP ALF so that their true outcome will never be known and overall survival is improved because of the use of liver grafting, as it should be. Because short-term survival after transplantation is more than 90% and mainly hinges on technical issues, such as graft quality, the impact of an intravenous medication is unlikely to affect overall outcome particularly in those with advanced hepatic failure, where death or transplant as outcomes occur quickly. We observed that 50% of coma III to IV patients achieved an outcome (death or transplant) by Day 4, whereas those with lesser coma grades only reached this threshold at Day 10 after admission to study. Thus, in retrospect, TFS is probably a better outcome measure than overall survival. It seems unlikely that patients with advanced coma grades would benefit so rapidly from NAC that they would not progress to an outcome as described. There were no safety issues and, using a Cox proportional hazards model, outcomes were better for the NAC Coma I to II group than all other categories (**Fig. 2**). The percent transplanted was significantly lower in the NAC group when follow-up extended out to 1 year. There was a trend toward shorter intensive care unit and hospital stays in favor of the NAC group, but this was not significant. The greatest improvement in TFS was seen in those treated with NAC (**Table 2**). For those with etiology as DILI TFS was 58% for NAC versus 27% for placebo, and for hepatitis B 40% for NAC versus 17% for placebo.

Two subsequent studies have focused on why NAC might have made a difference. Stravitz and colleagues measured levels at two time points of 10 cytokines, using a multiplex enzyme-linked immunosorbent assay on sera from 78 patients who participated in the NAC trial (William M. Lee, MD, unpublished data, 2013).

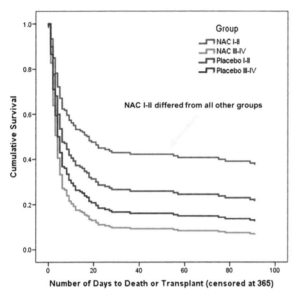

**Fig. 2.** Cox proportional hazards model by treatment and coma grade.

Treatment with NAC and low interleukin (IL)-17 levels were associated with improved outcomes in multivariate analysis. Among those with elevated IL-17 levels, 78% of the NAC-treated patients and 44% of the control subjects had undetectable IL-17 levels on Day 3 after admission to study. Thus, NAC may act by lowering IL-17 levels, thus averting ongoing liver damage at this crucial disease stage. In a second study, reviewing standard biochemistries from the NAC trial, Singh and colleagues[22] showed that patients with early coma grade who were treated with NAC showed significant improvement in bilirubin and alanine aminotransferase levels compared with the other three groups (maximum $P<.02$ for NAC 1–2 vs the three other treatments) when predicting death or transplantation. These two studies support the use of NAC in early stage hepatic coma caused by drug-related liver injury. To date, the Food and Drug Administration has not approved NAC for the indication of nonacetaminophen ALF.

| Table 2 NAC results by etiology | | | | |
|---|---|---|---|---|
| | Overall Survival | | Transplant-Free Survival | |
| | PLB | NAC | PLB | NAC |
| DILI | 17/26 | 15/19 | 7/26 | 11/19 |
| N = 45 | 65% | 79% | 27% | 58% |
| AIH | 10/15 | 7/11 | 4/15 | 1/11 |
| N = 26 | 67% | 64% | 27% | 9% |
| HBV | 6/12 | 19/25 | 2/12 | 10/25 |
| N = 37 | 50% | 76% | 17% | 40% |
| Indeterminate | 18/26 | 9/15 | 6/26 | 6/15 |
| N = 41 | 69% | 60% | 23% | 40% |

*Abbreviations:* AIH, autoimmune hepatitis; HBV, hepatitis B virus; PLB, placebo.

## Corticosteroid Use

Corticosteroid therapy has been proposed as treatment of DILI in the ALF setting but little evidence advanced to support it, and unlike alcoholic hepatitis, no controlled trials have been performed.[23] A recent analysis of the ALFSG database sought to provide circumstantial evidence for or against steroid use by reviewing outcomes for those who did and did not receive corticosteroid therapy for their ALF, regardless of cause (William M. Lee, MD, unpublished data, 2013). Of 131 patients with DILI ALF, 26 had received corticosteroids and 105 had not as shown in records examined. Survival was 50% for those receiving and 62% for those not receiving steroid therapy. This was uncontrolled and a bias toward treatment of desperately sick individuals may have been at play here.

### Hepatic Encephalopathy

Understanding the encephalopathy that occurs in ALF has been limited by the relative rarity of the condition. The role of ammonia as a causative agent has been debated. High ammonia levels correlate in a general way with the degree of encephalopathy but not that well, but do correlate more closely to the presence of cerebral edema. Acute kidney injury occurs in 70% of patients with acetaminophen-induced hepatic necrosis and encephalopathy. Recent data from ALFSG has established that high ammonia levels are virtually never seen in the absence of acute kidney injury. Hyperacute liver injury is closely associated with cerebral edema and this has been presumed to be related to the acuity of the injury; however, the most common cause of hyperacute ALF is acetaminophen and the presence of renal injury clearly plays a part in causing the high ammonia levels.

Use of lactulose and antibiotics in patients with ALF has been problematic, because colonic distention caused by lactulose is counterproductive in a surgical setting.[18] No proof of efficacy has been shown for either form of management classically used in encephalopathy caused by cirrhosis.

ALFSG is currently testing ornithine phenylacetate as an ammonia-trapping agent in an initial pilot study to evaluate safety and tolerability. Ammonia-lowering agents could represent a significant improvement in encephalopathy management and would demonstrate once and for all whether ammonia directly contributes to this condition.[24,25]

## TRANSPLANTATION AND PROGNOSIS

Transplantation provides a reliable rescue for patients when no signs of recovery are forthcoming. Only a small fraction of patients receive a liver graft: 24% of all patients with ALF, 9% of acetaminophen ALF, and 40% of patients with DILI ALF. For each patient, a careful assessment of need and appropriateness precedes listing so a prognostic score has long been considered a vital but elusive goal. Even when a patient is listed, organ availability determines ultimate outcome and patient candidacy can change from good to poor over hours. A review of transplantation data from the United Network for Organ Sharing registry disclosed that among patients undergoing liver transplantation between 1990 and 2002, a total of 2291 were considered to have acute hepatic necrosis, which is close to but may not be identical with ALF as described previously.[26] Of these, 357 (15%) were thought caused by DILI but including APAP. Thus, roughly half received a graft for APAP, the other half for idiosyncratic DILI. This suggests that despite the high morbidity of DILI once the threshold of ALF is reached, the number of patients actually undergoing transplantation for DILI remains small. It is important to point out that the United Network for Organ Sharing database only registers those listed for transplantation and receiving a graft, so this is a skewed group compared with the larger overall universe of patients with DILI that is more uniformly captured by ALFSG or DILIN. Once again, ALFSG only identifies those DILI cases meeting criteria of hepatic encephalopathy and prolonged INR, only 11% of all ALFSG enrolled patients and 9% of the all DILI patients (according to DILIN data).[13,14] Among ALFSG patients as noted, the slower evolution of disease and higher fatality rate or failure to improve has yielded a higher percentage of transplants undertaken in this group compared with those with acetaminophen-related hepatic failure. The higher number of acetaminophen cases results in similar total numbers of patients being transplanted for APAP and DILI.

When outcomes for the ALFSG group of 133 patients with DILI reviewed previously were examined, the Model for End Stage Liver Disease (MELD) score and coma grade on admission were the strongest predictors of liver transplantation.[14] Because most of these patients would have received a listing as Status 1, the highest priority, it is not clear whether MELD is relevant here. To date, robust prognostic scoring systems have not proved useful in ALF. Although Kings College Hospital (KCH) criteria have been used by some centers, it is evident that those reaching the threshold of Kings criteria are highly likely to require transplantation; those not reaching criteria still have a 50% mortality, indicating the limits of such a scoring system.[26,27] Other more global scores that reflect intensive care unit survival have not proved to be of any additional value. Cholongitas and colleagues[28] studied 125 consecutive patients with APAP, comparing Sequential Organ Failure Assessment (SOFA), MELD, Acute Physiologic and Chronic Health Assessment II (APACHE II), and KCH. They concluded that SOFA performed best of the four with an area under the receiver operator curve (AUC) of 0.79, whereas the AUCs for MELD, APACHE II, and KCH were 0.58, 0.72, and 0.65, respectively. This study applied only to APAP cases, suggesting that it may be necessary to develop a prognostic score for each ALF etiology. Taylor and colleagues[29] have developed a prognostic score with great accuracy for hepatitis A. More recently, an index was developed that outperformed MELD and KCH across the spectrum of ALF conditions.[30] In this system, M-30 antigen, a marker of apoptosis, was used in concert with coma grade, INR, bilirubin, and phosphorus and gave an AUC of 0.822 compared with MELD at 0.704 and KCH at 0.654. A direct comparison with SOFA was not made. The limitation of this index is that it requires a special test with limited availability to complete the index. M-30 did contribute to improving to the final score. Similarly, a study from Germany[31] substituted M-65 antigen levels for bilirubin in the MELD score to determine survival or need for transplantation or death in a wide spectrum of ALF where APAP constitute 13% and DILI 18%. In this study, the AUC for the modified MELD, referred to as M-MELD, was 0.87 on admission and better if maximum M-65 values were used; however, as a retrospective study one only knows what the maximum value obtained is after the study is completed. Similarly, the real value of a prognostic score must be on admission, when the decision to list is paramount. Outcomes later will become clarified and all prognostic scores will tend to improve. Further studies are under way to nail down a robust score that is applicable (or modified) for all etiologic groups and could be simplified to be developed as an "app," rendering it more user-friendly than current scores.

## GENOMICS AND THE FUTURE

Studies have tried to determine whether there is a specific host genomics signature that identifies increased susceptibility to catastrophic liver injury, because the ALF group of patients with DILI represents the tip of a much larger iceberg. For every isoniazid ALF patient, there are probably nine additional patients with alanine amino-transferase elevations not requiring and this was the original message in Hy law.[32] This is across a variety of drug groups and types. The question becomes: What makes one or another patient have a poor outcome with seemingly similar clinical features in other respects? Specific HLA haplotypes have been associated with certain drugs in genome-wide association studies.[11,12] However, a recent study analyzed whether there were keratin 8 and 18 host mutations that are considered to be cytoprotective that would possibly be underrepresented among a cohort of 344 patients with ALF. Indeed, keratin 8 variants in particular were overrepresented in white patients with ALF across etiologies.[33] This provides support for the concept that host increased susceptibility underlies conversion to ALF, although it is likely that this susceptibility is multifactorial. A further study has also suggested a specific acetaminophen UDP-glucuronosyltransferase enzyme polymorphism can explain the variable susceptibility of individuals to acetaminophen toxicity.[34]

Overall, it seems that genomic studies in the future will help identify those at greatest risk of unfavorable outcomes. Whether these assays turn out to be specific to drugs or are more global remains to be seen.

## SUMMARY

Although ALF caused by DILI comprises a small fraction of overall DILI, these patients require high resource use and have relatively poor outcomes. DILI caused by idiosyn-crasy more often leads to death or transplantation than does acetaminophen ALF, but the number of patients in each category receiving a graft is roughly the same. Efforts to improve outcomes should focus on more effective treatments and better methods to identify those that might experience poor outcomes.

## REFERENCES

1. Ostapowicz GA, Fontana RJ, Schiodt FV, et al. Results of a prospective study of acute liver failure at 17 tertiary care centers in the United States. Ann Intern Med 2002;137:945–54.
2. Schiødt FV, Atillasoy E, Shakil O, et al. Etiology and outcome for 295 patients with acute liver failure in the United States. Liver Transpl Surg 1999;5:29–34.
3. Bernal W, Auzinger G, Dhawan A, et al. Acute liver failure. Lancet 2010;376: 190–201.
4. Zimmerman HJ, Maddrey WC. Acetaminophen (paracetamol) hepatotoxicity with regular intake of alcohol: analysis of instances of therapeutic misadventure. Hepatology 1995;22:767–73.
5. Wootton FT, Lee WM. Acetaminophen hepatotoxicity in the alcoholic. South Med J 1990;83:1047–9.
6. Schiødt FV, Rochling FJ, Casey DL, et al. Acetaminophen toxicity in an urban county hospital. N Engl J Med 1997;337:1112–7.
7. Khandelwal N, James LP, Sanders C, et al, Acute Liver Failure Study Group. Un-recognized acetaminophen toxicity as a cause of indeterminate acute liver fail-ure. Hepatology 2011;53:567–76.
8. Kaplowitz N. Idiosyncratic drug hepatotoxicity. Nat Rev Drug Discov 2005;4: 489–99.
9. Tujios S, Fontana RJ. Mechanisms of drug-induced liver injury: from bedside to bench. Nat Rev Gastroenterol Hepatol 2011;8:202–11.
10. Lee WM, Senior JR. Recognizing drug-induced liver injury: current problems, possible solutions. Toxicol Pathol 2005;33:155–64.

11. Daly AK, Donaldson PT, Bhatnagar P, et al. HLA-B*5701 genotype is a major determinant of drug-induced liver injury due to flucloxacillin. Nat Genet 2009; 41:816–9.

12. Urban TJ. Whole-genome sequencing in pharmacogenetics. Pharmacogenomics 2013;14:345–8.

13. Chalasani N, Fontana RJ, Bonkovsky HL, et al. Causes, clinical features, and outcomes from a prospective study of drug induced liver injury in the United States. Gastroenterology 2008;135:1924–34.

14. Reuben A, Koch DG, Lee WM. Drug-induced acute liver failure: results of a U.S. multicenter, prospective study. Hepatology 2010;52:2065–76.

15. Brinker AD, Wassel RT, Lyndly J, et al. Telithromycin-associated hepatotoxicity: clinical spectrum and causality assessment of 42 cases. Hepatology 2009;49: 250–7.

16. Soreth J, Cox E, Kweder J, et al. Ketek: the FDA perspective. N Engl J Med 2007; 356:1675–6.

17. Jones DP, Lemasters JJ, Han D, et al. Mechanisms of pathogenesis in drug hepatotoxicity putting the stress on mitochondria. Mol Interv 2010;10:98–111.

18. Stravitz RT, Kramer AH, Davern T, et al, Acute Liver Failure Study Group. Intensive care of patients with acute liver failure: recommendations of the Acute Liver Failure Study Group. Crit Care Med 2007;35:2498–508.

19. Lee WM, Stravitz RT, Larson AM. Introduction to the revised American Association for the Study of Liver Diseases Position Paper on acute liver failure 2011. Hepatology 2012;55:965–7.

20. Davern TJ, Chalasani N, Fontana R, et al. Acute hepatitis E infection accounts for some cases of suspected drug-induced liver injury. Gastroenterology 2011;141: 1665–72.

21. Lee WM, Hynan LS, Rossaro L, et al. Intravenous N-acetylcysteine improves transplant-free survival in early stage non-acetaminophen acute liver failure. Gastroenterology 2009;137:856–64.

22. Singh S, Hynan LS, Lee WM, Acute Liver Failure Study Group. Improvements in hepatic serological biomarkers are associated with clinical benefit of intravenous N-acetylcysteine in early stage non-acetaminophen acute liver failure. Dig Dis Sci 2013;58(5):1397–402.

23. Ichai P, Duclos-Vallée J, Guettier C, et al. Usefulness of corticosteroids for the treatment of severe and fulminant forms of autoimmune hepatitis. Liver Transpl 2007;13:996–1003.

24. Jalan R, Wright G, Davies NA, et al. L-Ornithine phenylacetate (OP): a novel treatment for hyperammonemia and hepatic encephalopathy. Med Hypotheses 2007; 69:1064–9.

25. Lee WM, Jalan RV. Treatment of hyperammonemia in liver failure: a tale of two enzymes. Gastroenterology 2009;136:2048–51.

26. Larson AM, Fontana RJ, Davern TJ, et al, Acute Liver Failure Study Group. Acetaminophen-induced acute liver failure: results of a United States multicenter, prospective study. Hepatology 2005;42:1367–72.

27. Russo M, Galanko JA, Shrestha R, et al. Liver transplantation for acute liver failure from drug induced liver injury in the United States. Liver Transpl 2004;10: 1018–23.

28. Cholongitas E, Theocharidou E, Vasianopoulou P, et al. Comparison of the sequential organ failure assessment score with the king's college hospital criteria and the model for end-stage liver disease score for the prognosis of acetaminophen-induced acute liver failure. Liver Transpl 2012;18:405–12.

29. Taylor RM, Davern TJ, Munoz S, et al, Acute Liver Failure Study Group. Fulminant hepatitis A virus infection in the United States: incidence, prognosis, and outcomes. Hepatology 2006;44:1589–97.

30. Rutherford A, King LY, Hynan LS, et al, Acute Liver Failure Study Group. Development of an accurate index for predicting outcomes of patients with acute liver failure. Gastroenterology 2012;143:1237–43.

31. Bechmann LP, Jochum C, Kocabayoglu P, et al. Cytokeratin 18-based modification of the MELD score improves prediction of spontaneous survival after acute liver injury. J Hepatol 2010;53:639–47.

32. Temple R. Hy's law: predicting serious hepatotoxicity. Pharmacoepidemiol Drug Saf 2006;15:241–3.

33. Strnad P, Zhou Q, Hanada S, et al, Acute Liver Failure Study Group. Ethnic-specific keratin variants predispose to an adverse outcome in acute liver failure. Gastroenterology 2010;139:828–35.

34. Court MH, Freytsis M, Wang X, et al. The UDP-Glucuronosyltransferase (UGT) 1A polymorphism c.2042C>G (rs8330) is associated with increased human liver acetaminophen glucuronidation, increased UGT1A Exon 5a/5b splice variant mRNA ratio, and decreased risk of unintentional acetaminophen-induced acute liver failure. J Pharmacol Exp Ther 2013;345:297–307.

# Acetaminophen-related Hepatotoxicity

Chalermrat Bunchorntavakul, MD[a,b], K. Rajender Reddy, MD[a,*]

## KEYWORDS

- Acetaminophen • Hepatotoxicity • Overdose • Drug-induced liver injury
- Acute liver failure • N-acetylcysteine • Liver transplantation

## KEY POINTS

- Acetaminophen (APAP), a widely available antipyretic and analgesic, is the leading world-wide cause of drug overdose and acute liver failure (ALF).
- Single overdose ingestion and therapeutic misadventure may cause hepatotoxicity.
- Several factors, such as concomitant alcohol use or abuse, concurrent medications, genetic factors, and nutritional status, can influence the susceptibility and severity of APAP hepatotoxicity.
- Early manifestations of APAP hepatotoxicity are nonspecific, but require prompt recognition by physicians.
- Patients with repeated overdose tend to present late, and in such hepatotoxicity may have already evolved.
- The prognosis of patients with APAP-induced ALF is better than other causes of ALF; therefore, liver transplantation should be offered to those who are unlikely to survive and such assessment and decision to proceed with liver transplantation may be made based on the King's College criteria.

## INTRODUCTION

Acetaminophen (APAP or paracetamol or N-acetyl-p-aminophenol), a safe and effective antipyretic and analgesic, has been extensively used around the world since 1955. It is available as various formulations, as a single-ingredient medication (eg, immediate-release and extended-release tablets/capsules, suspensions, rectal suppositories, and for intravenous [IV] use) and also as a component of numerous

Conflict of Interest: The authors have nothing to disclose.
[a] Division of Gastroenterology and Hepatology, Department of Medicine, Hospital of the University of Pennsylvania, University of Pennsylvania, 2 Dulles, 3400 Spruce Street, Philadelphia, PA 19104, USA; [b] Division of Gastroenterology and Hepatology, Department of Medicine, Rajavithi Hospital, College of Medicine, Rangsit University, Rajavithi Road, Ratchathewi, Bangkok 10400, Thailand
* Corresponding author.
E-mail address: rajender.reddy@uphs.upenn.edu

Clin Liver Dis 17 (2013) 587–607
http://dx.doi.org/10.1016/j.cld.2013.07.005
1089-3261/13/$ – see front matter © 2013 Elsevier Inc. All rights reserved.

combination over-the-counter and prescription products used for pain and as an anti-pyretic. In the United States, more than 28 billion doses of APAP were distributed in 2003, and hydrocodone-APAP was the most commonly dispensed medication among 89 million out-patient prescriptions in 2005.[1,2]

Although APAP is generally considered to be safe at the usual therapeutic doses as recommended by the manufacturer (1–4 g/day), concerns have emerged over the past decade as APAP has been increasingly recognized as a major cause of acute liver failure (ALF) in adults in the United States and many other countries worldwide.[3–7] Single overdose ingestion usually follows attempted self-poisoning and exceeding 15 to 25 g may cause severe liver injury that is fatal in up to a quarter of the cases.[3,8,9] However, 30% to 50% of cases of APAP hepatotoxicity admitted to hospital nowadays result from a "therapeutic misadventure" wherein the daily dose may not have greatly exceeded the recommended safe limits but where specific risk factors are present.[3,8,9]

## EPIDEMIOLOGY

APAP has been a major cause of overdose and overdose-related ALF (~50% of cases) and death in the United States and in many other countries.[3–6] In the United States, APAP overdose is the leading reason for calls to the Poison Control Centers (>100,000 per year) and accounts annually for more than 56,000 emergency room visits, 2600 hospitalizations, and an approximate 450 deaths caused by ALF.[3] In the US ALF Multicenter Prospective Study, APAP accounted for 42% (275 of 662) of ALF cases; the annual percentage of APAP-related ALF rose during the study from 28% in 1998 to 51% in 2003.[8] Unintentional overdoses accounted for 48%; intentional (suicide attempts) 44%; and 8% were of unknown intent.[8] Most unintentional patients reported taking APAP for acute or chronic pain syndromes; 38% took two or more APAP preparations simultaneously, and 63% used narcotic-containing compounds.[8]

## PHARMACOLOGY AND HEPATOTOXICITY

The therapeutic dose of APAP is 325 to 1000 mg/dose (10–15 mg/kg/dose in children), given every 4 to 6 hours, with a maximum recommended daily dose of 4 g (80 mg/kg in children). Although the US Food and Drug Administration (FDA) Advisory Committee proposed a decrease in the maximum daily dose from 4000 to 3250 mg, this recommendation has not been implemented.[10] After oral ingestion, APAP is rapidly absorbed from the gastrointestinal tract with peak concentrations being achieved within 90 minutes.[1,11] Therapeutic serum concentrations range from 10 to 20 μg/mL. The presence of food in the stomach may delay the time to peak concentration, but not the extent of absorption.[1,11] With overdose ingestion, peak serum concentrations generally are achieved within 4 hours, but may be delayed beyond 4 hours after overdose of extended-release preparations or when drugs that delay gastric emptying time (eg, anticholinergics, opiates) are coingested.[12,13] Protein binding is minimal at therapeutic doses with a volume of distribution of approximately 0.9 L/kg.[11] The serum half-life of APAP is 2 to 2.5 hours; however, it is prolonged to more than 4 hours in patients with hepatic injury and chronic liver disease, and in those who ingested extended-release preparations.[1,11,14]

At therapeutic doses, approximately 85% to 90% of APAP undergoes phase II conjugation to sulfated and glucoronidated metabolites (about two-thirds through glucuronidation and one-third through sulfation in adults, whereas sulfation is predominant in children up to 12 years), which are then excreted in the urine.[1,11,15] About 2% of APAP is excreted in the urine unchanged. The remaining APAP (up to 10%) undergoes phase I oxidation by the hepatic cytochrome P-450 (CYP) pathway (primarily responsible by CYP2E1) to a toxic, highly reactive intermediate, N-acetyl-para-benzo-quinoneimine (NAPQI).[1,11,15] Small amount of NAPQI produced from normal doses of APAP is rapidly conjugated by hepatic glutathione (GSH), forming nontoxic mercaptate and cysteine compounds that are then excreted in the urine.[11,15,16] Small proportions of APAP are also oxidized by myeloperoxidase and cyclooxygenase-1, but the clinical significance of this pathway is unclear (**Fig. 1**).[15,16]

APAP is known to be a dose-related hepatotoxic agent. At toxic doses of APAP, sulfation and glucoronidation pathways become saturated and more APAP is metabolized through CYP2E1 to NAPQI.[1,15] An increased production of NAPQI eventually results in depletion of GSH, and when GSH stores are depleted by about 70% to 80%, NAPQI binds to hepatocytes causing cellular injury.[1,15,17] In the absence of GSH, NAPQI covalently binds to cysteine groups on hepatocyte molecules forming NAPQI-protein adducts (so-called APAP-protein adducts). This process is an irreversible step that leads to oxidative injury and hepatocellular necrosis.[1,15] Although unclear, mitochondrial damage, nuclear DNA fragmentation, and lipid peroxidation are likely to play an important role in APAP-induced hepatocellular damage.[15,18,19] GSH depletion further contributes to oxidative stress, activation of stress proteins and gene transcription mediators, and alterations in the liver's innate immune system.[1] There is a growing body of evidence suggesting a critical role of innate immunity and sterile inflammation in the progression and repair of APAP hepatotoxicity.[20,21] The early cell necrosis causes the release of various mediators, such as high-mobility group box 1 protein, DNA fragments, and heat shock proteins, and which enhance proinflammatory cytokine and chemokine formation from macrophages.[20] Although proinflammatory mediators recruit inflammatory cells (eg, neutrophils, monocytes, and natural killer cells) into the liver, neither the infiltrating cells nor the activated resident macrophages cause significant direct cytotoxicity. However, these proinflammatory mediators directly promote intracellular injury mechanisms by inducing nitric oxide synthase or inhibit cell death mechanisms by the expression of acute-phase proteins, which then promote hepatocyte proliferation.[20,21] Furthermore, the newly recruited macrophages, and possibly neutrophils, are involved in tissue repair through the removal of necrotic cell debris leading to resolution of the inflammation.[20]

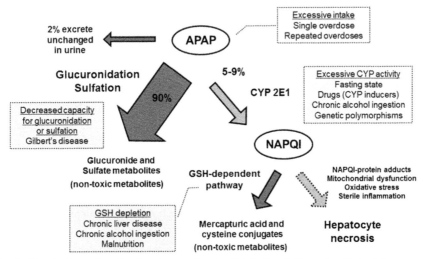

**Fig. 1.** Metabolism of acetaminophen and potential factors influencing its toxicity.

Zone 3 hepatocytes, which are most abundant in CYP2E1, are most vulnerable to injury, and this leads to the characteristic centrilobular pattern of hepatocellular necrosis observed in APAP hepatotoxicity.[1] Passive congestion and scattered infiltration of lymphocytes and neutrophils may also be observed.[15]

## FACTORS INFLUENCING APAP-RELATED HEPATOTOXICITY

The ingested dose of APAP seems to be the most important factor determining the development and severity of APAP hepatotoxicity. In addition, the pattern of use and various factors (eg, age, concurrent use of alcohol and certain medications, genetic factors, pre-existing liver disease, and nutritional status) can also influence the susceptibility to APAP hepatotoxicity through several mechanisms including decreased capacity for glucuronidation or sulfation, excessive CYP activity, and depletion of GSH stores (see **Table 1**).

### Dose and Pattern of Use

Although the FDA-labeled doses are clear, some users may ignore the directions and consume APAP amounts exceeding recommended doses, either by intention or by accident (therapeutic misadventure). A single acute ingestion of greater than or equal to 7.5 to 10 g in adults or 150 to 200 mg/kg in children older than 6 years (all APAP consumed within 8 hours) is likely to cause hepatotoxicity and requires prompt evaluation and therapeutic intervention.[1] Repeated overdoses of greater than or equal to 10 g in a 24-hour period or greater than or equal to 6 g per 24-hour period for greater than or equal to 48 hours may be associated with subsequent hepatotoxicity and the patient should undergo evaluation in a health care facility.[22] A lower threshold (4–10 g) for evaluation may be considered in a high-risk population (discussed later). Although most studies have reported safety of short-term and long-term use of APAP at the maximum recommended dose of 4 g,[23,24] a well-designed, randomized

| Table 1 | |
|---|---|
| **Factors influencing acetaminophen hepatotoxicity** | |
| **Factors** | **Potential Clinical Consequences** |
| Chronic alcohol ingestion | ↑ APAP hepatotoxicity, particularly with repeated overdoses |
| Medications and herbs that induce CYP2E1 (eg, INH, rifampicin, phenobarbital, and St. John's wort) | Possibly ↑ APAP hepatotoxicity |
| Medications that compete with hepatic glucorunidation (eg, zidovudine and trimethoprim-sulfamethoxazole) | Possibly ↑ APAP hepatotoxicity |
| Gilbert syndrome | Possibly ↑ APAP hepatotoxicity |
| Malnutrition | ↑ APAP hepatotoxicity, in alcoholics |
| Fasting state | ↑ APAP hepatotoxicity, in alcoholics |
| Chronic liver disease | ↑ APAP hepatotoxicity, particularly in alcoholics |
| Advanced age | Possibly ↑ APAP hepatotoxicity |
| Pregnancy | Potential for APAP hepatotoxicity in the fetus |

Abbreviations: APAP, acetaminophen; CYP, cytochrome P-450; INH, isoniazid.

placebo-controlled study of 145 healthy volunteers reported that the daily intake of APAP of 4 g for 14 days was associated with asymptomatic elevations of alanine aminotransferase (ALT) (>3 times the upper limits of normal) in up to 40% of subjects.[25] These elevations of ALT occurred despite APAP concentrations being within therapeutic limits, and resolved after APAP discontinuation, and without any clinical consequences.[25]

## Alcohol

The interaction between ethanol, a competitive substrate of CYP2E1, and APAP is complex. Acute alcohol ingestion is not a risk factor for APAP hepatotoxicity and may actually be protective by competing with APAP for CYP2E1.[26–28] In a prospective observational study of 362 patients presenting within 24 hours after acute APAP overdose, concurrent acute alcohol intake was reported by 49% of patients. The prevalence of hepatotoxicity was 5.1% (95% confidence interval, 2.6%–9.5%) in those who ingested ethanol, compared with 15.2% (95% confidence interval, 10.7%–21.2%) in those who did not ($P$ = .0027). Particularly, acute ethanol intake conferred a lower risk of hepatotoxicity in patients who had APAP concentrations above or below the "200-line" on the nomogram and was independent of the interval between ingestion and assessment.[28] In contrast, chronic alcohol ingestion may potentiate APAP hepatotoxicity by upregulating CYP2E1 and decreasing GSH synthesis.[9,15,26,29,30] Chronic alcohol ingestion enhances CYP2E1 activity about twofold by enzyme stabilization (half-life increases from 7 to 37 hours) and increased synthesis.[9,15,26] This effect lasts for up to 10 days and, interestingly, is maximal around 6 to 8 hours of abstinence suggesting that the risk of APAP hepatotoxicity is particularly increased in those recently abstinent from alcohol.[1,9,15,26,31] In addition, alcoholics are often malnourished, a state associated with depleted hepatic GSH stores thus further predisposing them to hepatotoxicity. Most available data have concluded that chronic alcohol consumption is associated with an increased risk of APAP hepatotoxicity in patients with repeated overdoses (therapeutic misadventure).[1,9,15,32] However, alcoholics do not seem to be at an increased risk of APAP liver injury at a therapeutic dose or in a single overdose setting, particularly if they are treated within 8 hours.[33,34] A review of more than 2000 cases in the literature indicates that the only reports linking alcohol and enhanced toxicity were retrospective reviews and case reports with no such link found in prospective reports.[35]

## Medications and Herbs

Concomitant use of medications that induce the CYP system, such as anticonvulsants (eg, phenobarbital, phenytoin, and carbamazepine) and antituberculosis agents (eg, isoniazid and rifampicin), may predispose to APAP hepatotoxicity by increased production of NAPQI by way of the oxidative pathway.[15,36,37] Severe APAP hepatotoxicity associated with the concurrent use of these medications has been anecdotally reported, although there are no compelling data that this occurs at a therapeutic dose.[36,37] Phenytoin is primarily metabolized by CYP3A4 and not CYP2E1 and as such there is an insignificant amount of APAP metabolite being produced. Thus, concomitant phenytoin use should not be considered a predisposing factor for APAP hepatotoxicity, but may in fact be protective in APAP overdose by way of enhanced glucuronidation.[35] Phenobarbital also does not significantly induce CYP2E1 but is rather a pleiotropic inducer of phase I and phase II reactions.[35] Some herbs and dietary supplements are inducers of CYP (eg, St. John's wort, garlic, grapefruit juice, and germander), and theoretically may potentiate APAP hepatotoxicity.[38] Zidovudine and trimethoprim-sulfamethoxazole may augment APAP hepatotoxicity by competitive use of the glucuronidation pathway and with subsequent increased metabolism toward CYP.[39]

### Genetic Factors

Genetic polymorphisms in the CYP isoenzymes can be associated with an excessive or diminished oxidative metabolism of APAP, but the clinical relevance to toxicity is unknown.[15,40,41] Impaired glucuronidation in patients with Gilbert syndrome seems to augment APAP toxicity.[42]

### Age

The metabolism of APAP is age-dependent, by which older patients are more susceptible to develop hepatotoxicity compared with young children after an acute overdose.[43,44]

### Nutritional Status

In the setting of chronic alcohol consumption, malnutrition and fasting state may potentiate APAP hepatotoxicity by reduced capacity for hepatic glucuronidation and because of depleted GSH stores.[15,45,46] Without chronic alcohol consumption, the effect of malnutrition and fasting on APAP hepatotoxicity is unclear. Although hepatic GSH stores are reduced by about 30% in patients with true protein-calorie malnutrition, such as anorexia nervosa, CYP2E1 and metabolic rates of drug metabolism are also decreased, possibly resulting in no change in the risk for APAP toxicity.[35,47]

### Chronic Liver Disease

Patients with cirrhosis have a higher area under the curve and lower clearance of APAP compared with healthy subjects.[48] In patients with cirrhosis, CYP activity is low or unchanged and does not seem to be inducible, whereas GSH stores may be depleted, but usually not to critical levels.[15,49] Although controversy exists, patients with chronic liver disease who do not regularly consume alcohol are not at significantly increased risk for developing APAP hepatotoxicity.[15,49] According to available data, less than 4 g/day of APAP seems safe for short-term dosing in patients with cirrhosis. Nevertheless, some experts have recommended less than 2 g/day, particularly for patients with decompensated disease or those who continue ingesting alcohol, given the small margin for error in a high-risk population.[49–51]

### Pregnancy

APAP is the most common drug overdose in pregnancy.[52] Although, the metabolism of APAP is altered (increased clearance caused by increased activity of glucorunidation and oxidative pathways) during pregnancy, there is insufficient evidence to suggest pregnancy as a predisposing factor for APAP hepatotoxicity. APAP has been demonstrated to cross the placenta and, at toxic doses, may harm maternal and fetal hepatocytes.[52,53] Although several cases of neonatal deaths and prematurity have been reported, most pregnancies with APAP overdose had normal outcomes, and APAP does not seem to increase adverse pregnancy outcome unless severe maternal toxicity develops.[52,53] Until available data on risk-stratification of toxicity to the fetus emerge, most physicians would consider pregnant women as a higher-risk group, in whom the strategy for antidote intervention should be more aggressive.

## CLINICAL MANIFESTATIONS

Early recognition of APAP overdose is likely to prevent subsequent morbidity and mortality. The early manifestations of APAP overdose are frequent, mild, and nonspecific, and include nausea, vomiting, malaise, and abdominal pain. In general, these symptoms do not reliably predict subsequent hepatotoxicity. However, a study of 291 patients suggested that an increase in episodes of vomiting at first presentation seems to be a risk marker of subsequent hepatotoxicity.[54] The clinical course of APAP hepatotoxicity in patients with single overdose can be classically divided into four sequential stages (see **Table 2**), but it should be noted that the course is variable and influenced by several factors, such as dose and formulation of APAP, coingested drug, and preexisting liver disease.

APAP hepatotoxicity is acute and characterized by marked elevation of serum aminotransferase (often >3000 IU/L), which typically starts increasing within 24 to 36 hours, and peaks around 72 hours after overdose.[55] The aspartate aminotransferase (AST) can be greater than 10,000 IU/L, and often more elevated than the ALT.[15] The degree of aminotransferase elevation correlates roughly with the degree of hepatocellular damage.[15] Maximal liver injury typically peaks between 3 and 5 days after ingestion, and may have features of jaundice, coagulopathy, and encephalopathy.[1] Prothrombin time that continues to increase beyond 4 seconds after overdose, and with a peak prothrombin time greater than or equal to 180 seconds are associated with approximately 90% mortality without liver transplantation (LT).[56] Patients may develop progressive central nervous system symptoms of lethargy, confusion, and coma, requiring intubation. Lactic acidosis is a poor prognostic marker in

**Table 2**
**Clinical manifestations of acetaminophen hepatotoxicity**

| | |
|---|---|
| Stage I (first 24 h) | Nausea, vomiting, malaise, lethargy, diaphoresis (some patients remain asymptomatic)<br>AST/ALT are typically normal (AST/ALT may begin to rise at 8–12 h after massive overdose) |
| Stage II (24–72 h) | Stage I symptoms usually improve or resolve (so-called latent period)<br>Subclinical AST/ALT elevation<br>In severe cases, RUQ pain, tender hepatomegaly, jaundice, and prolonged PT may be seen<br>Nephrotoxicity (elevated creatinine and oliguria) may become evident |
| Stage III (72–96 h) | Systemic symptoms of stage I reappear<br>AST/ALT elevation, typically peak at 72–96 h after ingestion (often >3000 IU/L)<br>Jaundice, encephalopathy, prolonged PT, and lactic acidosis may develop<br>ARF (10%–50%) and acute pancreatitis (0.3%–5%) may develop<br>Death often in this stage, usually from multiorgan system failure |
| Stage IV (96 h–2 wk) | Survivors of stage III enter recovery phase, which often lasts 1–2 wk, but may take several weeks in severe cases<br>Histologic recovery occurs slower than clinical recovery and may take up to 3 mo<br>When recovery occurs, it is complete; chronic hepatitis has not been reported |

*Abbreviations:* ALT, alanine aminotransferase; ARF, acute renal failure; AST, aspartate aminotransferase; PT, prothrombin time; RUQ, right upper quadrant.

APAP hepatotoxicity that can manifest as two scenarios: early onset after massive overdose and before the onset of hepatotoxicity in which large amount of NAPQI critically inhibits mitochondrial function; and later in course, usually after Day 2, resulting from tissue hypoxia together with decreased hepatic clearance of lactate in those with ALF.[57] Notably, central nervous system symptoms and metabolic acidosis early in the course of disease (stage I) are not common features of APAP toxicity, and other possible causes should be excluded, particularly coingestion of other substances.

Acute renal failure develops in 10% to 25% of patients with significant hepatotoxicity and is encountered in more than 50% of those with ALF.[58,59] It often becomes evident around 1 to 3 days after ingestion and often manifests as acute tubular necrosis, either alone or in combination with hepatic necrosis.[58,59] The mechanism of nephrotoxicity is thought to be related to the toxic metabolites of APAP oxidized by CYP in the kidney.[59] Acute renal failure is typically reversible, although it may worsen over 7 to 10 days and occasionally may require renal replacement therapy before the recovery occurs.[58,59] An elevated serum amylase is frequently seen in patients with APAP poisoning particularly in patients with ALF, whereas clinical acute pancreatitis occurs rarely (0.3%–5%).[60,61] Several cases of severe acute pancreatitis associated with APAP, however, have been reported,[60,61] and therefore the possibility of APAP poisoning should be kept in mind in patients presenting with ALF and pancreatitis.

Clinical presentation of patients with single overdose versus repeated overdoses is somewhat similar. Patients who unintentionally ingest above the therapeutic APAP doses are more likely to present late (when hepatotoxicity is already recognized clinically) and are more likely to have known risk factors for hepatotoxicity, especially chronic alcohol use.[32,62] In addition, this group of patient tends to have higher rates of morbidity and mortality than those who attempted suicide, even though the latter had taken higher total amount of APAP.[32,62,63]

## GENERAL APPROACH AND DIAGNOSTIC TOOLS

General approach promptly begins with careful history taking and physical examination. The precise time and amount of APAP intake, and 4-hour APAP level, or as soon thereafter as feasible, should be obtained. Other tests, such as hepatic biochemical tests, creatinine, and electrolytes, may also be useful, particularly in patients with repeated overdoses and those who present more than 8 hours after ingestion. Investigations for possible coingested substances and other causes of hepatitis may be required especially in those with an uncertain history.

Given the consequences of missed APAP poisoning, a screening for APAP seems reasonable in patients with unknown or possible drug overdose, or in those with indeterminate hepatitis and ALF.[1,64] Notably, interpretation of serum APAP levels should be done with caution in patients with serum bilirubin greater than 10 mg/dL because bilirubin interference can cause falsely positive or elevated APAP concentration measuring by enzymatic method.[65] Conversely, serum APAP concentration may already be negative at the time of established hepatotoxicity, thus not eliminating the possibility of APAP etiology for liver injury.

### Evaluations After Acute Single Overdose

The Rumack-Matthew nomogram is a valuable tool for handling patients with single acute ingestion who present to a health care facility within 24 hours (**Fig. 2**).[1,66–70] This nomogram was constructed in the 1970s to estimate the likelihood of hepatotoxicity caused by APAP for patients with a single ingestion at a known time.[1,66–70] To use the nomogram, patient's serum APAP concentration is plotted in line with time interval

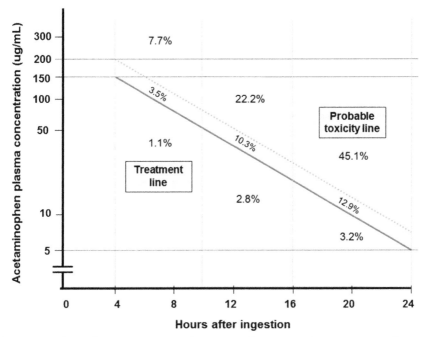

**Fig. 2.** Rumack-Matthew nomogram and outcome of treatment. Percentages are the number of cases with AST greater than 1000 IU/L at any time during their course taken from data from the US nationwide NAC study. (*Adapted from* Rumack BH. Acetaminophen misconceptions. Hepatology 2004;40:11; with permission.)

from ingestion. Patients with an APAP level above a line between 200 μg/mL at 4 hours and 25 μg/mL at 16 hours after ingestion, known as the "200 line" or the "probable toxicity line," are at risk for developing severe hepatotoxicity (defined as AST >1000 IU/L) in which N-acetylcysteine (NAC) treatment is recommended even in the absence of clinical or laboratory evidence for toxicity at the time.[1,66–71] Without NAC treatment, patients with APAP concentrations above the "200 line" have an approximate 60% incidence of severe hepatotoxicity with 5% mortality. Patients with APAP concentrations above the parallel "300 line" or "high toxicity line" have a subsequent 90% incidence of severe hepatotoxicity with 24% mortality.[66,71] After the generation of these data, the FDA then imposed an arbitrary 25% safety margin on the "200 line," which resulted in a parallel line staring at 150 μg/mL at 4 hours, known as the "150 line" or the "treatment line," and that has been most commonly used in the United States,[1,72,73] and in Australia and New Zealand.[74] Although controversy remains, this margin of safety was created to allow for possible errors in the estimated time of ingestion and variation in measured APAP concentration. Treatment outcomes using both the original "200" and the lower "150" lines in the US nationwide NAC study of more than 2500 patients demonstrated a very small rate of nomogram failure, especially with the "150 line."[35,72,73] In addition, the 25% safety margin is also likely to protect hepatotoxicity in high-risk populations, and there is no further convincing evidence to support lowering the treatment line. Thus, using a more conservative "100 line" significantly increases the number of patients being overtreated and also the overall associated cost.[75] In general, a single-time APAP concentration plot on the nomogram is adequate to justify NAC treatment. The caveat from this outcome nomogram is that a small change in historical timing can make a huge difference in which segment the patient is classified. If there is any question regarding the history, and the patient is anywhere close to the treatment line, NAC is indicated.[35]

It should be noted that the Rumack-Matthew nomogram was developed for single overdose with precise time of ingestion. Therefore, it cannot accurately assess risk after repeated overdoses, acute overdose of a sustained-release product, or when the time of ingestion is unknown or patients present beyond 24 hours, and these situations represent nearly half of APAP overdoses in the United States.[1,8,9,15,76]

### Evaluations After Repeated Overdoses

Patients with therapeutic misadventure often present after several days of ingestion with symptoms in which hepatotoxicity may have already begun. They are likely to develop hepatotoxicity if they have significant symptoms and clinical signs (eg, recurrent vomiting, confusion, liver tenderness, and jaundice) or have ingested an amount of APAP above the threshold (discussed previously). Serum APAP concentration should be measured, but the Rumack-Matthew nomogram is not applicable in this setting. Based on limited evidence, patients with supratherapeutic APAP levels of more than 20 µg/mL (or >10 µg/mL in patients with risk factors for toxicity) are at risk for developing subsequent hepatotoxicity, and therapy with NAC is suggested even if their ALT levels are normal.[1,15,69] Treatment with NAC seems unnecessary if serum APAP is undetectable or less than 10 µg/mL in asymptomatic patients with normal ALT. Patients with a history of excessive APAP intake and who have elevated ALT levels should receive NAC treatment even with undetectable serum APAP (**Box 1**).[1,15,69]

### Evaluations After Established Hepatotoxicity and Liver Failure

Cautious monitoring of clinical and laboratory parameters is vital, because greater than 90% of cases with APAP hepatotoxicity can be expected to resolve spontaneously.[15,77] However, patients with clinical signs indicating ALF (eg, encephalopathy, coagulopathy, and acidosis) should be transferred to an intensive care unit and a facility where LT is available.[78,79] Apart from a specific antidote, the general evaluation and management of ALF from APAP are not much different from ALF from other causes.[79–81] Although APAP-induced ALF is associated with more favorable outcomes compared with all other causes of ALF, it still has a high mortality (~30%) without LT.[6,8,15,77] LT-free survival rate seems to be similar between intentional and unintentional overdose groups.[8] To identify those patients with ALF who are unlikely to survive without LT, several clinical features and laboratory parameters have been evaluated and prognostic models have been developed. One of the most widely used prognostic models was developed at King's College in London, United Kingdom (**Box 2**).[15,81–83] Based on differences in prognosis, King's College criteria categorized patients into two groups: non-APAP and APAP-induced ALF. Without LT, patients with APAP-induced ALF who met the criteria had very high mortality (80%–90%)[15,82,83] and as such these patients deserve consideration of LT. Although it is the best prognostic model available to date wherein LT-free survival has been evaluated, it still suffers from a variability in its negative predictive value and sensitivity, and thus the challenge in the listing for LT. Several studies evaluating this criteria have shown positive predictive values ranging from 70% to 95% and negative predictive values ranging from 40% to 90%.[8,15,78,81–86] Overall, King's College criteria have proved to have acceptable specificity (<20%–30% of those who met the criteria survived spontaneously) but relatively low sensitivity to determine outcome, in that many patients who would ultimately require LT may be missed.[8,15,78,81–86] Nonetheless, it is still the most validated and

---

**Box 1**
**N-acetylcysteine: indications, dosing, and monitoring**

*Indications*

- Asymptomatic patients with single overdose: Serum APAP level above the "150 line" on Rumack-Matthew nomogram

- Asymptomatic patients with repeated overdoses: Serum APAP level above therapeutic range (>20 µg/mL) or above >10 µg/mL in patients with significant risk factors, such as chronic alcohol consumption

- Any patient with acute elevations of AST/ALT and a history of ingesting >4 g of APAP per day, irrespective of serum APAP level

*Standard dosing*

- IV regimen[a]: loading 150 mg/kg in 200-mL diluent in 1 hour, then 50 mg/kg in 500-mL diluent over 4 hours, and 100 mg/kg in 1000-mL diluent over 16 hours (IV NAC solution is hyperosmolar and is compatible with D5W, 0.45% NSS, and sterile water)

- Oral regimen: loading 140 mg/kg, then 70 mg/kg orally every 4 hours for 18 doses in total

- Dose adjustment in patients with moderate/severe renal or liver impairment is not required

*Monitoring*

- For patients with especially high risk for developing hepatotoxicity[b], rechecking APAP and ALT levels is recommended before completion of NAC. NAC can be stopped if APAP <10 µg/mL and normal ALT. If APAP ≥10 µg/mL or elevated ALT, NAC should be continued and be reevaluated after 12 hours

- For patients with severe hepatotoxicity or ALF, NAC infusion should be continued (6.25 mg/kg/h) until the patient receives LT or liver dysfunction reverses (ALT or AST have peaked and are improving, encephalopathy resolves, and INR <1.5) with undetectable APAP level.

*Abbreviations:* ALF, acute liver failure; ALT, alanine aminotransferase; APAP, acetaminophen; AST, aspartate aminotransferase; D5W, 5% dextrose in water; INR, international normalized ratio; IV, intravenous; NAC, N- acetylcysteine; NSS, normal saline solution; PT, prothrombin time.

[a] IV regimen is preferred for patients with ALF and those who have contraindications to oral administration (eg, coma, pancreatitis, bowel ileus or obstruction).

[b] Patients who present 8 hours after ingestion, have an elevated ALT before NAC treatment, or have a very high APAP concentration (>300 µg/mL).

---

**Box 2**
**King's College criteria for acetaminophen-induced acute liver failure**

*Indications*

- Arterial pH <7.3 or blood lactate >3 mg/dL (0.33 mmol/L); after adequate volume resuscitation, irrespective of the grade of encephalopathy

OR

- Blood lactate >3.5 mg/dL (0.39 mmol/L); after early volume resuscitation

OR three of the following

- Grade III or IV encephalopathy AND

- Prothrombin time >100 seconds (or INR >6.5) AND

- Serum creatinine >3.4 mg/dL (or >300 µmol/L)

clinically useful prognostic model for APAP-induced ALF and one that has been adopted by most transplant centers and by the American Association for the Study of the Liver.[8,15,78,81–86] The Model of End-stage Liver Disease (MELD) is also useful in APAP-induced ALF, but has not proved to be a better discriminator than the King's College criteria or international normalized ratio (INR) alone.[87] The sequential organ failure assessment score, originally designed for grading dysfunction of multiple organ systems, has been shown to be prognostically superior to the King's College and MELD criteria for APAP-induced ALF caused by single and repeated overdoses.[88–90] However, the use of sequential organ failure assessment score to justify LT requires further evaluation. Acute Physiology and Chronic Health Evaluation II score of greater than 15 on admission has been noted to be a sensitive tool to predict progression to ALF and was more sensitive than the King's College criteria on the day of admission.[8,91] A score of greater than 20 was associated with a lower LT-free survival.[8]

Apart from medical issues, psychiatric problems and family support should also be evaluated before offering LT, especially in patients with intentional APAP overdose, because there remains a concern of the risk of reattempting suicide after LT.

### Roles of APAP-protein Adducts

APAP-protein adducts are released into blood during hepatocyte lysis and the concentration of adducts in serum of overdose patients has correlated with toxicity.[92] The detection of serum APAP–protein adducts by using high-pressure liquid chromatography with electrochemical detection has reliably identified APAP hepatotoxicity and thus may be a useful diagnostic test for ALF of unknown cause or unclear history, and for patients who present more than 1 day after overdose.[64,92,93] Interestingly, up to 19% of indeterminate cases in the US-ALF study demonstrated adducts in serum suggesting that unrecognized APAP toxicity caused or contributed to ALF in these patients.[64,93] In addition to the application for diagnosis, the role of APAP-protein adducts for determining prognosis and for justifying intervention warrants further study. Unfortunately, the measurement of this adducts is sophisticated and is not yet routinely available in most centers.

## MANAGEMENT OF APAP OVERDOSE
### Gastrointestinal Decontamination

Activated charcoal is effective at limiting the absorption of APAP when given within 4 hours after overdose and is recommended in all patients who present early after APAP ingestion, unless there are contraindications (eg, unsecured airway or gastrointestinal tract injury).[94–97] Patients who present 4 hours after ingestion are unlikely to benefit from activated charcoal, except in those who ingested extended-release APAP preparations or coingested drugs that delayed gastric emptying time. Gastric lavage and induced emesis are not routinely recommended because they seem to be less effective and have no additional benefit when activated charcoal is given.[96,97]

### N-Acetylcysteine

NAC, a GSH precursor, is an established antidote for APAP poisoning and should be administered in all patients with APAP hepatotoxicity or in patients at significant risk for developing hepatotoxicity. The key to effective treatment is to initiate therapy before the onset of ALT elevation. When given early after acute APAP overdose, NAC provides cysteine for the replenishment and maintenance of hepatic GSH stores, thus providing more substrate for the detoxification of the reactive metabolites. Furthermore, it may also enhance sulfation pathway and directly reduce NAPQI back to APAP.[1,98,99] There has been no randomized placebo-controlled trial (such trials were considered unethical) evaluating the efficacy of NAC for APAP overdose.[100] Several case series have observed that severe hepatotoxicity was uncommon (<5%–10%) when NAC was administered within 8 hours after acute APAP overdose, whereas delays beyond 10 hours were associated with an increased risk of hepatotoxicity (20%–30%).[1,70,73,101] Patients with established liver injury may also benefit from NAC because it has been shown to improve LT-free survival among patients with APAP-induced ALF ($\sim$20%–30% reduction in mortality).[102,103] Instead of detoxifying NAPQI, the potential mechanisms of NAC in this state are of improving hepatic perfusion and oxygen delivery, scavenging reactive oxygen and nitrogen species, and refining mitochondrial energy production.[1,15] Apart from APAP hepatotoxicity, the beneficial effects of NAC have also been observed in patients with early coma-grade encephalopathy and with non-APAP ALF.[104]

NAC is available in oral and IV forms and their standard regimens (FDA-approved protocols) are different in the total dose and duration of treatment (see **Box 1**). The doses of NAC are calculated using patient body weight with a maximum of 110 kg for oral and 100 kg for IV therapy.[69] An observational study of APAP poisoning in patients weighing more than 100 kg found that maximum weight cut-off and actual weight-based NAC dose were safe, but clinicians preferred the latter and hepatotoxicity was similar (up to 33%) with both strategies.[105]

The choice of oral or IV administration depends on the clinical scenario, and a head-to-head comparison trial has not been performed in adults. Nevertheless, most available data suggest that both treatment strategies are safe and equally effective, and with minimal differences, in most circumstances.[1,15,69,106] Oral NAC has an unpleasant taste and smell and vomiting is common. Nausea and vomiting can be reduced by diluting NAC with soda or juice, holding one's breath while taking the medication, or administering by a nasogastric tube.[15] Eventually, about 5% of patients may not tolerate oral NAC and require IV therapy.[69] Anaphylactoid reactions (eg, rash, itching, angioedema, bronchospasm, tachycardia, and hypotension) develop in 10% to 20% of patients treated with IV NAC.[107,108] Patients with flushing alone or mild symptoms do not require intervention and the infusion can be continued with careful monitoring. Patients who develop urticaria, angioedema, hypotension, and bronchospasm should be treated with one or more medications of diphenhydramine, corticosteroids, and bronchodilators. The infusion should be stopped and can be restarted at a slower rate and with close monitoring.[69,109] In a randomized trial, slowing the initial infusion time from 15 minutes to 60 minutes had not compromised efficacy but also did not lower the incidence of anaphylactoid reactions.[108] IV regimen is preferred for patients with ALF and those who refuse, or have a contraindication to oral administration (eg, coma, pancreatitis, bowel ileus or obstruction).

Given the disparity between a prespecified treatment duration of the two regimens, alternative dosing schedules have been further studied; the 72-hour oral course seems to be too long and the 20-hour IV course may be too short.[69] Shorter courses of oral NAC (20–48 hours) have been evaluated and seem to be effective, particularly if a repeat APAP level is less than 10 µg/mL and there was no increase in serum ALT or INR after a minimum treatment duration of 20 hours.[110–114] Alternative 48-hour IV regimen (140 mg/kg loading followed by 12 doses of 70 mg/kg every 4 hours) is also effective in APAP overdose patients who present within 24 hours.[115] Some experts have recommended an individualized approach for IV NAC by repeating APAP and ALT levels at the end of a 16-hour infusion period and continuing treatment if the ALT was elevated or if APAP concentration was detectable. This strategy may be particularly important in the patient who presents 8 hours after ingestion; has an elevated ALT at the time NAC is started; or has a very high APAP concentration (>300 μg/mL).[69] The treatment guideline for single or repeated overdoses with severe hepatotoxicity or ALF is not well defined. However, most experts have advised a standard IV regimen while continuing a final infusion rate of 6.25 mg/kg/h until the patient receives LT or hepatotoxicity reverses (ALT or AST have peaked and are decreasing, encephalopathy resolves, and INR <1.5) with undetectable serum APAP concentration.[1,69,103,116]

### Liver Transplantation

LT is life-saving in those APAP overdose patients who progress to severe ALF. Several prognostic parameters or criteria have been identified to facilitate the decision-making with regard to the need for LT (discussed previously). A large experience of 1144 ALF cases (54% were APAP-related) from the US Acute Liver Failure Study Group has observed that APAP patients, compared with non-APAP patients, had better 2-year survival in those not transplanted but lower survival in those transplanted, indicating a good discriminatory ability of the physicians in observing versus transplanting those with APAP-ALF.[7] In this analysis, patients were classified into three groups: (1) not listed for LT (N = 697); (2) listed but not transplanted (N = 177); and (3) listed and transplanted (N = 270). The 2-year survival among non-APAP and APAP etiology in Groups 1, 2, and 3 was 34% and 31%, 83% and 59%, 53% and 72%, respectively.[7] Notably, a significant number of patients did not receive LT for a variety of reasons including milder disease and psychosocial disqualifiers.[7] In another experience of 858 patients admitted with APAP-induced hepatotoxicity in the United Kingdom, 60 of 95 patients listed for LT underwent the procedure.[6] Of 60 patients transplanted, 73% survived to discharge and 58% survived at an average of 9 years post-LT. When compared with patients who had LT from other causes of ALF, the incidence of psychiatric disease (principally depression) and 30-day mortality were greatest in the APAP group, but for those who survived beyond 30 days, there was no difference in long-term survival rates between APAP and non-APAP groups.[6] Adherence to follow-up appointments and compliance with immunosuppressive regimens were lower in the APAP overdose group, and was not predicted by any identifiable premorbid psychiatric conditions.[6]

### Other Treatment Modalities

Other potential treatment options for APAP hepatotoxicity have been evaluated chiefly by three main mechanisms of action: (1) modulation of APAP metabolism, (2) modulation of cytokines and chemokines and the innate immune system, and (3) modulation of oxidative stress-related injury. Cimetidine, an inhibitor of CYP enzymes, theoretically may decrease the formation of NAPQI. In animal models, protection against APAP hepatotoxicity using a combination of cimetidine and NAC was better than that found with either agent alone.[117] However, the use of cimetidine as an adjunct to NAC has shown no benefit in human studies.[118,119] Several biologic agents, such as inducible protein-10, macrophage inducible protein-2, interleukin-6, -11, -22, and anti–interferon-γ, have been demonstrated to decrease susceptibility for APAP toxicity in experimental models.[120,121] Telmisartan[122] and coenzyme Q10[123] can alleviate oxidative stress injury associated with APAP in animal models. However, to our knowledge, none of these agents have come to the clinical phase of study.

### REFERENCES

1. Hodgman MJ, Garrard AR. A review of acetaminophen poisoning. Crit Care Clin 2012;28(4):499–516.

2. Wysowski DK, Governale LA, Swann J. Trends in outpatient prescription drug use and related costs in the US: 1998-2003. Pharmacoeconomics 2006;24(3): 233-6.
3. Lee WM. Acetaminophen and the U.S. Acute Liver Failure Study Group: lowering the risks of hepatic failure. Hepatology 2004;40(1):6–9.
4. Ostapowicz G, Fontana RJ, Schiodt FV, et al. Results of a prospective study of acute liver failure at 17 tertiary care centers in the United States. Ann Intern Med 2002;137(12):947–54.
5. Ayonrinde OT, Phelps GJ, Hurley JC, et al. Paracetamol overdose and hepato-toxicity at a regional Australian hospital: a 4-year experience. Intern Med J 2005; 35(11):655–60.
6. Cooper SC, Aldridge RC, Shah T, et al. Outcomes of liver transplantation for paracetamol (acetaminophen)-induced hepatic failure. Liver Transpl 2009; 15(10):1351–7.
7. Reddy KR, Schilsky ML, Stravitz R, et al. Liver transplantation for acute liver fail-ure: results from the NIH Acute Liver Failure Study Group. Hepatology 2012; 56(Suppl 4):246A–7A.
8. Larson AM, Polson J, Fontana RJ, et al. Acetaminophen-induced acute liver fail-ure: results of a United States multicenter, prospective study. Hepatology 2005; 42(6):1364–72.
9. Zimmerman HJ, Maddrey WC. Acetaminophen (paracetamol) hepatotoxicity with regular intake of alcohol: analysis of instances of therapeutic misadventure. Hepatology 1995;22(3):767–73.
10. Krenzelok EP. The FDA Acetaminophen Advisory Committee Meeting: what is the future of acetaminophen in the United States? The perspective of a commit-tee member. Clin Toxicol (Phila) 2009;47(8):784–9.
11. Forrest JA, Clements JA, Prescott LF. Clinical pharmacokinetics of paracetamol. Clin Pharmacokinet 1982;7(2):93–107.
12. Bizovi KE, Aks SE, Paloucek F, et al. Late increase in acetaminophen concentra-tion after overdose of Tylenol Extended Relief. Ann Emerg Med 1996;28(5): 549–51.
13. Douglas DR, Sholar JB, Smilkstein MJ. A pharmacokinetic comparison of acet-aminophen products (Tylenol Extended Relief vs regular Tylenol). Acad Emerg Med 1996;3(8):740–4.
14. Schiodt FV, Ott P, Christensen E, et al. The value of plasma acetaminophen half-life in antidote-treated acetaminophen overdosage. Clin Pharmacol Ther 2002; 71(4):221–5.
15. Larson AM. Acetaminophen hepatotoxicity. Clin Liver Dis 2007;11(3):525–48, vi.
16. Graham GG, Scott KF, Day RO. Tolerability of paracetamol. Drug Saf 2005; 28(3):227–40.
17. Mitchell JR, Jollow DJ, Potter WZ, et al. Acetaminophen-induced hepatic necro-sis. IV. Protective role of glutathione. J Pharmacol Exp Ther 1973;187(1):211–7.
18. Knight TR, Fariss MW, Farhood A, et al. Role of lipid peroxidation as a mecha-nism of liver injury after acetaminophen overdose in mice. Toxicol Sci 2003; 76(1):229–36.
19. McGill MR, Sharpe MR, Williams CD, et al. The mechanism underlying acetaminophen-induced hepatotoxicity in humans and mice involves mitochon-drial damage and nuclear DNA fragmentation. J Clin Invest 2012;122(4):1574–83.
20. Jaeschke H, Williams CD, Ramachandran A, et al. Acetaminophen hepatotoxic-ity and repair: the role of sterile inflammation and innate immunity. Liver Int 2012; 32(1):8–20.

21. Liu ZX, Govindarajan S, Kaplowitz N. Innate immune system plays a critical role in determining the progression and severity of acetaminophen hepatotoxicity. Gastroenterology 2004;127(6):1760–74.

22. Dart RC, Erdman AR, Olson KR, et al. Acetaminophen poisoning: an evidence-based consensus guideline for out-of-hospital management. Clin Toxicol (Phila) 2006;44(1):1–18.

23. Temple AR, Benson GD, Zinsenheim JR, et al. Multicenter, randomized, double-blind, active-controlled, parallel-group trial of the long-term (6-12 months) safety of acetaminophen in adult patients with osteoarthritis. Clin Ther 2006;28(2): 222–35.

24. Temple AR, Lynch JM, Vena J, et al. Aminotransferase activities in healthy subjects receiving three-day dosing of 4, 6, or 8 grams per day of acetaminophen. Clin Toxicol (Phila) 2007;45(1):36–44.

25. Watkins PB, Kaplowitz N, Slattery JT, et al. Aminotransferase elevations in healthy adults receiving 4 grams of acetaminophen daily: a randomized controlled trial. JAMA 2006;296(1):87–93.

26. Lee WM. Drug-induced hepatotoxicity. N Engl J Med 2003;349(5):474–85.

27. Schmidt LE, Dalhoff K, Poulsen HE. Acute versus chronic alcohol consumption in acetaminophen-induced hepatotoxicity. Hepatology 2002;35(4):876–82.

28. Waring WS, Stephen AF, Malkowska AM, et al. Acute ethanol coingestion confers a lower risk of hepatotoxicity after deliberate acetaminophen overdose. Acad Emerg Med 2008;15(1):54–8.

29. Lauterburg BH, Velez ME. Glutathione deficiency in alcoholics: risk factor for paracetamol hepatotoxicity. Gut 1988;29(9):1153–7.

30. Zhao P, Slattery JT. Effects of ethanol dose and ethanol withdrawal on rat liver mitochondrial glutathione: implication of potentiated acetaminophen toxicity in alcoholics. Drug Metab Dispos 2002;30(12):1413–7.

31. Thummel KE, Slattery JT, Ro H, et al. Ethanol and production of the hepatotoxic metabolite of acetaminophen in healthy adults. Clin Pharmacol Ther 2000;67(6): 591–9.

32. Schiodt FV, Rochling FA, Casey DL, et al. Acetaminophen toxicity in an urban county hospital. N Engl J Med 1997;337(16):1112–7.

33. Dart RC, Kuffner EK, Rumack BH. Treatment of pain or fever with paracetamol (acetaminophen) in the alcoholic patient: a systematic review. Am J Ther 2000;7(2):123–34.

34. Kuffner EK, Dart RC, Bogdan GM, et al. Effect of maximal daily doses of acetaminophen on the liver of alcoholic patients: a randomized, double-blind, placebo-controlled trial. Arch Intern Med 2001;161(18):2247–52.

35. Rumack BH. Acetaminophen misconceptions. Hepatology 2004;40(1):10–5.

36. Bray GP, Harrison PM, O'Grady JG, et al. Long-term anticonvulsant therapy worsens outcome in paracetamol-induced fulminant hepatic failure. Hum Exp Toxicol 1992;11(4):265–70.

37. Nolan CM, Sandblom RE, Thummel KE, et al. Hepatotoxicity associated with acetaminophen usage in patients receiving multiple drug therapy for tuberculosis. Chest 1994;105(2):408–11.

38. Bunchorntavakul C, Reddy KR. Review article: herbal and dietary supplement hepatotoxicity. Aliment Pharmacol Ther 2013;37(1):3–17.

39. Shriner K, Goetz MB. Severe hepatotoxicity in a patient receiving both acetaminophen and zidovudine. Am J Med 1992;93(1):94–6.

40. Critchley JA, Nimmo GR, Gregson CA, et al. Inter-subject and ethnic differences in paracetamol metabolism. Br J Clin Pharmacol 1986;22(6):649–57.

41. Ueshima Y, Tsutsumi M, Takase S, et al. Acetaminophen metabolism in patients with different cytochrome P-4502E1 genotypes. Alcohol Clin Exp Res 1996; 20(Suppl 1):25A–8A.

42. de Morais SM, Uetrecht JP, Wells PG. Decreased glucuronidation and increased bioactivation of acetaminophen in Gilbert's syndrome. Gastroenterology 1992; 102(2):577–86.

43. Miller RP, Roberts RJ, Fischer LJ. Acetaminophen elimination kinetics in neonates, children, and adults. Clin Pharmacol Ther 1976;19(3):284–94.

44. Rumore MM, Blaiklock RG. Influence of age-dependent pharmacokinetics and metabolism on acetaminophen hepatotoxicity. J Pharm Sci 1992;81(3):203–7.

45. Price VF, Miller MG, Jollow DJ. Mechanisms of fasting-induced potentiation of acetaminophen hepatotoxicity in the rat. Biochem Pharmacol 1987;36(4):427–33.

46. Whitcomb DC, Block GD. Association of acetaminophen hepatotoxicity with fasting and ethanol use. JAMA 1994;272(23):1845–50.

47. Zenger F, Russmann S, Junker E, et al. Decreased glutathione in patients with anorexia nervosa. Risk factor for toxic liver injury? Eur J Clin Nutr 2004;58(2): 238–43.

48. Zapater P, Lasso de la Vega MC, Horga JF, et al. Pharmacokinetic variations of acetaminophen according to liver dysfunction and portal hypertension status. Aliment Pharmacol Ther 2004;20(1):29–36.

49. Benson GD, Koff RS, Tolman KG. The therapeutic use of acetaminophen in patients with liver disease. Am J Ther 2005;12(2):133–41.

50. Riley TR III, Bhatti AM. Preventive strategies in chronic liver disease. Part I. Alcohol, vaccines, toxic medications and supplements, diet and exercise. Am Fam Physician 2001;64(9):1555–60.

51. Chandok N, Watt KD. Pain management in the cirrhotic patient: the clinical challenge. Mayo Clin Proc 2010;85(5):451–8.

52. Wilkes JM, Clark LE, Herrera JL. Acetaminophen overdose in pregnancy. South Med J 2005;98(11):1118–22.

53. McElhatton PR, Sullivan FM, Volans GN. Paracetamol overdose in pregnancy analysis of the outcomes of 300 cases referred to the Teratology Information Service. Reprod Toxicol 1997;11(1):85–94.

54. Zyoud SH, Awang R, Sulaiman SA, et al. Assessing the impact of vomiting episodes on outcome after acetaminophen poisoning. Basic Clin Pharmacol Toxicol 2010;107(5):887–92.

55. Singer AJ, Carracio TR, Mofenson HC. The temporal profile of increased transaminase levels in patients with acetaminophen-induced liver dysfunction. Ann Emerg Med 1995;26(1):49–53.

56. Harrison PM, O'Grady JG, Keays RT, et al. Serial prothrombin time as prognostic indicator in paracetamol induced fulminant hepatic failure. BMJ 1990; 301(6758):964–6.

57. Shah AD, Wood DM, Dargan PI. Understanding lactic acidosis in paracetamol (acetaminophen) poisoning. Br J Clin Pharmacol 2011;71(1):20–8.

58. Blakely P, McDonald BR. Acute renal failure due to acetaminophen ingestion: a case report and review of the literature. J Am Soc Nephrol 1995;6(1):48–53.

59. Mazer M, Perrone J. Acetaminophen-induced nephrotoxicity: pathophysiology, clinical manifestations, and management. J Med Toxicol 2008;4(1):2–6.

60. Schmidt LE, Dalhoff K. Hyperamylasaemia and acute pancreatitis in paracetamol poisoning. Aliment Pharmacol Ther 2004;20(2):173–9.

61. Caldarola V, Hassett JM, Hall AH, et al. Hemorrhagic pancreatitis associated with acetaminophen overdose. Am J Gastroenterol 1986;81(7):579–82.

62. Gyamlani GG, Parikh CR. Acetaminophen toxicity: suicidal vs. accidental. Crit Care 2002;6(2):155–9.
63. Craig DG, Bates CM, Davidson JS, et al. Staggered overdose pattern and delay to hospital presentation are associated with adverse outcomes following paracetamol-induced hepatotoxicity. Br J Clin Pharmacol 2012;73(2):285–94.
64. Khandelwal N, James LP, Sanders C, et al. Unrecognized acetaminophen toxicity as a cause of indeterminate acute liver failure. Hepatology 2011;53(2): 567–76.
65. Beuhler MC, Curry SC. False positive acetaminophen levels associated with hyperbilirubinemia. Clin Toxicol (Phila) 2005;43(3):167–70.
66. Prescott LF, Illingworth RN, Critchley JA, et al. Intravenous N-acetylcystine: the treatment of choice for paracetamol poisoning. Br Med J 1979;2(6198): 1097–100.
67. Rumack BH, Matthew H. Acetaminophen poisoning and toxicity. Pediatrics 1975;55(6):871–6.
68. Rumack BH, Peterson RC, Koch GG, et al. Acetaminophen overdose. 662 cases with evaluation of oral acetylcysteine treatment. Arch Intern Med 1981; 141(3 Spec No):380–5.
69. Heard KJ. Acetylcysteine for acetaminophen poisoning. N Engl J Med 2008; 359(3):285–92.
70. Prescott LF. Treatment of severe acetaminophen poisoning with intravenous acetylcysteine. Arch Intern Med 1981;141(3 Spec No):386–9.
71. Prescott LF. Paracetamol overdosage. Pharmacological considerations and clinical management. Drugs 1983;25(3):290–314.
72. Rumack BH. Acetaminophen hepatotoxicity: the first 35 years. J Toxicol Clin Toxicol 2002;40(1):3–20.
73. Smilkstein MJ, Knapp GL, Kulig KW, et al. Efficacy of oral N-acetylcysteine in the treatment of acetaminophen overdose. Analysis of the national multicenter study (1976 to 1985). N Engl J Med 1988;319(24):1557–62.
74. Daly FF, Fountain JS, Murray L, et al. Guidelines for the management of paracetamol poisoning in Australia and New Zealand–explanation and elaboration. A consensus statement from clinical toxicologists consulting to the Australasian poisons information centres. Med J Aust 2008;188(5):296–301.
75. McQuade DJ, Dargan PI, Keep J, et al. Paracetamol toxicity: what would be the implications of a change in UK treatment guidelines? Eur J Clin Pharmacol 2012; 68(11):1541–7.
76. Bond GR, Hite LK. Population-based incidence and outcome of acetaminophen poisoning by type of ingestion. Acad Emerg Med 1999;6(11):1115–20.
77. Bernal W, Wendon J, Rela M, et al. Use and outcome of liver transplantation in acetaminophen-induced acute liver failure. Hepatology 1998;27(4): 1050–5.
78. Makin AJ, Wendon J, Williams R. A 7-year experience of severe acetaminophen-induced hepatotoxicity (1987-1993). Gastroenterology 1995;109(6):1907–16.
79. Stravitz RT, Kramer AH, Davern T, et al. Intensive care of patients with acute liver failure: recommendations of the U.S. Acute Liver Failure Study Group. Crit Care Med 2007;35(11):2498–508.
80. Lee WM. Acute liver failure. Semin Respir Crit Care Med 2012;33(1):36–45.
81. Polson J, Lee WM. AASLD position paper: the management of acute liver failure. Hepatology 2005;41(5):1179–97.
82. O'Grady JG, Alexander GJ, Hayllar KM, et al. Early indicators of prognosis in fulminant hepatic failure. Gastroenterology 1989;97(2):439–45.

83. O'Grady JG, Langley PG, Isola LM, et al. Coagulopathy of fulminant hepatic failure. Semin Liver Dis 1986;6(2):159–63.
84. Craig DG, Ford AC, Hayes PC, et al. Systematic review: prognostic tests of paracetamol-induced acute liver failure. Aliment Pharmacol Ther 2010;31(10): 1064–76.
85. Lee WM, Stravitz RT, Larson AM. Introduction to the revised American Association for the Study of Liver Diseases Position Paper on acute liver failure 2011. Hepatology 2012;55(3):965–7.
86. Bailey B, Amre DK, Gaudreault P. Fulminant hepatic failure secondary to acetaminophen poisoning: a systematic review and meta-analysis of prognostic criteria determining the need for liver transplantation. Crit Care Med 2003; 31(1):299–305.
87. Schmidt LE, Larsen FS. MELD score as a predictor of liver failure and death in patients with acetaminophen-induced liver injury. Hepatology 2007;45(3):789–96.
88. Cholongitas E, Theocharidou E, Vasianopoulou P, et al. Comparison of the sequential organ failure assessment score with the King's College Hospital criteria and the model for end-stage liver disease score for the prognosis of acetaminophen-induced acute liver failure. Liver Transpl 2012;18(4):405–12.
89. Craig DG, Reid TW, Wright EC, et al. The sequential organ failure assessment (SOFA) score is prognostically superior to the model for end-stage liver disease (MELD) and MELD variants following paracetamol (acetaminophen) overdose. Aliment Pharmacol Ther 2012;35(6):705–13.
90. Craig DG, Zafar S, Reid TW, et al. The sequential organ failure assessment (SOFA) score is an effective triage marker following staggered paracetamol (acetaminophen) overdose. Aliment Pharmacol Ther 2012;35(12):1408–15.
91. Mitchell I, Bihari D, Chang R, et al. Earlier identification of patients at risk from acetaminophen-induced acute liver failure. Crit Care Med 1998;26(2):279–84.
92. James LP, Letzig L, Simpson PM, et al. Pharmacokinetics of acetaminophen-protein adducts in adults with acetaminophen overdose and acute liver failure. Drug Metab Dispos 2009;37(8):1779–84.
93. Davern TJ II, James LP, Hinson JA, et al. Measurement of serum acetaminophen-protein adducts in patients with acute liver failure. Gastroenterology 2006;130(3):687–94.
94. Spiller HA, Krenzelok EP, Grande GA, et al. A prospective evaluation of the effect of activated charcoal before oral N-acetylcysteine in acetaminophen overdose. Ann Emerg Med 1994;23(3):519–23.
95. Spiller HA, Winter ML, Klein-Schwartz W, et al. Efficacy of activated charcoal administered more than four hours after acetaminophen overdose. J Emerg Med 2006;30(1):1–5.
96. Underhill TJ, Greene MK, Dove AF. A comparison of the efficacy of gastric lavage, ipecacuanha and activated charcoal in the emergency management of paracetamol overdose. Arch Emerg Med 1990;7(3):148–54.
97. Christophersen AB, Levin D, Hoegberg LC, et al. Activated charcoal alone or after gastric lavage: a simulated large paracetamol intoxication. Br J Clin Pharmacol 2002;53(3):312–7.
98. Lin JH, Levy G. Sulfate depletion after acetaminophen administration and replenishment by infusion of sodium sulfate or N-acetylcysteine in rats. Biochem Pharmacol 1981;30(19):2723–5.
99. Lauterburg BH, Corcoran GB, Mitchell JR. Mechanism of action of N-acetylcysteine in the protection against the hepatotoxicity of acetaminophen in rats in vivo. J Clin Invest 1983;71(4):980–91.

100. Brok J, Buckley N, Gluud C. Interventions for paracetamol (acetaminophen) overdose. Cochrane Database Syst Rev 2006;(2):CD003328.
101. Prescott LF, Park J, Ballantyne A, et al. Treatment of paracetamol (acetaminophen) poisoning with N-acetylcysteine. Lancet 1977;2(8035):432–4.
102. Harrison PM, Keays R, Bray GP, et al. Improved outcome of paracetamol-induced fulminant hepatic failure by late administration of acetylcysteine. Lancet 1990;335(8705):1572–3.
103. Keays R, Harrison PM, Wendon JA, et al. Intravenous acetylcysteine in paracetamol induced fulminant hepatic failure: a prospective controlled trial. BMJ 1991; 303(6809):1026–9.
104. Lee WM, Hynan LS, Rossaro L, et al. Intravenous N-acetylcysteine improves transplant-free survival in early stage non-acetaminophen acute liver failure. Gastroenterology 2009;137(3):856–64, 864.e1.
105. Varney SM, Buchanan JA, Kokko J, et al. Acetylcysteine for acetaminophen overdose in patients who weigh >100 kg. Am J Ther 2012. [Epub ahead of print].
106. Kanter MZ. Comparison of oral and i.v. acetylcysteine in the treatment of acetaminophen poisoning. Am J Health Syst Pharm 2006;63(19):1821–7.
107. Dawson AH, Henry DA, McEwen J. Adverse reactions to N-acetylcysteine during treatment for paracetamol poisoning. Med J Aust 1989;150(6):329–31.
108. Kerr F, Dawson A, Whyte IM, et al. The Australasian Clinical Toxicology Investigators Collaboration randomized trial of different loading infusion rates of N-acetylcysteine. Ann Emerg Med 2005;45(4):402–8.
109. Bailey B, McGuigan MA. Management of anaphylactoid reactions to intravenous N-acetylcysteine. Ann Emerg Med 1998;31(6):710–5.
110. Betten DP, Burner EE, Thomas SC, et al. A retrospective evaluation of shortened-duration oral N-acetylcysteine for the treatment of acetaminophen poisoning. J Med Toxicol 2009;5(4):183–90.
111. Betten DP, Cantrell FL, Thomas SC, et al. A prospective evaluation of shortened course oral N-acetylcysteine for the treatment of acute acetaminophen poisoning. Ann Emerg Med 2007;50(3):272–9.
112. Woo OF, Mueller PD, Olson KR, et al. Shorter duration of oral N-acetylcysteine therapy for acute acetaminophen overdose. Ann Emerg Med 2000;35(4):363–8.
113. Yip L, Dart RC. A 20-hour treatment for acute acetaminophen overdose. N Engl J Med 2003;348(24):2471–2.
114. Tsai CL, Chang WT, Weng TI, et al. A patient-tailored N-acetylcysteine protocol for acute acetaminophen intoxication. Clin Ther 2005;27(3):336–41.
115. Smilkstein MJ, Bronstein AC, Linden C, et al. Acetaminophen overdose: a 48-hour intravenous N-acetylcysteine treatment protocol. Ann Emerg Med 1991;20(10):1058–63.
116. Fontana RJ. Acute liver failure including acetaminophen overdose. Med Clin North Am 2008;92(4):761–94, viii.
117. Speeg KV Jr, Mitchell MC, Maldonado AL. Additive protection of cimetidine and N-acetylcysteine treatment against acetaminophen-induced hepatic necrosis in the rat. J Pharmacol Exp Ther 1985;234(3):550–4.
118. Burkhart KK, Janco N, Kulig KW, et al. Cimetidine as adjunctive treatment for acetaminophen overdose. Hum Exp Toxicol 1995;14(3):299–304.
119. Slattery JT, McRorie TI, Reynolds R, et al. Lack of effect of cimetidine on acetaminophen disposition in humans. Clin Pharmacol Ther 1989;46(5):591–7.
120. Kaplowitz N. Acetaminophen hepatoxicity: what do we know, what don't we know, and what do we do next? Hepatology 2004;40(1):23–6.

121. Scheiermann P, Bachmann M, Goren I, et al. Application of interleukin-22 mediates protection in experimental acetaminophen-induced acute liver injury. Am J Pathol 2013;182(4):1107–13.
122. Fouad AA, Al-Mulhim AS, Jresat I, et al. Therapeutic role of telmisartan against acetaminophen hepatotoxicity in mice. Eur J Pharmacol 2012;693(1–3):64–71.
123. Fouad AA, Jresat I. Hepatoprotective effect of coenzyme Q10 in rats with acetaminophen toxicity. Environ Toxicol Pharmacol 2012;33(2):158–67.

# Hepatotoxicity of Antibiotics
## A Review and Update for the Clinician

Jonathan G. Stine, MD, James H. Lewis, MD*

## KEYWORDS

- Drug-induced liver injury • Antibiotics • Drug safety • Monitoring

## KEY POINTS

- Antimicrobial agents head the list of drugs leading to acute drug-induced liver injury (DILI) among nonacetaminophen causes.
- Amoxicillin-clavulanate, nitrofurantoin, flucloxacillin, trimethoprim-sulfamethoxazole, and isoniazid and other antituberculosis drugs are the most commonly implicated, as reflected in large international DILI registries.
- Antibiotic-induced hepatotoxicity is often difficult to diagnose because it may be clinically similar to other causes of acute hepatitis and can be confounded by the hepatic manifestations of infectious disease being treated, as well as the presence of sepsis, multiple transfusions, hemolysis, and other causes of hepatic dysfunction and jaundice that can complicate the postoperative, intensive care unit, and a variety of outpatient settings.
- The delayed onset of hepatic injury after the discontinuation of agents such as amoxicillin-clavulanate can further complicate the diagnostic assessment.
- A high clinical index of suspicion will remain necessary until pharmacogenomic testing or other biomarkers become routinely available to predict or confirm that hepatotoxicity is related to a particular antibiotic.

## INTRODUCTION

Collectively, the various classes of antibiotics are a leading cause of drug-induced liver injury (DILI).[1,2] Indeed, among causes of nonacetaminophen-related acute DILI, antimicrobial agents lead the list in various worldwide registries, as well as heading the lists of drug causes of nonacetaminophen-related acute liver failure (ALF).[3–9] Acute antibiotic-associated DILI, however, can be difficult to diagnose, as the course of therapy is usually brief, ranging from a few days to a few weeks, and other confounding factors are often present. In some instances, as can be seen with amoxicillin-clavulanate, hepatic injury can be delayed until as many as 6 to 7 weeks after the course of therapy has been completed, further complicating causality assessment.

Division of Gastroenterology and Hepatology, Department of Medicine, Georgetown University Medical Center, 3800 Reservoir Road, NW Room M2408, Washington, DC 20007, USA
* Corresponding author.
E-mail address: lewisjh@gunet.georgetown.edu

Clin Liver Dis 17 (2013) 609–642
http://dx.doi.org/10.1016/j.cld.2013.07.008
1089-3261/13/$ – see front matter © 2013 Elsevier Inc. All rights reserved.

Moreover, antibiotic-associated hepatotoxicity can mimic nearly all forms of acute and chronic liver injury, adding to the difficulties in determining causation.[1] For example, when taken chronically, several antibiotics (eg, nitrofurantoin, minocycline) are known to cause liver disease with features of autoimmune hepatitis. Antituberculosis drugs (ATDs) may cause acute hepatocellular liver injury at any point during their 4- to 12-month duration of use. Finally, several antimicrobials are associated with a chronic cholestasis resulting from the vanishing bile duct syndrome (VBDS).[10]

In addition to the broad clinicopathologic spectrum of hepatotoxicity associated with the antimicrobials, the underlying infectious disease being treated may itself be associated with hepatic dysfunction and jaundice.[11] Illnesses such as Q fever, pneumococcal pneumonia, leptospirosis, and typhoid fever are among the classic infections leading to jaundice, making recognition of DILI more difficult. Similarly, sepsis and septic shock may lead to jaundice and can be significant confounders when antibiotic-related injury is being considered.

Several antibiotics seem to be particularly well suited to pharmacogenomic studies in determining an individual's susceptibility to injury. Following the example of abacavir, whereby human leukocyte antigen (HLA) B*5701 was demonstrated in the majority of patients who developed severe drug-induced skin injury (some of whom also demonstrated hepatotoxicity),[12] Daly and colleagues[13,14] have described specific HLA haplotypes that convey an increased risk of DILI for several antibiotics. The association of HLA B*5701 with hypersensitivity reactions with abacavir was sufficiently robust that recommendations for its testing in all patients due to receive the drug have been made by the Food and Drug Administration (FDA). Moreover, if the at-risk HLA phenotype is present, the agent is not prescribed.[15] However, to date the predictive accuracy of pharmacogenomic biomarkers for other antimicrobials has not been high enough to warrant withholding these antibiotics, especially when their planned use is short term and the benefits appear to outweigh any risk.[16]

This review provides summarized information on several classes of antimicrobial agents, highlighting new agents causing DILI and updating information on older agents.

## INCIDENCE OF ANTIBIOTIC DILI

With the appearance of several large international DILI registries, the incidence of severe DILI caused by antimicrobial agents can now be more precisely determined. As seen in **Table 1**, antimicrobials as the cause of ALF leading to transplant, as a percentage of all DILI cases, ranges from 13.5% to as much as 65% of cases seen in India.[3–9] Antimicrobials were the most common cause for nonacetaminophen (non-APAP) DILI ALF in the most recent US Acute Liver Failure Study Group (ALFSG) analysis (46% of the >60 drugs implicated), among which ATDs predominated.[5] Isoniazid (INH) was implicated in 21 cases, 15 as monotherapy and 6 when used in combination. Sulfa-containing drugs frequently caused ALF, with 9 reported cases of trimethoprim-sulfamethoxazole (TMP/SMX), 6 alone and 3 when used in combination with azithromycin, a statin, and/or antiretroviral compounds. Nitrofurantoin was implicated 12 times, with 11 individual cases, 1 in combination with a statin. Terbinafine and azole antifungal drugs were relatively common as well (n = 6). Among the causes of drug-induced ALF requiring transplantation,[6] antibiotics accounted for more than one-third of cases (21 of 56). Transplant-free survival was similar for the 14 cases of antimicrobial DILI in comparison with all drug classes (27% 3-week survival). Seventeen of an all-cause total of 41 patients with antimicrobial ALF died without transplant.

**Table 1**
**Summary of international DILI registries and antimicrobials**

| Authors,[Ref.] Year | Country and Years Covered | Antimicrobials as % of All DILI Cases | Comment |
|---|---|---|---|
| Bjornsson & Olsson,[3] 2005 | Sweden (1970–2004) | 32.3% (n = 252/784) | |
| Mindikoglu et al,[6] 2009 | USA (1987–2006) | 13.5% (n = 89/661) | ALF leading to OLT in UNOS database |
| Andrade et al,[4] 2005 | Spain (1994–2004) | 22.6% (n = 101/446) | |
| Devarbhavi et al,[7] 2010 | India (1997–2008) | 65.2% (n = 204/313) | Majority related to ATDs |
| Reuben et al,[5] 2010 | US Acute Liver Failure Study Group (1998–2007) | 39% (n = 52/133) | Drug-induced ALF cases |
| Chalasani et al,[8] 2008 | DILIN network USA (2003–2007) | 43.3% (n = 130/300) | |

*Abbreviations:* ALF, acute liver failure; ATD, antituberculosis drug; OLT, orthotopic liver transplantation; UNOS, United Network for Organ Sharing.

Among instances of non-ALF, registries in the United States, Spain, and other European centers also demonstrate that a large proportion of cases are due to antimicrobials.[3,4,8,9] The various classes represent between 30% and 40% of instances of severe DILI, and the individual antimicrobials implicated in these DILI registries are listed in **Table 2**. Multiple agents have been implicated, many in combination with either other antimicrobials or other classes of drugs, indicating the difficulty in separating out one possible etiologic agent from another. In the US DILI Network registry,[8] of the initial 217 subjects with suspected DILI from a single agent, antimicrobials accounted for 94 cases (43%), with the most common drugs being amoxicillin-clavulanate (n = 23), nitrofurantoin (n = 13), INH (n = 13), TMP/SMX (n = 9), ciprofloxacin and telithromycin (n = 5 each), and terbinafine and levofloxacin (n = 4 each).

Whereas amoxicillin-clavulanate leads the list of all-cause non-APAP DILI in the United States[8] as well as Spain[4] (59 of 446 = 13% overall; and 59% of all antimicrobials and 67% of all antibacterials for systemic use, respectively), other agents are more commonly implicated in other series, reflecting the regional nature of the infectious diseases being treated. For example, ATDs are the most commonly implicated agents in India,[7] both in terms of numbers of instances of DILI (58%) and fatal cases (21.5%). In Sweden, flucloxacillin was the most common antibiotic implicated in acute DILI, followed by erythromycin and TMP/SMX[3] Flucloxacillin was also among the most common causes of drug-induced jaundice in a large registry of DILI cases at a single Swedish center over a recent 10-year period.[9]

**Table 3** lists the antimicrobials in the World Health Organization safety database[17] and shows the most commonly implicated agents reported to cause acute hepatic injury, including ALF, as recorded between 1970 and 2008. This database lists 20 of the most commonly prescribed antibiotics worldwide, with flucloxacillin dominating the list along with INH and rifampin. Trovafloxacin, which is more widely used outside the United States, accounted for more than 15% of cases, as did erythromycin. Amoxicillin-clavulanate was also one of the more common agents, as was a relatively new agent, telithromycin, the first of the ketolide antibiotics.[17]

**Table 2**
**Individual antimicrobials implicated in various DILI registries**

| Authors,[Ref.] Year | Country (N) | Antibiotics Listed | Comments |
|---|---|---|---|
| Chalasani et al,[8] 2008 | DILI Network USA (N = 300) | Amoxicillin-clavulanate (n = 23)<br>Nitrofurantoin (n = 13)<br>Isoniazid (n = 13)<br>TMP/SMX (n = 9)<br>Ciprofloxacin (n = 5)<br>Telithromycin (n = 5)<br>Terbinafine (n = 4)<br>Levofloxacin (n = 4)<br>Azithromycin (n = 3)<br>Oxacillin (n = 3)<br>Minocycline (n = 3)<br>Amoxicillin (n = 2)<br>Doxycycline (n = 2)<br>Fluconazole (n = 2)<br>*One case each*:<br>Itraconazole<br>Linezolid<br>Moxifloxacin<br>Cephalexin<br>Cefazolin<br>Cefuroxime<br>Ceftriaxone<br>Gentamicin<br>Ketoconazole<br>Pyrazinamide<br>Cilastatin/imipenem<br>Clindamycin<br>Rifampin<br>*Combination therapy*:<br>TMP/SMX + levofloxacin<br>Nitrofurantoin + atorvastatin<br>Levofloxacin + valproate<br>Moxifloxacin, ciprofloxacin + amoxicillin/clavulanate<br>Levofloxacin + phenytoin<br>Levofloxacin + clindamycin<br>Nitrofurantoin + MVI<br>TMP/SMX + tetracycline<br>Ciprofloxacin + metronidazole<br>Cefuroxime + nystatin<br>Cephalexin + levofloxacin<br>Amoxicillin, Methyl 1-D, Cell-Tech<br>Azithromycin + ceftriaxone<br>Nitrofurantoin + azithromycin<br>Levofloxacin + escitalopram<br>Isoniazid + pyrazinamide<br>Telithromycin + doxycycline<br>Metronidazole + mercaptopurine<br>Telithromycin + nitrofurantoin<br>Isoniazid + fenofibrate<br>Telithromycin + amoxicillin/ clavulanate<br>Gatifloxacin + amoxicillin/clavulanate<br>Doxycycline + glibenclamide<br>Azithromycin + TMP/SMX<br>Clindamycin + diclofenac + lovastatin<br>Levofloxacin + valsartan | |

(*continued on next page*)

**Table 2**
*(continued)*

| Authors,[Ref.] Year | Country (N) | Antibiotics Listed | Comments |
|---|---|---|---|
| Bjornsson & Olsson,[3] 2005 | Sweden (N = 784) | Flucloxacillin (n = 129)<br>Erythromycin (n = 42)<br>TMP/SMX (n = 21)<br>Isoniazid (n = 7)<br>Ciprofloxacin (n = 7)<br>Dicloxacillin (n = 3)<br>Pivmecillinam (n = 3) | *Injury pattern:*<br>HC 76<br>Cholestatic/<br>  mixed 149<br>*Outcome:*<br>Death or OLT 16 |
| Andrade et al,[4] 2005 | Spain (N = 461) | Amoxicillin-clavulanate (n = 59)<br>Isoniazid + rifampin + pyrazinamide (n = 22)<br>Isoniazid (n = 9)<br>Erythromycin (n = 6)<br>Trovafloxacin (n = 5) | *Injury pattern:*<br>HC 34<br>Cholestatic 20<br>Mixed 25<br>*Outcome:*<br>65 hospitalized<br>5 ALF, 2 OLT, 7 death |
| Devarbhavi et al,[7] 2010 | India (N = 313) | Antituberculosis drugs (n = 181)<br>Dapsone (n = 17)<br>Amoxicillin–clavulanic acid (n = 3)<br>*Other antibiotics:*<br>Ceftriaxone<br>Fluconazole<br>Chloroquine | *Outcome (death):*<br>Antituberculosis drugs (n = 39)<br>Dapsone (n = 2)<br>Amoxicillin–clavulanic acid (n = 1) |
| Reuben et al,[5] 2010 | US ALFSG (N = 133) | *Antituberculosis drugs:*<br>Isoniazid (n = 15)<br>Isoniazid combined with 2 of 3:<br>  rifampicin, pyrazinamide,<br>  ethambutol (n = 6)<br>Rifampin and pyrazinamide with or<br>  without ethambutol (n = 3)<br>Dapsone (n = 1)<br>*Sulfur-containing drugs:*<br>TMP/SMX (n = 6)<br>TMP/SMX in combination with<br>  azithromycin, statin, and/or<br>  antiretroviral drugs (n = 3)<br>Sulfasalazine (n = 3)<br>*Other antibiotics:*<br>Nitrofurantoin (n = 11)<br>Nitrofurantoin with a statin (n = 1)<br>Amoxicillin (n = 2)<br>Doxycycline (n = 2)<br>Ciprofloxacin (n = 1)<br>Clarithromycin (n = 1)<br>Cefepime (n = 1)<br>*Antifungal agents:*<br>Terbinafine (n = 3)<br>Itraconazole (n = 1)<br>Ketoconazole (n = 1)<br>Ketoconazole with ezetimibe (n = 1) | All ALF cases |

*(continued on next page)*

**Table 2**
**(continued)**

| Authors,[Ref.] Year | Country (N) | Antibiotics Listed | Comments |
|---|---|---|---|
| Mindikoglu et al,[6] 2009 | UNOS US database (N = 661) | *Antituberculosis drugs:*<br>Isoniazid alone (n = 48)<br>Isoniazid with another antituberculosis drug (n = 2)<br>*Antibiotics:*<br>Nitrofurantoin (n = 12)<br>Ketoconazole (n = 8)<br>Amoxicillin and clavulanate (n = 5)<br>TMP/SMX (n = 5)<br>Minocycline (n = 7)<br>*Other antibiotics (n = 20):*<br>Terbinafine<br>Ciprofloxacin<br>Telithromycin<br>Levofloxacin<br>Itraconazole<br>Moxifloxacin | Causes of emergency liver transplant for drug-induced ALF |

*Abbreviations:* ALF, acute liver failure; ALFSG, Acute Liver Failure Multicenter Study Group; HC, hepatocellular; MVI, intravenous multivitamin concentrate; OLT, orthotopic liver transplantation; TMP/SMX, trimethoprim-sulfamethoxazole.

## INFECTIONS CAUSING JAUNDICE

Confounders to the diagnosis of antimicrobial-associated DILI are found in several settings, including infections themselves.[10,18] In the hospitalized patient, sepsis is a well-known cause of jaundice, especially when caused by urinary infections in children.[19] In a Japanese series, 33% of patients with sepsis-associated liver injury had jaundice.[20] Patients without underlying liver disease who have developed severe life-threatening sepsis, often requiring mechanical ventilation with positive end-expiratory pressure, have not only jaundice[21] but also significant necroinflammation, cholestasis, and steatosis, mimicking hepatitis on liver biopsy.[22] The jaundice associated with sepsis is usually cholestatic, with bilirubin levels often as high as 30 mg/dL, sometimes reaching 50 mg/dL or more. It generally resolves within a few weeks with appropriate supportive care in survivors.

Several other infections are also associated with jaundice. The association between pneumococcal pneumonia and clinical jaundice goes back decades.[23] Indeed, the presence of jaundice in various series ranged as high as 67% and may have been related to an increased frequency of hemolysis secondary to glucose-6-phosphate dehydrogenase deficiency.[23] Among gram-negative bacillary infections, typhoid fever caused by *Salmonella typhosa* is associated with jaundice in 10% to 15% of cases, and acute typhoid hepatitis may resemble acute viral hepatitis.[24]

In leptospirosis, jaundice may be present in more severe forms of the diagnosis (Weil disease), with a biphasic pattern of renal failure with hemorrhagic phenomenon and a high case-fatality rate. In a series from India, jaundice was a presenting feature in 17.6% of cases and was found in 74.5% overall.[25] Tuberculosis (TB), though very commonly involving the liver, only rarely leads to clinical jaundice.[26] Among the rickettsiae, Q fever caused by *Coxiella burnetii* usually is associated with a self-limited pneumonitis, with jaundice seen in up to 5% of cases. In pyogenic liver abscess, jaundice is reported to be a common manifestation in up to 20% to 40% of instances.[18]

**Table 3**
**Antimicrobial-related DILI and ALF in World Health Organization individual case safety report database (VigiBase)**

| Antibiotic | Total No. of Reports | Incidence of Liver-Related Events (%) | Incidence of ALF (%) |
|---|---|---|---|
| Amoxicillin | 30963 | 1.9 | 0.1 |
| Amoxicillin–clavulanic acid | 20761 | 16.7 | 0.4 |
| Azithromycin | 10577 | 5.9 | 0.6 |
| Cefuroxime | 8443 | 4.0 | 0.1 |
| Ciprofloxacin | 19915 | 6.1 | 0.4 |
| Cloxacillin | 7593 | 1.9 | 0.0 |
| Cotrimoxazole | 46689 | 4.9 | 0.2 |
| Doxycycline | 9149 | 3.9 | 0.3 |
| Erythromycin | 16436 | 15.3 | 0.2 |
| Flucloxacillin (foxacillin) | 4261 | 34.5 | 0.4 |
| Isoniazid | 8582 | 29.0 | 1.6 |
| Levofloxacin | 9953 | 4.5 | 0.7 |
| Minocycline | 6867 | 10.1 | 0.2 |
| Nitrofurantoin | 10854 | 10.5 | 0.7 |
| Norfloxacin | 6215 | 5.0 | 0.2 |
| Rifampicin (rifampin) | 7858 | 32.2 | 1.6 |
| Telithromycin | 2603 | 16.2 | 1.9 |
| Terbinafine | 14123 | 8.4 | 0.2 |
| Trimethoprim | 6114 | 2.9 | 0.1 |
| Trovafloxacin | 3877 | 15.4 | 2.6 |

*Data from* Suzuki A, Andrade RJ, Bjornsson E, et al. Drugs associated with hepatotoxicity and their reporting frequency of liver adverse events in VigiBase: unified list based on international collaborative work. Drug Saf 2010;33(6):503–22.

In the post–liver transplant (LT) setting, TMP/SMX[27] and antifungal agents[28] are among the most commonly identified drugs causing DILI, although assessing the cause of posttransplant hepatic dysfunction and rejection can be difficult. Instances of post-LT antibiotic-related DILI have also been reported with nafcillin, clarithromycin, daptomycin, and ertapenem.[27] Post-LT DILI is generally mild and the clinical course often self-limited, probably owing to the frequent liver-associated enzyme monitoring carried out in the post-LT period.

In the surgical setting, antibiotics are used both for preoperative prophylaxis and postoperative prevention of infection, and hepatotoxicity may be due to any number of other causes, including anesthetic-related liver injury, or jaundice from resorbing hematomas, the use of multiple blood product transfusions, and hemolysis, among others.[29]

Acute hepatitis E (HEV) is being found more commonly outside of the usual endemic areas and, not surprisingly, is being diagnosed as an alternative cause of DILI.[30–32] In a recent United Kingdom series, about 20% of suspected DILI cases were found to be due to acute HEV.[32] Similarly, in the US DILI Network,[31] several patients who were initially suspected as having antimicrobial-related DILI subsequently tested positive for acute HEV with positive immunoglobulin M serology (1 case each of suspected DILI from azithromycin, INH, and telithromycin were rediagnosed as acute HEV infection using stored sera). Just how often acute HEV might have been the true cause of other cases labeled as DILI is not known, but may be appreciable.

## PHARMACOGENOMICS, BIOMARKERS, AND ANTIBIOTIC DILI

Genome-wide association studies have detected specific HLA genotypes that can predict DILI caused by several agents, mainly flucloxacillin and amoxicillin-clavulanate.[13,14,33–35] Lucena and colleagues[33] identified both HLA class I and II antigens for amoxicillin-clavulanate, the most significant effect being with the HLA class II SNP rs9274407 ($P = 4.8 \times 10^{-14}$); however, given the low positive predictive values from their study, they found that there is limited utility for identifying HLA genotypes as predictive or biomarkers for DILI with amoxicillin-clavulanate at present,[33] echoing the findings of others.[16]

The various metabolic polymorphisms associated with ATDs suggest that slow acetylator status, reflected in NAT2 and CYP2E1, is an apparent risk factor for susceptibility to severe DILI.[36–39] However, in contrast to the situation with abacavir,[15] the authors are unaware of any studies with ATDs whereby these particular pharmacogenomic biomarkers have been used to withhold treatment.[40] Nonetheless, it is anticipated that the identification of more accurate, validated biomarkers to predict DILI before the development of elevated liver-associated enzymes (LAEs) will become available in the near future for many classes of agents, including antibiotics. Although a universally predictive biomarker has remained elusive,[40] several antibiotics remain at the center of pharmacogenomic study, and have brought us closer to identifying those at greatest risk of DILI. In this regard, tumor necrosis factor α, interferon-γ, interleukin-1α, and interleukin-6 have been identified as possible indicators of DILI induced by trovafloxacin and clarithromycin, and may offer potential for future use.[41]

Proteomic-based biomarkers, such as apolipoprotein E from stored sera in the US DILI Network, have been identified as potential candidates for several drugs, including several antibiotics. Bell and colleagues[42] examined samples from 74 DILI patients collected within 14 days of onset of acute DILI and compared them with the profiles of 40 healthy controls. The most commonly reported antibiotics in this series were INH (n = 5), amoxicillin-clavulanate (n = 3), nitrofurantoin (n = 3), minocycline, TMP/SMX, and telithromycin. Antifungal agents were implicated when prescribed in combination with another hepatotoxic medication. Apolipoprotein E expression was increased in those with acute DILI of all causes (not just antibiotics), and correctly identified DILI in 89% of samples (with an area under the receiver-operating characteristic curve of 0.97). Although apolipoprotein E is involved with acute-phase injury and inflammatory responses and appears to be a promising biomarker to identify patients who develop acute DILI, given the large number of different causative agents and the small number of patients exposed to any individual drug, these investigators were unable to determine whether there were any specific differences in the protein expression for the DILI caused by any of the specific medications, including antibiotics. **Table 4** provides a summary of potential DILI biomarkers for antibiotics.[43–52]

## INDIVIDUAL ANTIMICROBIAL AGENTS: WHAT'S NEW?
### Penicillins

Whereas native penicillins commonly lead to generalized hypersensitivity reactions, they are only rarely associated with hepatic injury, as attested to by very few instances of hepatotoxicity having been reported over several decades.[53–55] Several

**Table 4**
**Genetic risk factors for DILI**

| Drug | Proposed Mechanism/Genetic Risk Factor |
|---|---|
| Amoxicillin-clavulanate[33] | HLA class II SNP rs9274407 |
| Antituberculosis drugs[36,43–46] | NAT2 polymorphism<br>CYP2E1 polymorphisms<br>Drug transporter genes (ABCB1, SLCO1B1, ABCC2)<br>UGTA1 polymorphism<br>Pregnane X receptor (PXR) |
| Flucloxacillin[47–49,51] | PXR polymorphism (rs3814055; C-25385 T)<br>HLA B*5701 |
| Isoniazid[50] | Bcl-2 downregulation<br>CYP2E1 polymorphism<br>NAT2 polymorphism |
| Trovafloxacin[52] | Superoxide dismutase defect (SOD2) |

of the semisynthetic penicillin derivatives (eg, oxacillin, carbenicillin, and ampicillin) seem to produce jaundice or biochemical evidence of hepatic injury more commonly.[56–58] Cloxacillin, dicloxacillin, and floxacillin have led to multiple instances of cholestatic hepatitis.[59–61] Flucloxacillin seems to produce hepatic injury with a higher frequency,[62] and was the leading cause of antibiotic DILI in a Swedish registry.[3] Instances of cholestasis have persisted for up to 6 months, some complicated by VBDS.[63,64]

The combination drug amoxicillin-clavulanate is the most commonly listed cause of non-APAP DILI in the United States[8] and Spain (see **Table 2**).[4,65] It has been estimated to cause 1 case of jaundice for every 78,000 prescriptions.[66] In contrast to many other drug classes where females are at higher risk, older males may be predisposed to injury, with an incidence severalfold higher when 2 or more courses of therapy have been prescribed.[67] The mean onset of jaundice among 22 cases from Scotland was 17 days after the start of therapy,[66] but a delay of up to 6 to 7 weeks has been reported,[68] with hypersensitivity features present in up to two-thirds of cases. Interstitial nephritis and sialadenitis have accompanied some instances of injury.[69] Clavulanate is considered to be the hepatotoxic component, as the combination is more hepatotoxic than amoxicillin alone.[70]

Hepatic injury has also been reported with the combination of ticarcillin and clavulanate.[71] An immunoallergic mechanism seems likely, and a higher frequency of certain HLA haplotypes has been found as one possible predisposing factor (DRB1*1501/DRB5*0101/DQB1*0602).[66,69] Histologically, centrilobular cholestasis with a mixed portal inflammatory infiltrate, variable portal edema, and interlobular bile duct injury with bile duct proliferation has been described.[69] A case of granulomatous hepatitis also has been attributed to this combination drug.[72] Recovery usually occurs within 1 to 4 months, although fatal outcomes have been reported.[69]

### Cephalosporins

First-generation and second-generation cephalosporins are rarely associated with DILI, and only a few instances of cholestatic hepatic injury have been reported.[1] Ceftriaxone, a third-generation agent, is associated with formation of biliary sludge that can cause jaundice and symptoms of cholecystitis.[73,74] However, many cephalosporins are used regularly and safely in patients with cholangitis, biliary sepsis, and bacterial peritonitis, given their excellent coverage of gram-negative organisms.

### Fluoroquinolones

Injury by fluoroquinolones is uncommon, but may be either cholestatic or hepatocellular, likely because of hypersensitivity. Implicated drugs have included the first-generation agent nalidixic acid, the second-generation drugs norfloxacin, ciprofloxacin, and ofloxacin, and the third-generation products levofloxacin, moxifloxacin, and gatifloxacin (which has been reported to cause severe hepatocellular injury,[75,76] possibly associated with pancreatitis).[6,77] Granulomatous hepatitis has been described with norfloxacin,[78] and prolonged cholestasis is seen with ciprofloxacin.[79]

A fourth-generation agent, trovafloxacin, is associated with severe hepatic injury,[52,80–83] and its use in the United States has been restricted to inpatients under the direction of infectious disease experts. Reversible trovafloxacin-associated acute hepatocellular injury with peripheral and histologic eosinophilia has been described.[81,83] Liver biopsy findings have revealed perivenular and focal periportal necrosis with eosinophilic infiltration.[81,83] Trovafloxacin has a difluorophenyl substitution of position N-1 of the naphthyridone ring that is implicated in the development of hypersensitivity reactions.[82] A similar structure is seen with temafloxacin, which may account for its immunoallergic manifestations.[84] By contrast, the other quinolones have a different chemical structure and/or differences in P450 metabolism,[85] although eosinophilia has been described with their use as well.[86]

### Sulfonamides

These agents (sulfisoxazole, sulfamethoxazole) have been incriminated in hundreds of instances of hepatic injury.[1] Many have shown hepatic necrosis and hepatocellular jaundice, although reports of cholestatic injury and granulomas have been described. The hepatic injury pattern caused by sulfonamides appears to be mixed, and the mechanism involves hypersensitivity, including instances of Steven-Johnson syndrome.[87–89] Affected individuals may be predisposed by aberrant production and detoxification of hydroxylamine derivatives.[90,91] Prompt recurrence of injury is seen on rechallenge, and some patients have developed fulminant hepatitis.[92,93]

The potential for hepatotoxicity with TMP/SMX has been known for decades.[93] Toxicity often occurs with rash and various cytopenias.[94,95] Nevertheless, TMP/SMX is often used in the first 3 months after liver transplant to prevent *Pneumocystis carinii* pneumonia and, perhaps not unexpectedly, was the most commonly implicated agent in a cohort of post-LT DILI cases.[27]

TMP/SMX has led to several instances of acute cholestatic and hepatocellular injury (in some cases accompanied by pancreatitis),[96] although the injury appears to be more commonly cholestatic,[97,98] and instances of chronic cholestasis leading to VBDS have appeared.[99,100] Fulminant hepatic failure requiring LT has been reported, although the elevation of the enzymes (aspartate aminotransferase [AST] >23,000 and alanine aminotransferase [ALT] >11,000) suggests possible concurrent ischemic hepatitis.[93] Although the sulfonamide component has been implicated as the main cause of the disorder,[88] there is evidence that the trimethoprim can also contribute.[101] A significantly higher incidence of hypersensitivity reactions is found in HIV-positive patients receiving TMP/SMX compared with the general population (up to 70% vs 3%),[102] suggesting that care should be taken in this setting.

Sulfones, long used in the treatment of leprosy, seem to produce hepatic injury more often than do the sulfonamides.[1] The incidence has been reported to be about 2% to 5% in recipients of the prototypic compound dapsone.[103,104] Jaundice appears to be mixed hepatocellular, with histologic changes that include inflammation with sinusoidal beading and nonzonal necrosis. The mechanism for the hepatic injury is presumably hypersensitivity associated with a syndrome that includes an erythematous maculopapular skin eruption, fever, hepatomegaly, pruritus, lymphadenopathy, edema, and jaundice.[105] A latency of 2 to 7 weeks is seen after the start of treatment, and has led to fatal hepatitis.[105] Methemoglobinemia, hemolytic anemia, and hypoproteinemia may also be prominent features of the sulfone syndrome.[105]

### Tetracyclines

Tetracyclines characteristically caused microvesicular steatosis when given intravenously to pregnant women in a dose of 1.5 g/d or more, especially during the last trimester of pregnancy or in the setting of renal disease.[106] The hepatotoxicity was severe, resembling acute fatty liver of pregnancy or Reye syndrome,[107] and the lesion has been reproduced in experimental animals.[108] Although pregnancy seemed to enhance susceptibility to tetracycline-induced hepatic injury, nonpregnant females and males are also susceptible.[109] Hepatocytes contain innumerable small fat droplets that may be best seen on oil-red-O staining, and there is little or no necrosis and minimal cholestasis.[110] The clinical manifestations after intravenous tetracycline included nausea, vomiting, and abdominal pain, possibly related to the frequently associated pancreatitis. Jaundice was rarely severe, but most of the reported patients died.[106,109] Less severe cases may have been unrecognized or unrecorded. The mechanism is intrinsic hepatotoxicity caused by the inhibition of transport of lipid from the liver and impaired mitochondrial oxidation of fatty acids.[108,111] Tetracycline-induced microvesicular steatosis has lost its practical importance, because intravenous administration of the drug is nowadays rarely used. However, oral tetracycline has been implicated in chronic cholestasis accompanied by depletion of interlobular bile ducts (VBDS).[112]

Minocycline, a derivative of tetracycline often used to treat adolescent acne, can also produce steatosis, although it has been implicated in several dozen cases of hepatocellular injury, some acute and some with features of chronic hepatitis, and many with accompanying features of autoimmune hepatitis, including autoantibodies.[113–116] Three separate clinical presentations have been observed: a rapid-onset serum sickness–like illness associated with fever, myalgias, arthralgias, and rash occurring a mean of 15 days after administration; a hypersensitivity syndrome with exfoliative dermatitis and eosinophilia that occurs within 3 to 4 weeks of exposure; and a chronic drug-induced lupus-like syndrome that presents after a year or more of administration with jaundice, malaise, polyarthralgias, fever, and the presence of autoantibodies (usually antinuclear), with typical autoimmune hepatitis features on liver biopsy.[114,115] Women younger than 40 years are most susceptible, with a latency period about half as long as that seen in males.[115] Most cases resolve after the drug is discontinued, although corticosteroids or other immunosuppressive therapy have been required in some patients with autoimmune injury that fails to improve spontaneously.[116]

### Macrolides

Erythromycin estolate was considered for many years to be the only erythromycin derivative that produced jaundice.[97] It is now clear that several other erythromycin salts, including erythromycin ethylsuccinate, erythromycin propionate, and possibly erythromycin stearate, and even erythromycin base,[117–120] can produce the same syndrome and lesion. Jaundice occurs in about 1% to 2% of adults taking erythromycin estolate.[97] The jaundice is hepatocanalicular, with high values for alkaline phosphatase and modestly elevated aminotransferase values. Liver biopsy usually shows only bile casts and prominent portal inflammatory infiltration, often rich in eosinophils.[120] Erythromycin lactobionate, administered intravenously, has been incriminated in a case of severe hepatic necrosis.[121] Ultrastructural changes include dilatation and effacement of canaliculi and microvilli. Hyperplasia of the Golgi apparatus and smooth endoplasmic reticulum has also been demonstrated, as has mitochondrial injury.[120] The fever, rash, and blood and tissue eosinophilia in up to 60% of cases have led to the inference that erythromycin DILI is due to hypersensitivity[97]; however, the high incidence of hepatic dysfunction in patients taking erythromycin estolate, and in vitro and in vivo demonstrations of hepatocyte damage, suggest that intrinsic hepatotoxicity of the agent may also contribute to the injury.[110] The onset of symptoms generally occurs between 5 and 20 days after the start of therapy, with individuals who have been previously treated having a shortened latent period. About half of cases associated with erythromycin estolate were icteric, with bilirubin values as high as 50 mg/dL. Abdominal pain was common, and in some cases mimicked acute cholecystitis.[98,122] Jaundice usually subsided within 2 to 5 weeks after the drug was stopped, but prolonged cholestasis at the level of the bile canaliculus[123] and VBDS have been described.[97,98]

Azithromycin has been associated with intrahepatic cholestasis biochemically and histologically.[124,125] Roxithromycin and clarithromycin have also been reported to cause cholestatic hepatitis.[126,127] Triacetyloleandomycin (troleandomycin) is now largely of historical interest, but produced jaundice in 4% and biochemically detected hepatic dysfunction in more than 50% of patients who took 2 g daily for 2 or more weeks.[128] Characteristically the injury was mixed, with both cytotoxic and cholestatic features, the latter predominating. Patients taking both this drug and oral contraceptives seem more likely to develop jaundice than those taking either preparation alone.[129]

Telithromycin, the first of the ketolides, was associated with mild reversible cholestatic hepatitis in clinical trials.[130] In the postmarketing period, however, more than 200 instances of DILI occurred, including several severe reactions.[131] A safety signal of hepatotoxicity was evident soon after the drug was approved.[132–134] Brinker and colleagues[134] summarized the clinical features of 42 cases reviewed by the FDA. Latency was typically short (2–43 days; median 10 days), although injury was delayed even after the drug had been stopped in a few instances. Women outnumbered men by 2 to 1 and the median age was 50 (range 22–90) years. Abdominal pain was reported in 45%, fever in 29%, ascites in 17%, and jaundice in 60%, and eosinophilia was present in 19%. More than 75% of the patients were hospitalized, with 4 deaths and 1 case ending in LT. Histologic findings from 6 patients were reported as showing "toxic liver injury," with one biopsy showing cirrhosis in a patient who had been treated with a prolonged course of therapy. Although telithromycin was initially approved for the treatment of acute bacterial sinusitis, exacerbation of chronic bacterial bronchitis, and community-acquired pneumonia, the drug subsequently had its clinical indications pared back to only community-acquired pneumonia because of its adverse-event profile.[135]

### Other Antibiotics

Nitrofurantoin causes mainly acute hepatocellular injury, but it may be cholestatic or mixed,[136] and instances of ALF are reported in large registries.[3,4,8] In addition, the drug appears to have led to several instances of chronic hepatitis resembling autoimmune hepatitis with positive antinuclear and/or anti–smooth muscle antibodies,[116,137,138] and less often to a cholestatic injury or a granulomatous hepatitis.[136,139] Hypersensitivity features are often present. Withdrawal of the drug has not always led to resolution of the chronic injury, and corticosteroids have been required in some cases.[116,138] Combined toxicity leading to pneumonitis and hepatitis has developed in the same patient.[140]

Chloramphenicol jaundice has been reported, with the scant data available suggesting that both hepatic parenchymal necrosis and cholestasis can occur. The mechanism for the apparent hepatotoxicity is unclear,[1] with bone marrow toxicity, including aplastic anemia, being of much greater concern.[141]

Novobiocin, a naturally occurring cholestatic hepatotoxin, can produce unconjugated hyperbilirubinemia, apparently by interfering with the excretion of bilirubin.[1] Accordingly it should be categorized as a mild intrinsic hepatotoxin. Rare instances of hepatic necrosis attributable to idiosyncrasy have been described, although it is now little used.[97]

## ANTITUBERCULOSIS DRUGS

The most important members of this group with respect to liver injury are INH[142] and pyrazinamide (PZA).[143] Rifampin has been implicated in a few cases of acute hepatic injury,[144,145] but, more importantly, appears to potentiate the hepatotoxicity of INH as well as PZA.[146] Streptomycin and dihydrostreptomycin appear to be free of hepatotoxic potential, but para–aminosalicylic acid (PAS) can cause liver damage.[147] Ethambutol leads to very rare instances of cholestatic jaundice.[148] Hepatobiliary involvement by mycobacteria can present a diagnostic challenge, complicating the recognition and diagnosis of hepatotoxicity of ATDs.[26,149,150]

### Isoniazid

Although regarded today as one of the most common causes of severe hepatotoxicity among all classes of drugs, this agent showed only a slight potential for producing serious hepatic injury during its first 2 decades of clinical use.[151,152] Despite the large number of patients receiving INH, before 1972 only a few instances of jaundice were attributed to its administration, and these were usually in individuals who were also taking other potentially hepatotoxic drugs. Garibaldi and colleagues[153] were among the first to recognize its significant hepatotoxic potential when they reported 19 instances of hepatocellular injury, most accompanied by jaundice, from among 2321 patients taking INH for chemoprophylaxis. These investigators also cited several other previously unreported instances of INH hepatotoxicity described to them by other physicians. Since then, numerous additional reports have appeared,[154] although the rate of overt hepatotoxicity from INH given for the treatment of latent TB infection (LTBI) remains low: for example, 0.10% among 11,000 patients starting treatment and 0.15% for those completing treatment in a Seattle–Kings County TB Clinic,[155] and 2.75 to 7.2 per 1000 patients in a large public health department clinic study involving 3377 individuals.[156]

### Clinical features of INH DILI

Between 10% and 20% of patients treated with INH alone for LTBI develop low-level, asymptomatic elevations in aminotransferases during the first several months of therapy, most of which do not progress to more severe injury,[151,157] a process termed hepatic adaptation or tolerance.[158] Fatigue, anorexia nausea, vomiting, and abdominal pain are the most commonly reported symptoms (in 50%–75% of cases) with fever and rash in 5% to 10% of individuals who develop more severe DILI, with jaundice, coagulopathy and hypoglycemia heralding the development of acute or subacute liver failure. The case-fatality rate is in excess of 10% of icteric cases with fulminant hepatitis, with INH being responsible for more LTs after DILI than for all other medications except acetaminophen.[5–7,159]

Liver biopsy specimens have revealed diffuse degeneration and necrosis similar to changes seen with acute viral hepatitis, with fatal cases demonstrating massive necrosis.[110,151,154] In a few patients, changes consistent with chronic hepatitis have been noted, although there are too few cases to confirm that true chronic injury develops.[154]

## Mechanism of INH DILI

INH is a hydrazine metabolized to hepatotoxic intermediates by N-acetyltransferase. Genetic polymorphisms of the N-acetyltransferase 2 (NAT2) gene correlate with rapid and slow acetylation, and several cytochrome P450 microsomes and other enzyme systems are also involved with its disposition.[40,160] Huang and colleagues[160] demonstrated that in addition to older age, a slow acetylator phenotype (whereby a larger percentage [33%] of INH is excreted unchanged [compared with <10% in rapid acetylators]) places individuals at increased risk of liver injury. In their series of 224 patients, 15% developed hepatotoxicity overall, more than twice as many having a slow acetylator phenotype (26% vs 11%). Higher aminotransferase levels were also seen in the slow acetylators.[160] INH monotherapy for 6 to 12 months is better tolerated in both human immunodeficiency virus (HIV)-positive and non–HIV-infected patients with latent TB, compared with short-course multidrug regimens involving rifampicin and pyrazinamide.[161,162]

The clinical features and experimental animal data have traditionally supported the view that metabolic idiosyncrasy leading to a toxic acetylhydrazine metabolite is responsible for the cytotoxic injury of INH.[142] However, Metushi and colleagues[163] have recently suggested that possible immune-mediated mechanisms may also play a role in some cases, based on the findings that rechallenge cases lead to injury within hours; autoantibodies and a lupus-like syndrome can be induced; significant eosinophilia may be present on biopsy; and INH can activate macrophages. Rifampicin is thought to enhance the hepatotoxicity of INH via enzyme induction.[164] Building on the knowledge that pregnane X receptors (PXR) are involved, Li and colleagues[46] have suggested that cotherapy with rifampicin and INH leads to accumulation of protoporphyrin IX, an endogenous hepatotoxin, owing to altered heme biosynthesis mediated by PXR.

## Rifampin

Severe liver injury with jaundice resulting from rifampin alone is rare.[144,145,165] Compared with those patients taking rifampin in combination with INH[166] and/or PZA,[146] enhancement of INH toxicity is reported to be due to rifampin induction of P-450 cytochromes, p-glycoprotein transporters, and uridine diphosphate–glucuronosyl transferases.[167,168] Of note, the increased risk of hepatotoxicity seen with rifampicin and PZA in the general population with LTBI was not observed among HIV-positive individuals.[169] Presumably unrelated to hepatocellular injury is the ability of rifampin to produce conjugated hyperbilirubinemia via inhibition of the major bile-salt exporter pump.[97,170] Early studies also showed that rifampin also competes with bilirubin for clearance at the level of sinusoidal and canalicular membranes.[171,172] Hepatic injury caused by rifampin monotherapy usually appears during the first 2 to 4 weeks of therapy,[144] whereas injury from INH alone or in combination is seen after the first 1 to 2 months.[142]

Rifabutin, a semisynthetic derivative of rifamycin, is used both alone and in combination with macrolides for the primary prophylaxis and treatment of Mycobacterium tuberculosis and Mycobacterium avium complex infections. Elevations of aminotransferases have been reported in 6% to 8% of patients with AIDS.[173] Rifabutin induces hepatic microsomal enzymes to a lesser extent than rifampicin.[174]

## Pyrazinamide

The nicotinic acid derivative PZA has a risk of inducing hepatotoxicity equal to or greater than that from INH.[165] Most instances of DILI are seen with PZA in combination with other TB agents. Indeed, owing to several reports of severe liver injury (including hospitalization, the need for LT, and case fatalities) seen with the combination of PZA and rifampicin, the Centers for Disease Control and Prevention (CDC) has cautioned against the use of this regimen as treatment of latent TB.[143,165] In addition, the American Thoracic Society (ATS) and the Infectious Diseases Society of America joined the CDC in recommending that this combination not be used except as part of a multidrug combination for active TB.[165] The risk of hepatitis from PZA plus rifampin has been found to be 3-fold higher than that of INH.[143,175]

The mechanism of injury appears to be a combination of dose-dependent hepatotoxicity, formation of reactive metabolites, and hypersensitivity, the latter suggested by eosinophilia and hepatic granuloma formation.[165] The authors have reported a patient who developed acute reversible autoimmune hepatitis and thyroiditis after the start of prophylactic therapy with PZA and rifampin for a documented purified protein derivative (PPD) conversion.[176] PZA requires activation by amidase to form pyrazinoic acid (PA), which is then hydroxylated by xanthine oxidase (XO) to form 5-hydroxypyrazinoic acid (5-OH-PA). PZA can also be directly oxidized to form 5-OH-PZA. Allopurinol, an XO inhibitor, reduces the clearance of PZA,[177] and has increased the hepatotoxicity of PZA in vitro.[178] Shih and colleagues[179] recently confirmed that the 5-OH-PA metabolite is responsible for PZA-induced hepatotoxicity in both animals and humans, and that both PA and 5-OH-PA levels in the urine were significantly correlated with hepatotoxicity.

### Para–Aminosalicylic Acid

Owing to a high incidence of drug-induced hypersensitivity, PAS is currently relegated to second-line treatment of multidrug-resistant *Mycobacterium tuberculosis*.[180] Hepatic injury is seen as part of the generalized immunoallergic reaction, which occurs in 0.3% to 5% of patients taking the drug. PAS-associated DILI appears after 1 to 5 weeks of therapy; and includes fever, rash, eosinophilia, lymphadenopathy, and often atypical circulating lymphocytes (giving rise to the term pseudomononucleosis).[147] Approximately 25% of patients with this generalized hypersensitivity developed jaundice and biochemical evidence of mixed hepatocellular hepatic injury. The histologic changes included prominent inflammation, with sinusoidal beading accompanying the diffuse degeneration, necrosis, and cholestasis. Necrosis was massive in fatal cases. In some nonfatal cases there was striking periportal necrosis.[1]

### Monitoring for ATD-associated DILI

The ATS guidelines from 2006 remain the most widely followed.[181] Although frequent ALT monitoring, as often as twice weekly for the first 2 weeks and then monthly, was recommended by some groups based on their experience with severe hepatotoxicity,[164] more recent series place the general risk of severe DILI at from less than 1% to 4%, and monitoring for the development of clinical symptoms is usually all that is considered necessary.[165,181] The ATS recommends ALT monitoring only for patients at high risk of DILI from INH, namely chronic alcohol users, HIV-positive patients, those with chronic viral hepatitis or other causes of elevated LAEs, and pregnant or postpartum females (within 3 months of delivery).[181] Patients older than 35 years are also considered at higher risk, and may benefit from ALT monitoring as well. For those without these risk factors, several reports document its safe use with only clinical monitoring.[181] Indeed, a recent report from the United States noted that of 10 severe adverse events (SAEs) that occurred between 2004 and 2008 among patients treated with INH for LTBI, all were prompted by symptoms rather than laboratory abnormalities.[182] It is worth noting, however, that most of those SAEs were diagnosed by health care providers other than the original ATD prescribers, and several patients delayed their medical evaluation until the development of clinical jaundice, which eventuated in the need for liver transplant in some cases.

### Risk Factors for ATD DILI

In contrast to most other drugs causing hepatic injury, the risk of INH DILI is clearly age related, with older patients at higher risk.[165,181] Kunst and Khan[183] also found INH risk to be related to age, with a rate of 1.7% for those older than 35 years compared with 0.2% for a younger population. In a large public health department study of 1100 individuals, the number of hepatotoxic events (AST >5 times the upper limit of normal) per 1000 patients was 4.4 for ages 25 to 34 years; 8.54 between ages 35 and 49; and 20.83 for those aged 50 and older.[156] No apparent gender difference has been seen with the exception of pregnant and postpartum women.[184] Alcohol abuse has long been considered a significant risk factor.[1] Sharma and colleagues[185] and Singla and colleagues[186] demonstrated that hypoalbuminemia (<3.5 g/dL) was a positive predictor of DILI, placing patients at nearly 3 times the risk. Warmelink and colleagues[187] showed that weight loss of 2 kg or more within 4 weeks of beginning treatment was an important risk factor for DILI. Historically, higher doses of ATDs, specifically regimens including pyrazinamide, were associated with higher rates of adverse reactions. However, a recent meta-analysis of 29 studies found that high-dose pyrazinamide (60 mg/kg) did not significantly increase the risk of hepatotoxicity when compared with medium-dose (40 mg/kg) and low-dose (30 mg/kg) regimens, consistent with its predominantly idiosyncratic mechanism of injury.[188]

Initially, chronic viral hepatitis and HIV were thought to convey an increased risk for ATD DILI.[189] More recent studies suggest that the risk of hepatotoxicity caused by these viral infections may not be significantly increased.[181,190,191]

### Pharmacogenomics of ATDs

Several genomic factors influence susceptibility to ATD DILI (see **Table 4**). Slow acetylator status for the NAT2 gene (discussed earlier), and several other genetic polymorphisms involving the cytochrome P450 system and other factors affecting metabolic disposition of ATDs, seem to be the most important.[44,192–194] However, not all investigators have found a positive correlation between DILI and certain genetic polymorphisms of ATDs.[195] Perhaps because of such conflicting results, to the authors' knowledge none of these purported risk factors have been invoked as a reason to withhold treatment.[40] However, certain groups have successfully used the information garnered from phenotype analyses to guide therapy to prevent both treatment failures and toxicity.[196]

### Reintroduction of ATD After Liver Injury

For patients who develop hepatic injury and are required to discontinue ATDs, the ATS guidelines[181] currently recommend a staggered reintroduction of rifampin, INH, and pyrazinamide before restarting maximum dosing of all 3 agents (**Table 5**).[197,198] Sharma and colleagues[185] performed a randomized controlled trial whereby they started patients on maximum doses of these 3 agents from day 1, and found no statistically significant difference between DILI recurrence when comparing the immediate maximum dosing group with groups following ATS recommendations on incremental dosing. For patients with severe DILI from INH and pyrazinamide requiring transplant, alternative TB regimens including quinolones and ethambutol have been successfully reintroduced,[199] although in this French series rifampin led to episodes of acute rejection, and was not recommended by the investigators.

**Table 5**
**Recommendations for drug reintroduction in DILI patients undergoing TB therapy**

| Authors,[Ref.] Year | Recommendations |
|---|---|
| American Thoracic Society,[181,197] 2006, 2010 | Rechallenged patients who had reached a treatment limiting threshold should have clinical and biochemical monitoring at 2- to 4-wk intervals |
| | After ALT returns to less than 2 times the ULN, rifampin may be restarted with or without ethambutol |
| | After 3–7 d isoniazid may be reintroduced, subsequently rechecking ALT |
| | If symptoms recur or ALT increases, the last drug added should be stopped |
| | For those who have experienced prolonged or severe hepatotoxicity, but tolerate reintroduction with rifampin and isoniazid, rechallenge with pyrazinamide may be hazardous |
| | In this circumstance, pyrazinamide may be permanently discontinued, with treatment extended to 9 mo |
| | Although pyrazinamide can be reintroduced in some milder cases of hepatotoxicity, the benefit of a shorter treatment course likely does not outweigh the risk of severe hepatotoxicity from pyrazinamide rechallenge |
| Sharma et al,[185] 2010 | Isoniazid, rifampicin, and pyrazinamide can be reintroduced simultaneously at full dosage safely from day 1 |
| | Treatment should not be delayed secondary to fears of hepatotoxicity in patients with bilateral extensive pulmonary tuberculosis |
| Senousy et al,[198] 2010 | Reintroduction should not be attempted until liver function is normal, liver tests are at less than 2 times the ULN, and it is more than 2 wk since the disappearance of jaundice |
| | Staged reintroduction starting with Rifampin, then isoniazid then pyrazinamide, unless patients had severe liver dysfunction, in which case pyrazinamide should be avoided |
| | Each drug should be given for 3–7 d before the next medication is added |
| | Medications should be reintroduced at doses lower than what was used in initial therapy, and doses should be gradually titrated up to the therapeutic range |

*Abbreviations:* ALT, alanine aminotransferase; ULN, upper limit of normal.

## Prevention of ATD DILI

In addition to identifying host risk factors that influence the type and degree of clinical and biochemical monitoring, several cytoprotective compounds have been used to prevent ATD hepatotoxicity. While *N*-acetylcysteine (NAC) has traditionally been used to treat paracetamol (acetaminophen)-induced ALF, new data are emerging that support its use in preventing hepatotoxicity from ATDs.[200] Baniasadi and colleagues performed a randomized controlled trial in 60 patients aged 60 years or older that compared a traditional 4-drug regimen (INH, rifampin, pyrazinamide, ethambutol) with the same drug regimen in combination with NAC (600 mg twice a day orally). At the end of the first week, the group without NAC had ALT and AST values elevated 3- to 4-fold higher than those receiving NAC, suggesting a hepatoprotective role of NAC in older patients. A hepatoprotective role in the prevention ATD-induced DILI is also under study for various herbal and antioxidant compounds, including silymarin.[201–204]

## Latent Tuberculosis and Liver Transplantation

Detecting and managing latent TB in the LT patient is problematic. Early INH chemoprophylaxis after LT is often poorly tolerated and is frequently discontinued before a complete course of treatment.[205] In a series of 420 patients from the United States, 6% (n = 25) were diagnosed with latent TB, with clinical detection rates being similar for both PPD and QuantiFERON gold.[205] Of the patients treated for latent TB, 8 subjects discontinued therapy because of untoward side effects; however, none of these patients developed TB reactivation after transplantation, and 3-year survival rates were similar between the 25 patients with latent TB and the 296 patients without latent TB (78.7% vs 74.6%).[205] In a Spanish series of 53 patients diagnosed with latent TB by PPD and treated for 6 months with INH, zero cases of TB reactivation were reported at 52 months after LT.[206] Four patients had minor elevations in LAEs that resolved with withdrawal of INH; no graft dysfunction was observed, and no patients were retransplanted because of DILI.[206] A recent Brazilian series demonstrated that INH was safe to use in LT candidates.[207] Among 33 LT candidates with an average Model for End-Stage Liver Disease (MELD) score of 20 with latent TB identified by PPD, 27 patients were treated with INH.[207] Eighteen patients (66.6%) completed the 6 months of prophylaxis, 8 patients were transplanted between 2 and 4 months while still on INH; and 1 patient stopped INH owing to decompensation from spontaneous bacterial peritonitis (SBP) in the absence of LAE elevation. No patient experienced clinical decompensation or significant elevations in LAEs from INH,[207] which confirmed similar findings from other solid organ transplant (SOT) centers.[208] TB complicated about 1% of 2001 SOT recipients (including 7 of 701 with LT) in a Spanish series from January 2000 to December 2011, none of whom received antituberculous prophylaxis.[209] The mean time to diagnosis was 64 (range 2–169) months, with 28% developing active TB within the first year after transplantation. Fifty percent had pulmonary TB, 39% disseminated infections, with 11% confined to lymph nodes. All patients were treated with INH, most receiving a 3-drug regimen. Seven patients (5 liver recipients and 2 kidney recipients) developed hepatotoxicity, and 1 developed rejection without allograft loss. The mortality during the period of ATD treatment was 17% (3 of 18).

## ANTIFUNGAL AGENTS

Ketoconazole, an azole derivative, has been reported to lead to more than 100 instances of hepatocellular injury and a much smaller number of cases of apparent cholestatic injury.[210–212] The incidence of jaundice appears to be low; based on apparent usage; it has been estimated to range from 0.01% to 0.1%.[211] Minor abnormalities of liver function tests occur in about 10% of recipients,[211] but fatalities in those with severe hepatotoxicity were up to 10%.[210] Fluconazole can lead to a 15% to 20% incidence of elevated aminotransferase and to rare cases of jaundice and severe hepatitis.[213,214] Itraconazole has led to hepatocellular and cholestatic injury,[215,216] and is a more potent hepatotoxin than fluconazole in animals.[217] Voriconazole, the newest of the azoles, also has been reported to cause hepatotoxicity, likely through an idiosyncratic mechanism, as supratherapeutic drug levels have not been associated with increased DILI.[218] In an observational series from Kings College Hospital, of 29 patients with severe liver dysfunction treated with voriconazole, 69% had liver injury, 35% had elevated aminotransferases, 15% cholestasis, and 45% mixed.[219] Caution is advised when using voriconazole in patients with severe liver dysfunction, and alternative agents such as amphotericin B, which rarely causes hepatic injury,[220] should be used instead.

Fluocytosine is converted to 5-fluorouracil, a transformation on which its antifungal activity depends. Data on the hepatic effects of this drug are scant; it appears to lead to transient elevations of serum aminotransferase levels in 10% of recipients, and has been incriminated in hepatic necrosis.[1,221]

Terbinafine, a synthetic antimycotic agent of the alylamine class, has been reported to lead to cholestatic injury, including VBDS, a mixed hepatocellular-cholestatic injury, and submassive hepatocellular necrosis with liver failure.[222–225] Injury has been linked to the allylic aldehyde metabolite of the compound (7,7-dimethylhept-2-ene-4-ynal).[226] Chronic hepatitis B may be a risk factor in a case with autoimmune features.[227]

## ANTIVIRAL AGENTS

Highly active antiretroviral therapy drugs are discussed elsewhere in this issue by Douglas Dieterich and colleagues.

A trial of fialuridine (fluoroiodoarabinofuranosyluracil), a nucleoside analogue for the treatment of chronic hepatitis B, was halted because of the sudden development of hepatic failure, lactic acidosis, and death in 5 patients.[228] Histopathologic changes included diffuse microvesicular steatosis, glycogen depletion, cholestasis, and ductular proliferation. Similarly to other antiretroviral agents producing liver toxicity, mitochondrial injury was noted ultrastructurally.[228]

Interferon-$\alpha$ therapy as part of regimens to treat chronic hepatitis C has only rarely been associated with acute heptotoxicity.[229,230] In some cases, the liver injury may be due to exacerbation of unsuspected autoimmune hepatitis.[231] Granulomatous hepatitis has been reported in association with interferon-$\alpha$,[232] but has also been found in a small percentage of patients regardless of therapy.[233,234] In the post-LT setting, acute VBDS has been described in patients treated for recurrent hepatitis C infection.[235] In patients with chronic hepatitis B, fatal hepatic decompensation has been reported following treatment with interferon-$\alpha$,[236] and autoimmune hepatitis also has been noted.[237]

## ANTIPROTOZOAL AND ANTHELMINTIC AGENTS

Amodiaquine, an antimalarial, has led to several instances of severe hepatitis, several of which were fatal.[238] Pentamidine, used for the treatment of P carinii pneumonia in patients with AIDS, has led to a 30% incidence of elevated aminotransferase levels.[239] Metronidazole has been implicated in a few instances of cholestatic hepatitis confirmed by rechallenge.[240]

Chlorinated hydrocarbons and organic antimonials used as anthelmintics are known to cause hepatic injury.[1] Hycanthone, used for the treatment of schistosomiasis, has also been found to produce hepatocellular injury and, in some cases, fatal necrosis.[241] Thiabendazole has produced intrahepatic cholestasis, in some instances progressing to VBDS[242] and even cirrhosis.[243] Niclofolan has been incriminated in cholestatic jaundice.[244] Piperazine has been reported to cause acute hepatocellular injury.[245] Albendazole[246] and mebendazole[247] also have been reported to produce hepatic injury. Praziquantel does not appear to be hepatotoxic.[248]

## ANTIBIOTIC USE IN CIRRHOSIS (INCLUDING TREATMENT OF SPONTANEOUS BACTERIAL PERITONITIS)

Cirrhosis presents a set of unique challenges when dealing with drug metabolism and disposition, and most drugs have either not been formally assessed in this setting or have been evaluated in only short-duration pharmacokinetic/pharmacodynamic studies in a limited number of subjects.[249] Nevertheless, antibiotics are among the most commonly used agents in the management of patients with complications of cirrhosis and portal hypertension. In patients with acute variceal hemorrhage, antibiotic prophylaxis is associated with improved survival and a lower mortality.[250,251]

Fluoroquinolones are the most commonly used antibiotics in cirrhosis, especially to treat and prevent SBP, as well as for prophylaxis when performing endoscopic or surgical procedures. In a recent review of prospective studies and meta-analyses, the investigators concluded that norfloxacin as secondary prophylaxis significantly decreased the occurrence of SBP, but not mortality rates.[250] The use of ciprofloxacin (given as daily or weekly regimens) is less well studied but also appears to be effective.[252]

No significant changes in plasma levels or half-life have been seen with ciprofloxacin, and no dosing adjustments are necessary in patients with cirrhosis[253] or ascites.[254] Although ofloxacin metabolism is altered by renal dysfunction in patients with ascites,[254,255] the penetration of ofloxacin into ascitic fluid is excellent, achieving therapeutic levels even in the setting of renal dysfunction.[254,256] However, fluoroquinolones are known to prolong QTc intervals in cirrhotics, related to decreased CYP 3A4 activity, and in patients who have undergone transjugular intrahepatic portosystemic shunt.[257]

Macrolide antibiotics, including erythromycin, azithromycin, clindamycin, and chloramphenicol, should be avoided in cirrhotic patients.[249,258] Tetracycline has a prolonged half-life, which corresponds to dose-related hepatotoxicity and should also be avoided.[258] β-Lactam antibiotics should be used with caution given their propensity for leukopenia, as cirrhotics are predisposed to infection from impaired reticular endothelial cell function and phagocytosis that can lead to ineffective hepatic destruction of bacteria.[258] Aminoglycosides and vancomycin are generally contraindicated given their relatively high risk of inducing or worsening renal failure.[258] **Table 6** provides a complete list of antibiotics to be used with caution or avoided in cirrhotics.

The recommendations for the use of ATDs in cirrhosis are based largely on the known risk of hepatotoxicity in patients with chronic liver disease (CLD).[249,259] Rifampicin is eliminated in the bile and can cause elevations in bilirubin, owing to competitive inhibition of excretory pathways. As a result, it can potentially worsen jaundice in a cirrhotic; its risk of hepatotoxicity is increased when used concomitantly with INH, and caution is advised in cirrhosis.[260] In patients with CLD, ofloxacin has been used safely as a substitute for rifampicin and may be less hepatotoxic than rifampin and pyrazinamide when combined with pyrazinamide.[197] INH has an increased risk of DILI in

**Table 6**
**Antibiotics or antifungals to be avoided or used with caution in liver failure**

| Drug | Reason |
|------|--------|
| Macrolides (azithromycin, erythromycin) | QTc prolongation |
| β-Lactams (cephalosporins, pipericillin) | Leukopenia |
| Aminoglycosides | Renal failure |
| Vancomycin | Renal failure |
| Nitrofurantoin (chronic use) | Drug-induced autoimmune hepatitis |
| Tetracycline | Prolonged half-life may lead to acute liver failure |
| Rifampin | Worsening jaundice |

*Data from* Stine JG, Lewis JH. Review article: use of medications in patients with cirrhosis. Aliment Pharmacol Ther 2013;37(12):1132–56; and Amarapurkar DN. Prescribing medications in patients with decompensated liver cirrhosis. Int J Hepatol 2011;2011:1–5.

cirrhotics with specific polymorphisms (eg, slow acetylators), which leads to increased plasma levels and untoward clinical effects.[261] Although generally contraindicated in severe liver disease,[249] INH has been used safely with frequent (every 2–4 weeks) liver enzyme monitoring in cirrhotic patients awaiting LT,[262] and has been successfully used to treat posttransplant tuberculosis.[205,263] Pyrazinamide has an increased half-life in hepatic impairment,[261] leading to increased hepatotoxicity.[264] Current recommendations suggest the Child-Pugh Class A cirrhotics be treated in the same manner as noncirrhotic patients; however, pyrazinamide should be avoided in Class B disease.[258] Ethambutol, a fluoroquinolone and a second-line agent, may be used in Child-Pugh Class C disease.[258] In contrast to these studies, Park and colleagues[265] did not find that cirrhosis was an independent risk factor for hepatotoxicity, and that ATDs can be used safely in patients with CLD. Stucchi and colleagues[207] confirmed the safe use of INH in a series of 27 pretransplant cirrhotic patients with a positive PPD and a mean MELD score of 20. Two-thirds of this group completed a 6-month course of prophylaxis, with several others treated for up to 4 months before receiving their transplant. Mean values for aminotransferases before and after INH were similar among those treated. Only 1 patient stopped therapy because of decompensation from SBP.

Antifungal agents including ketoconazole, miconazole, fluconazole, and itraconazole should be used with caution in cirrhosis, largely because of the variable effects on cytochrome P450 enzyme activity.[258] Voriconazole must be dose-reduced for Child-Pugh Class A and B disease; however, it has not been studied in Class C patients.[249]

## SUMMARY

Antimicrobial agents head the list of drugs leading to acute DILI among nonacetaminophen causes. Amoxicillin-clavulanate, nitrofurantoin, flucloxacillin, TMP/SMX, and INH and other ATDs are the most commonly implicated, as reflected in large international DILI registries. Antibiotic-induced hepatotoxicity is often difficult to diagnose because it may be clinically similar to other causes of acute hepatitis and can be confounded by the hepatic manifestations of infectious disease being treated, as well as the presence of sepsis, multiple transfusions, hemolysis, and other causes of hepatic dysfunction and jaundice that can complicate the postoperative and intensive care unit settings, as well as a variety of outpatient venues. The delayed onset of hepatic injury after the discontinuation of agents such as amoxicillin-clavulanate can further complicate the diagnostic assessment. A high clinical index of suspicion will remain necessary until pharmacogenomic testing or other biomarkers become routinely available to predict or confirm that hepatotoxicity is related to a particular antibiotic.

## REFERENCES

1. Zimmerman HJ. Hepatotoxicity: the adverse effects of drugs and other chemicals on the liver. 2nd edition. Philadelphia: Lippincott Williams and Wilkins; 1999.
2. Andrade RJ, Tulkens PM. Hepatic safety of antibiotics used in primary care. J Antimicrob Chemother 2011;66(7):1431–46.
3. Bjornsson E, Olsson R. Outcome and prognostic markers in severe drug-induced liver disease. Hepatology 2005;42:481–9.
4. Andrade RJ, Lucena MI, Fernandez MC, et al. Drug-induced liver injury: an analysis of 461 instances submitted to the Spanish Registry over a 10-year period. Gastroenterology 2005;129:512–21.

5. Reuben A, Koch DG, Lee WM. Acute liver failure study group. drug-induced acute liver failure: results of a U.S. multicenter, prospective study. Hepatology 2010;52(6):2065–76. http://dx.doi.org/10.1002/hep.23937.

6. Mindikoglu AL, Magder LS, Regev A. Outcome of liver transplantation for drug-induced acute liver failure in the United States: analysis of the United Network for Organ Sharing database. Liver Transpl 2009;15(7):719–29 [Erratum in Liver Transpl 2010;16(12):1446].

7. Devarbhavi H, Dierkhising R, Kremers WK, et al. Single-center experience with drug-induced liver injury from India: causes, outcome, prognosis, and predictors of mortality. Am J Gastroenterol 2010;105(11):2396–404.

8. Chalasani N, Fontana RJ, Bonkovsky HL, et al. Drug Induced Liver Injury Network (DILIN). Causes, clinical features, and outcomes from a prospective study of drug-induced liver injury in the United States. Gastroenterology 2008; 135(6):1924–34.

9. De Valle MB, Av Klinteberg V, Alem N, et al. Drug-induced liver injury in a Swedish University hospital out-patient hepatology clinic. Aliment Pharmacol Ther 2006;24(8):1187–95.

10. Reau NS, Jensen DM. Vanishing bile duct system. Clin Liver Dis 2008;12(1): 203–17.

11. Talwani R, Gilliam BL, Howell C. Infectious diseases and the liver. Clin Liver Dis 2011;15(1):111–30.

12. Mallal S, Phillips E, Carosi G, et al. HLA-B*5701 screening for hypersensitivity to abacavir. N Engl J Med 2008;358(6):568–79.

13. Daly AK. Using genome-wide association studies to identify genes important in serious adverse drug reactions. Annu Rev Pharmacol Toxicol 2012;52:21–35.

14. Daly AK, Donaldson PT, Bhatnagar P. HLA-B*5701 genotype is a major determinant of drug-induced liver injury due to flucloxacillin. Nat Genet 2009;41:816–9.

15. Phillips E, Mallal S. Successful translation of pharmacogenetics into the clinic: the abacavir example. Mol Diagn Ther 2009;13(1):1–9.

16. Krawczyk M, Mullenbach R, Weber S, et al. Genome-wide association studies and genetic risk assessment of liver diseases. Nat Rev Gastroenterol Hepatol 2010;7(12):669–81.

17. Suzuki A, Andrade RJ, Bjornsson E, et al. Drugs associated with hepatotoxicity and their reporting frequency of liver adverse events in VigiBase: unified list based on international collaborative work. Drug Saf 2010;33(6):503–22.

18. Cunha BA. Systemic infections affecting the liver. Some cause jaundice, some do not. Postgrad Med 1988;84(5):161–3.

19. Shahian M, Rashtian P, Kalani M. Unexplained neonatal jaundice as an early diagnostic sign of urinary tract infection. Int J Infect Dis 2012;16(7):e487–90.

20. Kobashi H, Toshimori J, Yamamoto K. Sepsis-associated liver injury: incidence, classification and the clinical significance. Hepatol Res 2013;43(3):255–66.

21. Brienza N, Dalfino L, Cinnella G, et al. Jaundice in critical illness: promoting factors of a concealed reality. Intensive Care Med 2006;32(2):267–74.

22. Koskinas J, Gomatos IP, Tiniakos DG, et al. Liver histology in ICU patients dying from sepsis: a clinico-pathological study. World J Gastroenterol 2008;14(9): 1389–93.

23. Tugwell P, Williams AO. Jaundice associated with lobar pneumonia. A clinical, laboratory and histological study. Q J Med 1977;46(181):97–118.

24. Ahmed A, Ahmed B. Jaundice in typhoid patients: differentiation from other common causes of fever and jaundice in the tropics. Ann Afr Med 2010;9(3): 135–40.

25. Datta S, Sarkar RN, Biswas A, et al. Leptospirosis: an institutional experience. J Indian Med Assoc 2011;109(10):737–8.
26. Taylor TH, Lewis JH. Tuberculosis of the liver, biliary tract and pancreas. In: Schlossberg D, editor. Tuberculosis and nontuberculosis mycobacterial infections. 6th edition. Washington, DC: ASM Press; 2011. p. 373–408.
27. Sembera S, Lammert C, Talwalkar JA, et al. Frequency, clinical presentation and outcomes of drug-induced liver injury after liver transplantation. Liver Transpl 2012;18(7):803–10.
28. Zhenglu W, Hui L, Shuying ZH, et al. A clinical-pathological analysis of drug-induced hepatic injury after liver transplantation. Transplant Proc 2007;39: 3287–91.
29. Faust TW, Reddy KR. Postoperative jaundice. Clin Liver Dis 2004;8(1): 151–66.
30. Chen EY, Baum K, Collins W, et al. Hepatitis E masquerading as drug-induced liver injury. Hepatology 2012;56(6):2420–3.
31. Davern TJ, Chalasani N, Fontana RJ, et al. Acute hepatitis E infection accounts for some cases of suspected drug-induced liver injury. Gastroenterology 2011; 141(5):1665–72.
32. Dalton HR, Fellows HJ, Stableforth W, et al. The role of hepatitis E virus testing in drug-induced liver injury. Aliment Pharmacol Ther 2007;26(10):1429–35.
33. Lucena MI, Molokhia M, Shen Y, et al. Susceptibility to amoxicillin-clavulanate-induced liver injury is influenced by multiple HLA class I and II alleles. Gastroenterology 2011;141(1):338–47.
34. Donaldson PT, Daly AK, Henderson J, et al. Human leucocyte antigen class II genotype in susceptibility and resistance to co-amoxiclav-induced liver injury. J Hepatol 2010;53(6):1049–53.
35. Daly AK, Day CP. Genetic association studies in drug-induced liver injury. Drug Metab Rev 2012;44(1):116–26.
36. Lee SW, Chung LS, Huang HH, et al. NAT2 and CYP2E1 polymorphisms and susceptibility to first-line anti-tuberculosis drug-induced hepatitis. Int J Tuberc Lung Dis 2010;14(5):622–6.
37. Tang SW, Lv XZ, Zhang Y, et al. CYP2E1, GSTM1 and GSTT1 genetic polymorphisms and susceptibility to antituberculosis drug-induced hepatotoxicity: a nested case-control study. J Clin Pharm Ther 2012;37(5):588–93.
38. An HR, Wu XQ, Wang ZY, et al. NAT2 and CYP2E1 polymorphisms associated with antituberculosis drug-induced hepatotoxicity in Chinese patients. Clin Exp Pharmacol Physiol 2012;39(6):535–43.
39. Teixeira RL, Morato RG, Cabello PH, et al. Genetic polymorphisms of NAT2, CYP2E1 and GST enzymes and the occurrence of antituberculosis drug-induced hepatitis in Brazilian TB patients. Mem Inst Oswaldo Cruz 2011; 106(6):716–24.
40. Hawkins MT, Lewis JH. Latest advances in predicting DILI in humans: focus on biomarkers. Expert Opin Drug Metab Toxicol 2012;8(12):1521–30.
41. Cosgrove B, Alexopoulos L, Hang T. Cytokine-associated drug toxicity in human hepatocytes is associated with signaling network dysregulation. Mol Biosyst 2010;6:1195–206.
42. Bell L, Vuppalanchi R, Watkins P. Serum proteomic profiling in patients with drug-induced liver injury. Aliment Pharmacol Ther 2012;35:600–12.
43. Kim SH, Kim SH, Lee JH, et al. Polymorphisms in drug transporter genes (ABCB1, SLCO1B1 and ABCC2) and hepatitis induced by antituberculosis drugs. Tuberculosis (Edinb) 2012;92(1):100–4.

44. Wang T, Wang W, Wang ZY, et al. Association of P450–2E1 and GSTM1 genetic polymorphisms with susceptibility to antituberculosis drug-induced hepatotoxicity. Zhonghua Jie He He Hu Xi Za Zhi 2009;32(8):585–7 [in Chinese].

45. Chang JC, Liu EH, Lee CN, et al. UGT1A1 polymorphisms associated with risk of induced liver disorders by anti-tuberculosis medications. Int J Tuberc Lung Dis 2012;16(3):376–8.

46. Li F, Lu J, Cheng J, et al. Human PXR modulates hepatotoxicity associated with rifampicin and isoniazid co-therapy. Nat Med 2013;19(4):418–20.

47. Andrews E, Armstrong M, Tugwood J, et al. A role for the pregnane X receptor in flucloxacillin-induced liver injury. Hepatology 2010;51(5):1656–64.

48. Phillips EJ, Mallal SA. HLA-B*5701 and flucloxacillin associated drug-induced liver disease. AIDS 2013;27(3):491–2.

49. Monshi M, Faulkner L, Gibson A, et al. HLA-B*57:01-restricted activation of drug-specific T-cells provides the immunological basis for flucloxacillin-induced liver injury. Hepatology 2013;57(2):727–39.

50. Bhadauria S, Mishra R, Kanchan R, et al. Isoniazid-induced apoptosis in HepG2 cells: generation of oxidative stress and Bcl-2 down-regulation. Toxicol Mech Methods 2010;20(5):242–51.

51. Daly AK, Day CP. Genetic association studies in drug-induced liver injury. Semin Liver Dis 2009;29:400–11.

52. Hsiao CJ, Younis H, Boelsterli UA. Trovafloxacin, a fluoroquinolone antibiotic with hepatotoxic potential, causes mitochondrial peroxynitrite stress in a mouse model of underlying mitochondrial dysfunction. Chem Biol Interact 2010;188(1): 204–13.

53. Goldstein LI, Ishak KG. Hepatic injury associated with penicillin therapy. Arch Pathol 1974;98:114–7.

54. Onate J, Monejo M, Aguirrebenogoa K, et al. Hepatotoxicity associated with penicillin V therapy. Clin Infect Dis 1995;20:474–5.

55. Williams CN, Malatjalian DA. Severe penicillin-induced cholestasis in a 91 year old woman. Dig Dis Sci 1981;26:470–3.

56. Dismukes WE. Oxacillin-induced hepatic dysfunction. JAMA 1973;226:881–3.

57. Knirsch AK, Gralla EJ. Abnormal serum transaminase levels after parenteral ampicillin and carbenicillin administration. N Engl J med 1970;282:1081–2.

58. Wilson FM, Belamaric J, Lauter CB, et al. Anicteric carbenicillin hepatitis. Eight episodes in four patients. JAMA 1975;232:818–21.

59. Bengtsson F, Floren CH, Hagerstrand I, et al. Flucloxacillin-induced cholestatic liver damage. Scand J Infect Dis 1985;17:125–8.

60. Kleinman MS, Presberg JE. Cholestatic hepatitis after dicloxacillin-sodium therapy. J Clin Gastroenterol 1986;8:77–8.

61. Victorino RM, Maria VA, Correia AP, et al. Floxacillin-induced cholestatic hepatitis with evidence of lymphocyte sensitization. Arch Intern Med 1987;147: 987–9.

62. Derby LE, Jick H, Henry DA, et al. Cholestatic hepatitis associated with flucloxacillin. Med J Aust 1993;158:596–600.

63. Miros M, Kerlin P, Walker N, et al. Flucloxacillin induced delayed cholestatic hepatitis. Aust N Z J Med 1990;20:251–3.

64. Turner IB, Eckstein RP, Riley JW, et al. Prolonged hepatic cholestasis after flucloxacillin therapy. Med J Aust 1989;151(11–12):701–5.

65. Lucena MI, Andrade RJ, Kaplowitz N, et al. Phenotypic characterization of idiosyncratic drug-induced liver injury: the influence of age and sex. Hepatology 2009;49(6):2001–9.

66. O'Donohue J, Oien KA, Donaldson P, et al. Co-amoxiclav jaundice: clinical and histological features and HLA class II association. Gut 2000;47:717–20.
67. Garcia Rodriguez LA, Stricker BH, Zimmerman HJ. Risk of acute liver injury associated with the combination of amoxicillin and clavulanic acid. Arch Intern Med 1996;156:1327–32.
68. Mari JY, Guy C, Beyens MN, et al. Delayed drug-induced hepatic injury. Evoking the role of amoxicillin-clavulanic acid combination. Therapie 2000;55:699–704 [in French].
69. Hautekeete ML, Brenard R, Horsmans Y, et al. Liver injury related to amoxicillin-clavulanic acid: interlobular bile duct lesions and extrahepatic manifestations. J Hepatol 1995;22:71–7.
70. Caballero Plasencia AM, Valenzuela Barranco M, Martin Ruiz JL, et al. Hepato-toxicity caused by amoxicillin, clavulanic acid or both? Gastroenterol Hepatol 1997;20:45–6 [in Spanish].
71. Sweet JM, Jones MP. Intrahepatic cholestasis due to ticarcillin-clavulanate. Am J Gastroenterol 1995;90:675–6.
72. Silvain C, Fort E, Levillain P, et al. Granulomatous hepatitis due to combination of amoxicillin and clavulanic acid. Dig Dis Sci 1992;37:150–2, 596.
73. Bor O, Dinleyici EC, Kebapci M, et al. Ceftriaxone-associated biliary sludge and pseudocholelithiasis during childhood: a prospective study. Pediatr Int 2004;46:322–4.
74. Bickford CL, Spencer AP. Biliary sludge and hyperbilirubinemia associated with ceftriaxone in an adult: case report and review of the literature. Pharmaco-therapy 2005;25:1389–95.
75. Coleman CI, Spencer JV, Chung JO, et al. Possible gatifloxacin-induced fulmi-nant hepatic failure. Ann Pharmacother 2002;36(7–8):1162–7.
76. Henann NE, Zambie MF. Gatifloxacin-associated acute hepatitis. Pharmaco-therapy 2001;21:1579–82.
77. Cheung O, Chopra K, Yu T, et al. Gatifloxacin-induced hepatotoxicity and acute pancreatitis. Ann Intern Med 2004;140:73–4.
78. Bjornsson E, Olsson R, Remotti H. Norfloxacin-induced eosinophilic necrotizing granulomatous hepatitis. Am J Gastroenterol 2000;95:3662–4.
79. Bataille L, Rahier J, Geubel A. Delayed and prolonged cholestatic hepatitis with ductopenia after long-term ciprofloxacin therapy for Crohn's disease. J Hepatol 2002;37:696–9.
80. Lazarczyk DA, Goldstein NS, Gordon SC. Trovafloxacin hepatotoxicity. Dig Dis Sci 2001;46:925–6.
81. Lucena MI, Andrade RJ, Rodrigo L, et al. Trovafloxacin-induced acute hepatitis. Clin Infect Dis 2000;30:400–1.
82. Garey KW, Amsden GW. Trovafloxacin: an overview. Pharmacotherapy 1999;19:21–34.
83. Chen HJ, Bloch KJ, MacLean JA. Acute eosinophilic hepatitis from trovafloxa-cin. N Engl J Med 2000;342:359–60.
84. Blum MD, Graham DJ, McCloskey CA. Temafloxacin syndrome: review of 95 cases. Clin Infect Dis 1994;18:946–50.
85. Ball P, Mandell L, Niki Y, et al. Comparative tolerability of the newer fluoroquino-lone antibacterials. Drug Saf 1999;21:407–21.
86. Gonzalez Carro P, Huidobro ML, Zabala AP, et al. Fatal subfulminant hepatic fail-ure with ofloxacin. Am J Gastroenterol 2000;95:1606.
87. Azinge NO, Garrick GA. Stevens-Johnson syndrome (erythema multiforme) following ingestion of trimethoprim-sulfamethoxazole on two separate

occasions in the same person: a case report. J Allergy Clin Immunol 1978;62: 125–6.

88. Dujovne CA, Chan CH, Zimmerman HJ. Sulfonamide hepatic injury. Review of the literature and report of a case due to sulfamethoxazole. N Engl J Med 1967;277:785–8.

89. Mainra RR, Card SE. Trimethoprim-sulfamethoxazole-associated hepatotoxicity – part of a hypersensitivity syndrome. Can J Clin Pharmacol 2003;10:175–8.

90. Farrell J, Naisbitt DJ, Drummond NS, et al. Characterization of sulfamethoxazole and sulfamethoxazole metabolite-specific T-cell responses in animals and humans. J Pharmacol Exp Ther 2003;306:229–37.

91. Naisbitt DJ, Gordon SF, Pirmohamed M, et al. Antigenicity and immunogenicity of sulphamethoxazole: demonstration of metabolism-dependent haptenation and T-cell proliferation in vivo. Br J Pharmacol 2001;133:295–305.

92. Rubin R. Sulfasalazine-induced fulminant hepatic failure and necrotizing pancreatitis. Am J Gastroenterol 1994;89:789–91.

93. Zaman F, Ye G, Abreo KD, et al. Successful orthotopic liver transplantation after trimethoprim-sulfamethoxazole associated fulminant liver failure. Clin Transplant 2003;17:461–4.

94. Munoz SJ, Martinez-Hernandez A, Maddrey WC. Intrahepatic cholestasis and phospholipidosis associated with the use of trimethoprim-sulfamethoxazole. Hepatology 1990;12:342–7.

95. Carson JL, Strom BL, Duff A, et al. Acute liver disease associated with erythromycins, sulfonamides, and tetracyclines. Ann Intern Med 1993;119(Pt 1):576–83.

96. Brett AS, Shaw SV. Simultaneous pancreatitis and hepatitis associated with trimethoprim-sulfamethoxazole. Am J Gastroenterol 1999;94:267–8.

97. Lewis JH, Zimmerman HJ. Drug- and chemical-induced cholestasis. Clin Liver Dis 1999;3:433–64.

98. Mohi-ud-din R, Lewis JH. Drug- and chemical-induced cholestasis. Clin Liver Dis 2004;8:95–132.

99. Yao F, Behling CA, Saab S, et al. Trimethoprim-sulfamethoxazole-induced vanishing bile duct syndrome. Am J Gastroenterol 1997;92:167–9.

100. Kowdley KV, Keeffe EB, Fawaz KA. Prolonged cholestasis due to trimethoprim sulfamethoxazole. Gastroenterology 1992;102:2148–50.

101. Tanner AR. Hepatic cholestasis induced by trimethoprim. Br Med J (Clin Res Ed) 1986;293:1072–3.

102. van der Ven AJ, Vree TB, Koopmans PP, et al. Adverse reactions to co-trimoxazole in HIV infection: a reappraisal of the glutathione-hydroxylamine hypothesis. J Antimicrob Chemother 1996;37(Suppl B):55–60.

103. Johnson DA, Cattau EL Jr, Kuritsky JN, et al. Liver involvement in the sulfone syndrome. Arch Intern Med 1986;146:875–7.

104. Sheen YS, Chu CY, Wang SH, et al. Dapsone hypersensitivity syndrome in non-leprosy patients: a retrospective study of its incidence in a tertiary referral center in Taiwan. J Dermatolog Treat 2009;20:340–3.

105. Agrawal S, Agarwalla A. Dapsone hypersensitivity syndrome: a clinicoepidemiological review. J Dermatol 2005;32:883–9.

106. Kunelis CT, Peters JL, Edmondson HA. Fatty liver of pregnancy and its relationship to tetracycline therapy. Am J Med 1965;38:359–77.

107. Combes B, Whalley PJ, Adams RH. Tetracycline and the liver. Prog Liver Dis 1972;4:589–96.

108. Breen K, Schenker S, Heimberg M. The effect of tetracycline on the hepatic secretion of triglyceride. Biochim Biophys Acta 1972;270:74–80.

109. Peters RL, Edmondson HA, Mikkelsen WP, et al. Tetracycline-induced fatty liver in nonpregnant patients. A report of six cases. Am J Surg 1967;113:622–32.
110. Lewis JH, Kleiner DE. Hepatic injury due to drugs, herbal compounds, chemicals and toxins. In: Burt AD, Portmann BC, Ferrell LD, editors. MacSween's pathology of the liver. 6th edition. Edinburgh (United Kingdom): Churchill Livingstone Elsevier; 2012. p. 645–760.
111. Freneaux E, Labbe G, Letteron P, et al. Inhibition of the mitochondrial oxidation of fatty acids by tetracycline in mice and in man: possible role in microvesicular steatosis induced by this antibiotic. Hepatology 1988;8:1056–62.
112. Hunt CM, Washington K. Tetracycline-induced bile duct paucity and prolonged cholestasis. Gastroenterology 1994;107:1844–7.
113. Gough A, Chapman S, Wagstaff K, et al. Minocycline induced autoimmune hepatitis and systemic lupus erythematosus-like syndrome. Br Med J 1996;312: 169–72.
114. Knowles SR, Shapiro L, Shear NH. Serious adverse reactions induced by minocycline. Report of 13 patients and review of the literature. Arch Dermatol 1996; 132:934–9.
115. Lawrenson RA, Seaman HE, Sundstrom A, et al. Liver damage associated with minocycline use in acne: a systematic review of the published literature and pharmacovigilance data. Drug Saf 2000;23:333–49.
116. Cjara AJ. Drug-induced autoimmune-like hepatitis. Dig Dis Sci 2011;56(4): 958–76.
117. Diehl AM, Latham P, Boitnott JK, et al. Cholestatic hepatitis from erythromycin ethylsuccinate. Report of two cases. Am J Med 1984;76:931–4.
118. Hosker JP, Jewell DP. Transient, selective factor X deficiency and acute liver failure following chest infection treated with erythromycin BP. Postgrad Med J 1983; 59:514–5.
119. Inman WH, Rawson NS. Erythromycin estolate and jaundice. Br Med J (Clin Res Ed) 1983;286:1954–5.
120. Zafrani ES, Ishak KG, Rudzki C. Cholestatic and hepatocellular injury associated with erythromycin esters: report of nine cases. Dig Dis Sci 1979;24:385–96.
121. Gholson CF, Warren GH. Fulminant hepatic failure associated with intravenous erythromycin lactobionate. Arch Intern Med 1990;150:215–6.
122. Degott C, Feldmann G, Larrey D, et al. Drug-induced prolonged cholestasis in adults: a histological semiquantitative study demonstrating progressive ductopenia. Hepatology 1992;15:244–51.
123. Trauner M, Meier PJ, Boyer JL. Molecular pathogenesis of cholestasis. N Engl J Med 1998;339(17):1217–27.
124. Chandrupatla S, Demetris AJ, Rabinovitz M. Azithromycin-induced intrahepatic cholestasis. Dig Dis Sci 2002;47:2186–8.
125. Suriawinata A, Min AD. A 33-year-old woman with jaundice after azithromycin use. Semin Liver Dis 2002;22:207–10.
126. Pedersen FM, Bathum L, Fenger C. Acute hepatitis and roxithromycin. Lancet 1993;341:251–2.
127. Wallace RJ Jr, Brown BA, Griffith DE. Drug intolerance to high-dose clarithromycin among elderly patients. Diagn Microbiol Infect Dis 1993;16:215–21.
128. Zimmerman HJ. Intrahepatic cholestasis. Arch Intern Med 1979;139:1038–45.
129. Haber I, Hubens H. Cholestatic jaundice after triacetyloleandomycin and oral contraceptives. The diagnostic value of gamma-glutamyl transpeptidase. Acta Gastroenterol Belg 1980;43(11–12):475–82.
130. Spiers KM, Zervos MJ. Telithromycin. Expert Rev Anti Infect Ther 2004;2:685–93.

131. Clay KD, Hanson JS, Pope SD, et al. Brief communication: severe hepatotoxicity of telithromycin: three case reports and literature review. Ann Intern Med 2006; 144(6):415–20.

132. Chen Y, Guo JJ, Healy DP, et al. Risk of hepatotoxicity associated with the use of telithromycin: a signal detection using data mining algorithms. Ann Pharmacother 2008;42(12):1791–6.

133. Dore DD, DiBello JR, Lapane KL. Telithromycin use and spontaneous reports of hepatotoxicity. Drug Saf 2007;30(8):697–703.

134. Brinker AD, Wassel RT, Lyndly J, et al. Telithromycin-associated hepatotoxicity: clinical spectrum and causality assessment of 42 cases. Hepatology 2009; 49(1):250–7.

135. Gleason PP, Walters C, Heaton AH, et al. Telithromycin: the perils of hasty adoption and persistence of off-label prescribing. J Manag Care Pharm 2007;13(5):420–5.

136. Goldstein LI, Ishak KG, Burns W. Hepatic injury associated with nitrofurantoin therapy. Am J Dig Dis 1974;19:987–98.

137. Sharp JR, Ishak KG, Zimmerman HJ. Chronic active hepatitis and severe hepatic necrosis associated with nitrofurantoin. Ann Intern Med 1980;92:14–9.

138. Amit G, Cohen P, Ackerman Z. Nitrofurantoin-induced chronic active hepatitis. Isr Med Assoc J 2002;4:184–6.

139. Sippel PJ, Agger WA. Nitrofurantoin-induced granulomatous hepatitis. Urology 1981;18:177–8.

140. Koulaouzidis A, Bhat S, Moschos J, et al. Nitrofurantoin-induced lung- and hepatotoxicity. Ann Hepatol 2007;6:119–21.

141. Feder H. Chloramphenicol: what we have learned in the last decade. South Med J 1986;79(9):1129–34.

142. Fernandez-Villar A, Sopena B, Fernandez-Villar J, et al. The influence of risk factors on the severity of anti-tuberculosis drug-induced hepatotoxicity. Int J Tuberc Lung Dis 2004;8:1499–505.

143. McNeill L, Allen M, Estrada C, et al. Pyrazinamide and rifampin vs isoniazid for the treatment of latent tuberculosis: improved completion rates but more hepatotoxicity. Chest 2003;123:102–6.

144. Scheuer PJ, Summerfield JA, Lal S, et al. Rifampicin hepatitis. A clinical and histological study. Lancet 1974;1:421–5.

145. Fountain FF, Tolley EA, Jacobs AR, et al. Rifampin hepatotoxicity associated with treatment of latent tuberculosis infection. Am J Med Sci 2009;337(5):317–20. http://dx.doi.org/10.1097/MAJ.0b013e31818c0134.

146. Stout JE. Safety of rifampin and pyrazinamide for the treatment of latent tuberculosis infection. Expert Opin Drug Saf 2004;3(3):187–98.

147. Sochocky S. Acute hepatitis due to para-aminosalicylic acid. Br J Clin Pract 1971;25:179–82.

148. Gulliford M, Mackay AD, Prowse K. Cholestatic jaundice caused by ethambutol. Br Med J (Clin Res Ed) 1986;292:866.

149. Chong VH, Lim KS. Hepatobiliary tuberculosis. Singapore Med J 2010;51(9): 744–51.

150. Amarapurkar DN, Patel ND, Amarapurkar AD. Hepatobiliary tuberculosis in western India. Indian J Pathol Microbiol 2008;51(2):175–81.

151. Mitchell JR, Zimmerman HJ, Ishak KG, et al. Isoniazid liver injury: clinical spectrum, pathology, and probable pathogenesis. Ann Intern Med 1976;84(2):181–92.

152. Byrd RB, Horn BR, Solomon DA, et al. Toxic effects of isoniazid in tuberculosis chemoprophylaxis. Role of biochemical monitoring in 1,000 patients. JAMA 1979;241(12):1239–41.

153. Garibaldi RA, Drusin RE, Ferebee SH, et al. Isoniazid-associated hepatitis. Report of an outbreak. Am Rev Respir Dis 1972;106:357–65.
154. Black M, Mitchell JR, Zimmerman HJ, et al. Isoniazid-associated hepatitis in 114 patients. Gastroenterology 1975;69:289–302.
155. Nolan CM, Goldberg SV, Buskin SE. Hepatotoxicity associated with isoniazid preventive therapy: a 7-year survey from a public health tuberculosis clinic. JAMA 1999;281:1014–8.
156. Fountain FF, Tolley E, Chrisman CR, et al. Isoniazid hepatotoxicity associated with treatment of latent tuberculosis infection: a 7-year evaluation from a public health tuberculosis clinic. Chest 2005;128(1):116–23.
157. Scharer L, Smith JP. Serum transaminase elevations and other hepatic abnormalities in patients receiving isoniazid. Ann Intern Med 1969;71:1113–20.
158. Lewis JH. The adaptive response (drug tolerance) helps to prevent drug-induced liver injury. Gastroenterol Hepatol (N Y) 2012;8(5):333–6.
159. Ostapowicz G, Fontana RJ, Schiodt FV, et al. Results of a prospective study of acute liver failure at 17 tertiary care centers in the United States. Ann Intern Med 2002;137:947–54.
160. Huang YS, Chern HD, Su WJ, et al. Polymorphism of the N-acetyltransferase 2 gene as a susceptibility risk factor for antituberculosis drug-induced hepatitis. Hepatology 2002;35:883–9.
161. Gao XF, Wang L, Liu GJ, et al. Rifampicin plus pyrazinamide versus isoniazid for treating latent tuberculosis infection: a meta-analysis. Int J Tuberc Lung Dis 2006;10(10):1080–90.
162. Akolo C, Adetifa I, Shepperd S, et al. Treatment of latent tuberculosis infection in HIV infected persons. Cochrane Database Syst Rev 2010;(1):CD000171. http://dx.doi.org/10.1002/14651858.CD000171.pub3.
163. Metushi IG, Cai P, Zhu X, et al. A fresh look at the mechanism of isoniazid-induced hepatotoxicity. Clin Pharmacol Ther 2011;89(6):911–4.
164. Durand F, Jebrak G, Pessayre D, et al. Hepatotoxicity of antitubercular treatments. Rational for monitoring liver status. Drug Saf 1996;15(6):394–405.
165. American Thoracic Society/CDC. Update: adverse event data and revised American Thoracic Society/CDC recommendations against the use of rifampin and pyrazinamide for treatment of latent tuberculosis infection – United States, 2003. MMWR Morb Mortal Wkly Rep 2003;52:735–9.
166. Steele MA, Burk RF, DesPrez RM. Toxic hepatitis with isoniazid and rifampin: a meta-analysis. Chest 1991;99:465–71.
167. Pessayre D. Present views on isoniazid and isoniazid-rifampicin hepatitis. Agressologie 1982;23:13–5.
168. Rae JM, Johnson MD, Lippman ME, et al. Rifampin is a selective, pleiotropic inducer of drug metabolism genes in human hepatocytes: studies with cDNA and oligonucleotide expression assays. J Pharmacol Exp Ther 2001;229:849–57.
169. Gordin FM, Cohn DL, Matts JP, et al. Hepatotoxicity of rifampin and pyrazinamide in the treatment of latent tuberculosis infection in HIV-infected persons: is it different than in HIV-uninfected persons? Clin Infect Dis 2004;39(4):561–5.
170. Byrne JA, Strautnieks SS, Mieli-Vergani G, et al. The human bile salt export pump: characteristics of substrate specificity and identification of inhibitors. Gastroenterology 2002;123:1649–58.
171. Capelle P, Dhumeaux D, Mora M, et al. Effect of rifampicin on liver function in man. Gut 1972;13:366–71.

172. Grosset J, Leventis S. Adverse effects of rifampicin. Rev Infect Dis 1983;5: S440–50.

173. Benson CA, Williams PL, Cohn DL, et al. Clarithromycin or rifabutin alone or in combination for primary prophylaxis of Mycobacterium avium complex disease in patients with AIDS: a randomized, double-blind, placebo-controlled trial. The AIDS Clinical Trials Group 196/Terry Beirn Community Programs for Clinical Reasearch on AIDS 009 Protocol Team. J Infect Dis 2000;181(4):1289–97.

174. Aristoff PA, Garcia GA, Kirchhoff PD. Hollis Showalter HD. Rifamycins—obstacles and opportunities. Tuberculosis (Edinb) 2010;90(2):94–118.

175. Chang KC, Leung CC, Yew WW, et al. Hepatotoxicity of pyrazinamide: cohort and case-control analyses. Am J Respir Crit Care Med 2008;177:1391–6.

176. Khokhar O, Gange C, Clement S, et al. Autoimmune hepatitis and thyroiditis associated with rifampin and pyrazinamide prophylaxis: an unusual reaction. Dig Dis Sci 2005;50:207–11.

177. Lacroix C, Guyonnaud C, Chaou M, et al. Interactions between allopurinol and pyrazinamide. Eur Respir J 1988;1:807–11.

178. Tostmann A, Aamoutse RE, Peters WH, et al. Xanthine oxidase inhibition by allopurinol increases in vitro pyrazinamide-induced hepatotoxicity in HepG2 cells. Drug Chem Toxicol 2010;33(3):325–8.

179. Shih TY, Pai CY, Yang P, et al. A novel mechanism underlies the hepatotoxicity of pyrazinamide. Antimicrob Agents Chemother 2013;57(4):1685–90. http://dx.doi.org/10.1128/AAC.01866-12.

180. Prasad R, Verma SK, Sahai S, et al. Efficacy and safety of kanamycin, ethionamide, PAS and cycloserine in multidrug-resistant pulmonary tuberculosis patients. Indian J Chest Dis Allied Sci 2006;48(3):183–6.

181. Saukkonen JJ, Cohn DL, Jasmer RM, et al, ATS (American Thoracic Society) Hepatotoxicity of Antituberculosis Therapy Subcommittee. An official ATS statement: hepatotoxicity of antituberculosis therapy. Am J Respir Crit Care Med 2006;174:935–52.

182. Centers for Disease Control and Prevention. Severe isoniazid-associated liver injuries among persons being treated for latent tuberculosis infection — United States, 2004–2008. MMWR Morb Mortal Wkly Rep 2010;59(8):224–9.

183. Kunst H, Khan KS. Age-related risk of hepatotoxicity in the treatment of latent tuberculosis infection: a systematic review. Int J Tuberc Lung Dis 2010;14(11): 1374–81.

184. Franks AL, Binkin NJ, Snider DE Jr, et al. Isoniazid hepatitis among pregnant and postpartum Hispanic patients. Public Health Rep 1989;104(2):151–5.

185. Sharma SK, Singla R, Sarda P, et al. Safety of 3 different reintroduction regimens of antituberculosis drugs after development of antituberculosis treatment-induced hepatotoxicity. Clin Infect Dis 2010;50(6):833–9.

186. Singla R, Sharma SK, Mohan A, et al. Evaluation of risk factors for antituberculosis treatment induced hepatotoxicity. Indian J Med Res 2010;132:81–6.

187. Warmelink I, Ten Hacken NH, van der Werf TS, et al. Weight loss during tuberculosis treatment is an important risk factor for drug-induced hepatotoxicity. Br J Nutr 2010;28:1–9.

188. Pasipanodya JG, Gumbo T. Clinical and toxicodynamic evidence that high-dose pyrazinamide is not more hepatotoxic than the low doses currently used. Antimicrob Agents Chemother 2010;54(7):2847–54.

189. Ungo JR, Jones D, Ashkin D, et al. Antituberculosis drug-induced hepatotoxicity. The role of hepatitis C virus and the human immunodeficiency virus. Am J Respir Crit Care Med 1998;157(6 Pt 1):1871–6.

190. Nader LA, de Mattos AA, Picon PD, et al. Hepatotoxicity due to rifampicin, isoniazid and pyrazinamide in patients with tuberculosis: is anti-HCV a risk factor? Ann Hepatol 2010;9(1):70–4.
191. Sirinak C, Kittikraisak W, Pinjeesekikul D, et al. Viral hepatitis and HIV-associated tuberculosis: risk factors and TB treatment outcomes in Thailand. BMC Public Health 2008;8:245.
192. Huang YS, Chern HD, Su WJ, et al. Cytochrome P450 2E1 genotype and the susceptibility to antituberculosis drug-induced hepatitis. Hepatology 2003; 37(4):924–30.
193. Tang N, Deng R, Wang Y, et al. GSTM1 and GSTT1 null polymorphisms and susceptibility to anti-tuberculosis drug-induced liver injury: a meta-analysis. Int J Tuberc Lung Dis 2013;17(1):17–25. http://dx.doi.org/10.5588/ijtld.12.0447.
194. Forestiero FJ, Cecon L, Hirata MH, et al. Relationship of NAT2, CYP2E1 and GSTM1/GSTT1 polymorphisms with mild elevation of liver enzymes in Brazilian individuals under anti-tuberculosis drug therapy. Clin Chim Acta 2013;415: 215–9. http://dx.doi.org/10.1016/j.cca.2012.10.030.
195. Tang SW, Lv XZ, Chen R, et al. Lack of association between genetic polymorphisms of CYP3A4, CYP2C9, CYP2C19 and anti-tuberculosis drug-induced liver injury in community-based Chinese population. Clin Exp Pharmacol Physiol 2013;40(5):326–32. http://dx.doi.org/10.1111/1440-1681.12074.
196. Azuma J, Ohno M, Kubota R, et al. NAT2 genotype guided regimen reduces isoniazid-induced liver injury and early treatment failure in the 6-month four-drug standard treatment of tuberculosis: a randomized controlled trial for pharmacogenetics-based therapy. Eur J Clin Pharmacol 2013;69(5):1091–101.
197. Saukkonen J. Challenges in reintroducing tuberculosis medications after hepatotoxicity. Clin Infect Dis 2010;50(6):840–2.
198. Senousy BE, Belal SI, Draganov PV. Hepatotoxic effects of therapies for tuberculosis. Nat Rev Gastroenterol Hepatol 2010;7(10):543–56.
199. Ichai P, Saliba F, Antoun F, et al. Acute liver failure due to antitubercular therapy: Strategy for antitubercular treatment before and after liver transplantation. Liver Transpl 2010;16(10):1136–46.
200. Baniasadi S, Eftekhari P, Tabarsi P, et al. Protective effect of N-acetylcysteine on antituberculosis drug-induced hepatotoxicity. Eur J Gastroenterol Hepatol 2010; 22(10):1235–8.
201. Li J, Lin WF, Pan YY, et al. Protective effect of silibinin on liver injury induced by antituberculosis drugs. Zhonghua Gan Zang Bing Za Zhi 2010;18(5):385–6 [in Chinese].
202. Yue J, Dong G, He C, et al. Protective effects of thiopronin against isoniazid-induced hepatotoxicity in rats. Toxicology 2009;264(3):185–91.
203. Singh M, Sasi P, Gupta VH, et al. Protective effect of curcumin, silymarin and N-acetylcysteine on antitubercular drug-induced hepatotoxicity assessed in an in vitro model. Hum Exp Toxicol 2012;31(8):788–97.
204. Samuel AJ, Mohan S, Chellappan DK, et al. Hibiscus vitifolius (Linn) root extract shows potent protective action against anti-tubercular drug induced hepatotoxicity. J Ethnopharmacol 2012;141(1):396–402.
205. Jafri SM, Singal AG, Kaul D, et al. Detection and management of latent tuberculosis in liver transplant patients. Liver Transpl 2011;17(3):306–14.
206. Fábrega E, Sampedro B, Cabezas J, et al. Chemoprophylaxis with isoniazid in liver transplant recipients. Liver Transpl 2012;18(9):1110–7.
207. Stucchi RS, Boin IF, Angerami RN, et al. Is isoniazid safe for liver transplant candidates with latent tuberculosis? Transplant Proc 2012;44(8):2406–10.

208. Yehia BR, Blumberg EA. Mycobacterium tuberculosis infection in liver transplantation. Liver Transpl 2010;16(10):1129–35.

209. Bodro M, Sabé N, Santín M, et al. Clinical features and outcomes of tuberculosis in solid organ transplant recipients. Transplant Proc 2012;44(9):2686–9.

210. Lewis JH, Zimmerman HJ, Benson GD, et al. Hepatic injury associated with ketoconazole therapy. Analysis of 33 cases. Gastroenterology 1984;86:503–13.

211. Lake-Bakaar G, Scheuer PJ, Sherlock S. Hepatic reactions associated with ketoconazole in the United Kingdom. Br Med J (Clin Res Ed) 1987;294:419–22.

212. Stricker BH, Blok AP, Bronkhorst FB, et al. Ketoconazole-associated hepatic injury. A clinicopathological study of 55 cases. J Hepatol 1986;3:399–406.

213. Bronstein JA, Gros P, Hernandez E, et al. Fatal acute hepatic necrosis due to dose-dependent fluconazole hepatotoxicity. Clin Infect Dis 1997;25:1266–7.

214. Ikemoto H. A clinical study of fluconazole for the treatment of deep mycoses. Diagn Microbiol Infect Dis 1989;12(Suppl 4):239S–47S.

215. Gupta AK, Chwetzoff E, Del Rosso J, et al. Hepatic safety of itraconazole. J Cutan Med Surg 2002;6:210–3.

216. Talwalkar JA, Soetikno RE, Carr-Locke DL, et al. Severe cholestasis related to itraconazole for the treatment of onychomycosis. Am J Gastroenterol 1999;94:3632–3.

217. Somchit N, Norshahida AR, Hasiah AH, et al. Hepatotoxicity induced by antifungal drugs itraconazole and fluconazole in rats: a comparative in vivo study. Hum Exp Toxicol 2004;23:519–25.

218. Chu HY, Jain R, Xie H, et al. Voriconazole therapeutic drug monitoring: retrospective cohort study of the relationship to clinical outcomes and adverse events. BMC Infect Dis 2013;13(1):105.

219. Solís-Muñoz P, López JC, Bernal W, et al. Voriconazole hepatotoxicity in severe liver dysfunction. J Infect 2013;66(1):80–6.

220. Miller MA. Reversible hepatotoxicity related to amphotericin B. Can Med Assoc J 1984;131:1245–7.

221. Vermes A, Guchelaar HJ, Dankert J. Flucytosine: a review of its pharmacology, clinical indications, pharmacokinetics, toxicity and drug interactions. J Antimicrob Chemother 2000;46:171–9.

222. Anania FA, Rabin L. Terbinafine hepatotoxicity resulting in chronic biliary ductopenia and portal fibrosis. Am J Med 2002;112:741–2.

223. Fernandes NF, Geller SA, Fong TL. Terbinafine hepatotoxicity: case report and review of the literature. Am J Gastroenterol 1998;93:459–60.

224. Lazaros GA, Papatheodoridis GV, Delladetsima JK, et al. Terbinafine-induced cholestatic liver disease. J Hepatol 1996;24:753–6.

225. Lovell MO, Speeg KV, Havranek RD, et al. Histologic changes resembling acute rejection in a liver transplant patient treated with terbinafine. Hum Pathol 2003;34:187–9.

226. Ajit C, Suvannasankha A, Zaeri N, et al. Terbinafine-associated hepatotoxicity. Am J Med Sci 2003;325:292–5.

227. Paredes AH, Lewis JH. Terbinafine-induced acute autoimmune hepatitis in the setting of hepatitis B virus infection. Ann Pharmacother 2007;41(5):880–4.

228. Kleiner DE, Gaffey MJ, Sallie R, et al. Histopathologic changes associated with fialuridine hepatotoxicity. Mod Pathol 1997;10:192–9.

229. Cervoni JP, Degos F, Marcellin P, et al. Acute hepatitis induced by alpha-interferon, associated with viral clearance, in chronic hepatitis C. J Hepatol 1997;27:1113–6.

230. Lock G, Reng CM, Graeb C, et al. Interferon-induced hepatic failure in a patient with hepatitis C. Am J Gastroenterol 1999;94:2570–1.
231. Papo T, Marcellin P, Bernuau J, et al. Autoimmune chronic hepatitis exacerbated by alpha-interferon. Ann Intern Med 1992;116:51–3.
232. Veerabagu MP, Finkelstein SD, Rabinovitz M. Granulomatous hepatitis in a patient with chronic hepatitis C treated with interferon-alpha. Dig Dis Sci 1997; 42:1445–8.
233. Goldin RD, Levine TS, Foster GR, et al. Granulomas and hepatitis C. Histopathology 1996;28:265–7.
234. Lewis JH. Granulomas of the liver. In: Schiff ER, Sorrell MF, Maddrey WC, editors. Schiff's diseases of the liver. 11th edition. Baltimore (MD): Lippincott Williams and Wilkins; 2011. p. 1034–58.
235. Dousset B, Conti F, Houssin D, et al. Acute vanishing bile duct syndrome after interferon therapy for recurrent HCV infection in liver-transplant recipients. N Engl J Med 1994;330:1160–1.
236. Janssen HL, Brouwer JT, Nevens F, et al. Fatal hepatic decompensation associated with interferon alfa. European concerted action on viral hepatitis (Eurohep). Br Med J 1993;306:107–8.
237. Cianciara J, Laskus T. Development of transient autoimmune hepatitis during interferon treatment of chronic hepatitis B. Dig Dis Sci 1995;40:1842–4.
238. Bernuau J, Larrey D, Campillo B, et al. Amodiaquine-induced fulminant hepatitis. J Hepatol 1988;6:109–12.
239. Wharton JM, Coleman DL, Wofsy CB, et al. Trimethoprim-sulfamethoxazole or pentamidine for *Pneumocystis carinii* pneumonia in the acquired immunodeficiency syndrome. A prospective randomized trial. Ann Intern Med 1986;105: 37–44.
240. Bjornsson E, Nordlinder H, Olsson R. Metronidazole as a probable cause of severe liver injury. Hepatogastroenterology 2002;49:252–4.
241. Farid Z, Smith JH, Bassily S, et al. Hepatotoxicity after treatment of schistosomiasis with hycanthone. Br Med J 1972;2:88–9.
242. Manivel JC, Bloomer JR, Snover DC. Progressive bile duct injury after thiabendazole administration. Gastroenterology 1987;93:245–9.
243. Roy MA, Nugent FW, Aretz HT. Micronodular cirrhosis after thiabendazole. Dig Dis Sci 1989;34:938–41.
244. Reshef R, Lok AS, Sherlock S. Cholestatic jaundice in fascioliasis treated with niclofolan. Br Med J (Clin Res Ed) 1982;285:1243–4.
245. Hamlyn AN, Morris JS, Sarkany I, et al. Piperazine hepatitis. Gastroenterology 1976;70:1144–7.
246. Jagota SC. Jaundice due to albendazole. Indian J Gastroenterol 1989;8:58.
247. Junge U, Mohr W. Mebendazole-hepatitis. Z Gastroenterol 1983;21:736–8 [in German].
248. Ebeid F, Farghali H, Botros S, et al. Praziquantel did not exhibit hepatotoxicity in a study with isolated hepatocytes. Trans R Soc Trop Med Hyg 1990;84(2): 262–4.
249. Stine JG, Lewis JH. Review article: use of medications in patients with cirrhosis. Aliment Pharmacol Ther 2013;37(12):1132–56.
250. Segarra-Newnham M, Henneman A. Antibiotic prophylaxis for prevention of spontaneous bacterial peritonitis in patients without gastrointestinal bleeding. Ann Pharmacother 2010;44(12):1946–54.
251. Chavez-Tapia NC, Barrientos-Gutierrez T, Tellez-Avila FI, et al. Antibiotic prophylaxis for cirrhotic patients with upper gastrointestinal bleeding. Cochrane

Database Syst Rev 2010;(9):CD002907. http://dx.doi.org/10.1002/14651858. CD002907.pub2.

252. Terg R, Fassio E, Guevara M, et al. Ciprofloxacin in primary prophylaxis of spontaneous bacterial peritonitis: a randomized, placebo-controlled study. J Hepatol 2008;48(5):774–9.

253. Dixit RK, Satapathy SK, Kumar R, et al. Pharmacokinetics of ciprofloxacin in patients with liver cirrhosis. Indian J Gastroenterol 2002;21:62–3.

254. Montay G, Gaillot J. Pharmacokinetics of fluoroquinolones in hepatic failure. J Antimicrob Chemother 1990;26(Suppl B):61–7.

255. Silvain C, Bouquet S, Breux JP, et al. Oral pharmacokinetics and ascitic fluid penetration of ofloxacin in cirrhosis. Eur J Clin Pharmacol 1989;37(3):261–5.

256. Sambatakou H, Giamarellos-Bourboulis EJ, Galanakis N, et al. Phramacokinetics of fluoroquinolones in uncompensated cirrhosis: the significance of penetration in the ascetic fluid. Int J Antimicrob Agents 2001;18:441–4.

257. Vuppalanchi R, Juluri R, Ghabril M, et al. Drug-induced QT prolongation in cirrhotic patients with transjugular intrahepatic portosystemic shunt. J Clin Gastroenterol 2011;45(7):638–42.

258. Amarapurkar DN. Prescribing medications in patients with decompensated liver cirrhosis. Int J Hepatol 2011;2011:1–5.

259. Cho YJ, Lee SM, Yoo CG, et al. Clinical characteristics of tuberculosis in patients with liver cirrhosis. Respirology 2007;12:401–5.

260. Gupta NK, Lewis JH. Review article: the use of potentially hepatotoxic drugs in patients with liver disease. Aliment Pharmacol Ther 2008;28:1021–41.

261. Saito A, Nagayama N, Yagi O, et al. Tuberculosis complicated with liver cirrhosis. Kekkaku 2006;81:457–65.

262. Jahng AW, Tran T, Bui L, et al. Safety of treatment of latent tuberculosis infection in compensated cirrhotic patients during transplant candidacy period. Transplantation 2007;83:1557–62.

263. Holty JE, Gould MK, Meinke L, et al. Tuberculosis in liver transplant recipients: a systematic review and meta-analysis of individual patient data. Liver Transpl 2009;15:894–906.

264. Kaneko Y, Nagayama N, Kawabe Y, et al. Drug-induced hepatotoxicity caused by anti-tuberculosis drugs in tuberculosis patients complicated with chronic hepatitis. Kekkaku 2008;83:13–9.

265. Park WB, Kim W, Lee KL, et al. Antituberculosis drug-induced liver injury in chronic hepatitis and cirrhosis. J Infect 2010;61(4):323–39.

# Nonsteroidal Anti-Inflammatory Drug–Induced Hepatoxicity

Alberto Unzueta, MD[a], Hugo E. Vargas, MD[b],*

## KEYWORDS

- Nonsteroidal anti-inflammatory drugs • Drug-induced liver injury • Acute liver injury
- Liver transplantation • Idiosyncratic hepatotoxicity • Hy's law • Drug safety
- Drug surveillance

## KEY POINTS

- The mechanism of hepatotoxicity associated with NSAIDs is mainly idiosyncratic and has a very low incidence compared with the widespread use of NSAIDs worldwide.
- Surveillance and monitoring after approval of new medications and NSAIDs is extremely important to detect severe cases of hepatotoxicity.
- Among currently approved NSAIDs the safety profile for severe hepatotoxicity is equivalent with some evidence of cross-reactivity among some NSAIDs. A higher incidence of DILI has been described with diclofenac and sulindac.
- A genetic predisposition to develop DILI has been found with some NSAIDs (diclofenac and lumiracoxib). Pharmacogenomic studies are a promising way to evaluate individuals or populations with predisposition to DILI.
- Use of NSAIDs in patients with coexisting liver or renal disease and who are taking other potential hepatotoxic medications must be avoided because this could increase the potential for severe hepatotoxicity.

## INTRODUCTION

Since recognition of the first cases of nonsteroidal anti-inflammatory drug (NSAIDs)–induced hepatotoxicity the incidence has been considered very rare, mainly because of the idiosyncratic cause of drug-induced liver injury (DILI). With the more widespread use of these prescription and over-the-counter medications, well-described DILI with acute liver failure (ALF) leading to transplantation and death in relationship to these agents has been reported. However, most of the cases associated with DILI caused by NSAIDs (N-DILI) are asymptomatic or mild, and only in a minority of cases has severe hepatotoxicity been described.

[a] Division of Hospital Internal Medicine, Mayo Clinic, 5777 East Mayo Boulevard, Phoenix, AZ 85054, USA; [b] Division of Hepatology, Mayo Clinic, 5777 East Mayo Boulevard, Phoenix, AZ 85054, USA
* Corresponding author.
*E-mail address:* vargas.hugo@mayo.edu

Clin Liver Dis 17 (2013) 643–656
http://dx.doi.org/10.1016/j.cld.2013.07.009
1089-3261/13/$ – see front matter © 2013 Elsevier Inc. All rights reserved.

Several cases of NSAIDs withdrawn from the market (bromfenac, benoxaprofen, and lumiracoxib) illustrate the relevance of postmarketing monitoring to detect severe cases of liver injury. The incremental regulations and restrictions applied by some countries in the use of NSAIDs, such as nimesulide, are relevant to prevent new cases of severe hepatotoxicity. Most of these regulations are based on reports of isolated cases because epidemiologic studies have not clearly revealed evidence of severe hepatotoxicity with most NSAIDs.

The development of cyclooxygenase-2 (COX-2) inhibitors opened a promising era for NSAIDs because of the significant decrease in gastrointestinal side effects. However, the evidence of severe cardiovascular events led to the withdrawal of rofecoxib in 2004 and significantly limited the use of celecoxib with a "boxed warning" by the Food and Drug Administration (FDA). DILI is a rare event but currently is the most common cause of ALF in the United States, hence the diagnosis of N-DILI is of clinical relevance.

## DRUG-INDUCED LIVER INJURY

Idiosyncratic DILI is defined as an unexpected hepatic adverse drug reaction of an individual to the pharmacologic action of a drug. DILI has been recognized as the most common cause of ALF in the United States.[1] Acetaminophen is responsible for approximately half of cases and nonacetaminophen DILI is implicated in 7% to 15% of cases in the United States and Europe.[2–4] The most common drugs associated with DILI are antibiotics, antiepileptic drugs, and NSAIDs.[5,6] Hepatotoxicity is also one of the main reasons for nonapproval of new medications by the FDA. The incidence of DILI has been calculated in a prospective population study in France as 14 cases in 100,000 people with a rate of 6% fatality[7]; however, the true incidence is unknown because of underreporting and lack of diagnostic standards. Hospitalizations associated with DILI are rare but the mortality associated with ALF is significant.[8]

### Diagnostic Criteria for DILI

An international DILI Expert Working Group has recently published guidelines for the diagnosis and classification of DILI.[9] One of the following criteria need to be present: (1) greater than or equal to 5 × Upper Limit of Normal (ULN) level for alanine aminotransferase (ALT); (2) greater than or equal to 2 × ULN for alkaline phosphatase (AP); or (3) greater than or equal to 3 × ULN for ALT and greater than 2 × ULN for bilirubin. These criteria aim to guide the standardization of research in DILI and also to help diagnose drug hepatotoxicity.

### Clinical Patterns of DILI

Three types of liver damage based on ALT, AP, and bilirubin levels are currently considered. Hepatocellular is the most common followed by mixed and cholestatic. Liver biopsy is not necessary for diagnosis in most cases because there are not specific histologic criteria for diagnosis of DILI. The pattern of liver injury is defined by R value, where $R = (ALT/ULN)(ALP/ULN)$, hepatocellular pattern: $R \geq 5$, mixed pattern: $R > 2$ and $< 5$, cholestatic pattern: $R \leq 2$.[9]

### Hy's Law and Severity of Hepatotoxicity

A clinical observation made by the late Hyman Zimmerman,[10–12] considered the founding father of the study of drug hepatotoxicity, has been validated in several population studies as a marker of severe DILI.[5,13] Fulfillment of Hy's law or a

Hy's case consists of hepatocellular damage with increase in bilirubin and clinical jaundice with minimal elevation of AP (elevations of aminotransferases >3 × ULN and serum bilirubin >2 × ULN). This has been associated with ALF and approximately 10% mortality or need for liver transplantation.[5] It is considered a safety biomarker by the FDA that identifies a subgroup of patients with high risk of liver injury.[14] The grading of the severity of DILI has been recently proposed as mild, moderate, severe, and fatal or transplantation based on common laboratory values that assess liver disease.[9]

### Clinical Resources

*Liver tox* (http://livertox.nih.gov) is a comprehensive World Wide Web–based resource created in 2012 by the DILI network that provides current clinical information regarding approximately 600 drugs currently approved by the FDA in the United States. It provides illustrative clinical cases and can also generate causality assessment scores of individual cases based on RUCAM diagnostic instrument.[15] A compilation of drugs that have been associated with ALF reported to major registries and other databases has been created.[16]

### SEVERE HEPATOTOXICITY ASSOCIATED WITH NSAIDS
#### The Bromfenac, Benoxaprofen, and Lumiracoxib Cases

The history of bromfenac illustrates the challenges involved in detecting N-DILI. Bromfenac, a phenylaceticacid-derivative NSAID, was approved by the FDA in 1997 for the management of acute orthopedic pain, with recommended use of no more than 10 days. During the 4 months after its approval, numerous individual reports and case series were published that documented resultant ALF requiring liver transplantation or causing death.[17–20] A systematic review of NSAIDs withdrawn from the US and UK market (bromfenac, ibufenac, and benoxaprofen) found no published clinical trials of bromfenac before its approval.[21] The preapproval public FDA database included three clinical trials with 1195 subjects. Transaminase elevations greater than 3X ULN were detected in 2.8% of subjects, most of whom had flu-like symptoms beforehand. In June 1998, the manufacturer voluntarily withdrew bromfenac less than 1 year after its approval after reports of four deaths and eight cases of ALF necessitating liver transplantation.[21]

The bromfenac case illustrates nonallergic, idiosyncratic drug-related hepatotoxicity.[22] Hepatocyte necrosis was associated with cumulative doses of this NSAID.[23] In the preapproval trials, one case of possible hepatocellular injury associated with jaundice was detected, leading to a projected incidence of ALF of 1 per 10,000 (Hy's law).[21] In hindsight, questions arose about whether the detection of even one case that invoked Hy's law (severe hepatocellular jaundice) and the presence of symptomatic hepatitis in other cases might have prevented approval of the drug and the subsequent postapproval morbidity and mortality.[24] It is also relevant that severe hepatotoxicity developed in most patients who took the medication for a longer time than the FDA guidelines and that labeling instructions for short-term use were not followed by physicians or patients.[12] Because the incidence of idiosyncratic severe hepatotoxicity with NSAIDs is rare, the number of afflicted subjects required in the preapproval process to trigger concerns of severe hepatotoxicity is an important fact to consider.

The relevance of surveillance and monitoring programs, and the report of single cases by physicians (FDA MEDWATCH), is crucial in the evaluation of drugs with potentially severe hepatotoxicity. This is exemplified by a cautionary footnote from the editors of the *British Medical Journal* in a letter to the editor reporting two cases of benoxaprofen-related fatal cholestatic jaundice[25]:

> We have received several other letters describing side effects of benoxaprofen but for reasons of space we suggest that further case reports should be forwarded to the Committee on Safety of Medicines.[25]
>
> —ED, BMJ

A previous report of five elderly women with cholestatic jaundice and ALF associated with benoxaprofen had been published by the journal.[26] Benoxaprofen is an NSAID that was approved in the United States in April 1982 and was withdrawn from the market 4 months later, after numerous reports of severe hepatotoxicity in the United States and United Kingdom. Although there were no case reports published in the United States, the FDA received numerous reports of liver injury associated with benoxaprofen.[27]

Lumiracoxib is a selective COX-2 inhibitor structurally related to diclofenac. It is the latest NSAID withdrawn from the market because of association with severe DILI. It was never approved for use in the United States. Lumiracoxib illustrates, as in the case with bromfenac and benoxaprofen, the importance of postmarketing monitoring to detect severe cases of N-DILI that were not expected in preapproval clinical trials.[28] The Therapeutic Arthritis Research and Gastrointestinal Event Trial, a randomized clinical trial comparing lumiracoxib with naproxen and ibuprofen, found elevations of aminotransferases greater than three times ULN that was significant between lumiracoxib (2.57%; N = 230) and NSAIDs (0.63%; N = 56); odds ratio, 3.97 (confidence interval [CI], 2.96–5.32). Six cases of clinical hepatitis were detected in the lumiracoxib group; all of them improved after the drug was stopped and no reports of liver failure were seen.[29,30] During clinical trials lumiracoxib showed a promising cardiovascular and gastrointestinal safety profile. However, the drug was withdrawn in Europe and Australia (2007) because of reports of approximately 20 cases of severe hepatotoxicity that included 14 cases with ALF with two deaths and three liver transplants.[28,31,32] A genome-wide association study found an increased risk for DILI in lumiracoxib users with the HLA-DQA1*0102 allele.[33] There is an increasing number of drugs that have been linked to human leukocyte antigen genotypes.[34] In the future, the use of pharmacogenetic studies could play a meaningful role in the evaluation of the hepatotoxicity of drugs by the identification of genetic risk factors for susceptible populations.[35]

### Nimesulide: A Case of Incremental Regulation to Prevent Hepatotoxicity

Nimesulide is an NSAID that belongs to the class of the sulphonanilides (the only NSAID in this group). It was initially approved in Italy in 1985 and is available in more than 50 countries.[36] Some countries, such as the United States, Canada, England, Japan, Australia, and New Zealand, never approved its use. Several other European countries, such as Finland, Spain, Ireland, Portugal, and a handful in other parts of the world (Argentina, Uruguay, and Singapore) withdrew the medication secondary to concerns of severe hepatotoxicity based on published reports.[36,37] Nimesulide has continued to be prescribed widely and is commonly used in Italy and other countries.[38] Epidemiologic population-based reports have not confirmed an increased risk of severe hepatotoxicity compared with other commonly used NSAIDs.[39] A Consensus Report Group on nimesulide in 2005 found a positive risk-benefit ratio in terms of gastrointestinal side effects and hepatotoxicity.[40] However, in 2007, the European Medicines Agency issued restrictions for prescription of nimesulide as a second-line therapy. In 2011, new European restrictions limited nimesulide for use in acute pain and primary dysmenorrhea because of concerns that long-term use will increase the risk of liver injury.[41]

## EPIDEMIOLOGY OF NSAID-INDUCED HEPATOTOXICITY

In part because of the heterogeneity of this drug class and the relative safety of these agents, the incidence of N-DILI in several population-based studies has been estimated to be low and ranging from 0.29 to 9 per 100,000 patient-years.[42]

A prospective double-blind trial of diclofenac (N = 17,289 patients) versus etoricoxib (N = 17,412 patients) for rheumatoid arthritis (RA) or osteoarthritis (OA) with a mean follow-up of 18 months found no increased incidence in hospitalizations or mortality associated with either NSAID.[43] There were four cases of liver injury (0.023%) and two cases of severe hepatocellular jaundice (0.012%), but no cases of liver failure, transplantation, or death. Patients with preexisting liver disease or alcohol abuse were excluded from the study.

A postmarketing surveillance study from the reimbursement database of National Health Insurance in Taiwan reported 4519 hospitalizations associated with acute hepatitis (viral and other hepatobiliary pathology excluded). This led the investigators to conclude that there was an increased incidence of hospitalizations associated with N-DILI (acute/subacute necrosis, toxic hepatitis) from 2001 to 2004.[44] The odds ratios for nimesulide-, diclofenac-, ibuprofen-, and celecoxib-related DILI were considerably increased.

A case/noncase study that analyzed the databases of the US FDA and the World Health Organization for the proportion of reports of events associated with N-DILI found an increased rate of hepatotoxicity associated with nimesulide (16.7% vs 14.4%), bromfenac (12% vs 20.7%), diclofenac (8.1% vs 4.7%), and sulindac (6.1% vs 9.9%), compared with that of other NSAIDs.[45]

A comparison of pharmacovigilance databases from Spain and France from 1982 to 2001 using a case/noncase method revealed differences in NSAID hepatotoxicity.[46] The Spanish database included 2114 (3.38%) out of 62,456 reports of patients with liver injury and the French database had 27,372 (13.68%) out of 200,046 cases of liver injury. In the Spanish database, the drugs droxicam, sulindac, and nimesulide showed a significant association with hepatotoxicity. In the French database, significant risk was associated with clometacin and sulindac. The difference in the reported DILI was attributed to different prescription uses, reporting patterns, and possible genetic differences.

A systematic review of the literature of epidemiologic population studies evaluating NSAID liver injury associated with hospitalization or death showed an incidence of hospitalization ranging from 3.1 to 23.4 per 100,000 patient-years of current use of NSAIDs.[47] No deaths were reported.

Another systematic review of randomized controlled trials of NSAIDs used for management of OA or RA revealed that diclofenac (3.55%; CI, 3.12%–4.03%) had increased aminotransferases greater than 3X ULN compared with placebo (0.29%; CI, 0.17%–0.51%) and other NSAIDs (except for rofecoxib: 1.80%; CI, 1.52%–2.13%).[48] Only one hospitalization (among 37,671 patients) and one death were reported (among 51,942 patients) in a patient taking naproxen.

Risk factors associated with N-DILI are genetic, nongenetic, and environmental. Among nongenetic factors age, gender, use of other hepatotoxic drugs, and other conditions, such as chronic liver diseases, OA, RA, or human immunodeficiency infection, have been implicated.[49,50] A predisposition of N-DILI in patients with metabolic syndrome and steatosis has been proposed.[51] Genetic factors of N-DILI have been identified for diclofenac and lumiracoxib.[33,52]

### Characteristics of NSAIDs Associated with Hepatotoxicity

#### Propionic acid derivatives

**Ibuprofen** The hepatotoxicity associated with ibuprofen has been considered to be the lowest among commonly used NSAIDs (**Fig. 1, Table 1**).[42,48,53] The most common type of liver injury caused by ibuprofen is hepatocellular and cholestatic. It has been associated with prolonged cholestasis and vanishing bile duct syndrome.[54,55] Cases of hepatocellular damage with significant elevation of transaminases and resolution of abnormalities after stopping ibuprofen have been described in patients with hepatitis C.[35,56] The rates of ALF and death have been consistently rare in several series.[46,48,57] Overall, ibuprofen seems to have one of the best hepatotoxic safety profiles.[42]

**Naproxen** Naproxen is a propionic acid derivative that has a longer half-life than other frequently used NSAIDs, allowing twice-a-day dosing. In the United States it is available by prescription and over the counter. More than 10 million prescriptions are filled every year. Among more than 6000 cases of NSAID-induced hepatotoxicity, naproxen has been associated in 11% of those cases.[58] The pattern of serum enzyme abnormalities is hepatocellular and cholestatic. Immune-allergic hypersensitivity reactions are uncommon. Abnormal liver enzymes have been described in approximately 4% of cases, symptomatic liver disease in 9 to 12 cases per 100,000 patients, and ALF in 3.8 per 100,000 patient-years of use.[59,60] Symptomatic hepatitis can occur starting after 1 week up to 12 weeks of initiation of the drug.[61,62] Cross-hepatotoxicity causing acute hepatitis with hepatocellular pattern between naproxen and fenoprofen, another propionic acid derivative, has been described.[61] The specific mechanism of liver injury has not been identified but most likely is idiosyncratic because of a toxic metabolite. Intrinsic toxicity has not been seen after accidental overdose.[63] Recovery usually occurs after discontinuation of medication but it can take from 1 to 5 months.[61,62]

#### Acetic acid derivatives

**Diclofenac** Diclofenac is another of the most commonly used NSAIDs in the United States and throughout the rest of the world.[64] Its widespread use correlates with a high rate of liver-associated adverse drug effects, although most of the hepatotoxicity

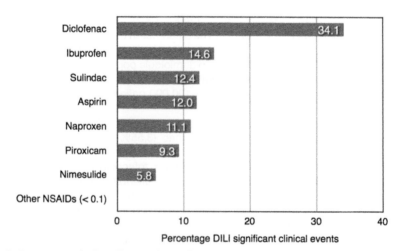

**Fig. 1.** Frequency of clinically significant liver injury associated with NSAIDs. (*Data from* Agundez JA, Lucena MI, Martinez C, et al. Assessment of nonsteroidal anti-inflammatory drug-induced hepatotoxicity. Expert Opin Drug Metab Toxicol 2011;7(7):817–28.)

**Table 1**
**Characteristics of most common NSAIDs associated with hepatotoxicity**

| NSAID Class | Serologic Pattern Liver Damage | Clinical Phenotype | Proposed Mechanism of DILI-Genetic Risk Factors Variants |
|---|---|---|---|
| Acetic acid derivatives | | | |
| Diclofenac | Hepatocellular | Acute hepatitis, autoimmune like-hepatitis | Metabolic-idiosyncratic, mitochondrial dysfunction |
| | | | Increased toxic metabolite formation |
| | | | Oxidoreductase enzymes[52] |
| | | | CYP2C8 *4 |
| | | | Conjugation enzymes[52] |
| | | | UGT2B7 *2 |
| | | | Cytokines regulating inflammation-immune reactions[70] |
| | | | Interleukin-4 590T |
| | | | Interleukin-10 627A |
| | | | Decreased biliary excretion toxic metabolites |
| | | | Transporters[52] |
| | | | MRP2 ABCC2 C-24T |
| Sulindac | Cholestatic Mixed | Immunoallergic hepatitis | Hypersensitivity |
| Propionic acid derivatives | | | |
| Ibuprofen | Hepatocellular | Acute hepatitis Vanishing bile duct syndrome | Metabolic-idiosyncratic Mitochondrial dysfunction |
| Naproxen | Cholestatic Hepatocellular | Cholestatic hepatitis Immunoallergic hepatitis | Metabolic-idiosyncratic Hypersensitivity |
| Salicylates | | | |
| Aspirin | Hepatocellular | Acute hepatitis | Intrinsic toxicity-dose dependent |
| | Reye syndrome | Acute fatty liver with microvesicular steatosis | Mitochondrial dysfunction |
| Oxicams | | | |
| Piroxicam | Hepatocellular Cholestatic | Immunoallergic hepatitis | Hypersensitivity |
| Sulfonanilides | | | |
| Nimesulide | Hepatocellular Cholestatic | Acute hepatitis Acute hepatic necrosis | Metabolic-idiosyncratic Mitochondrial dysfunction |

is not severe and the safety profile based on the number of prescriptions filled annually (approximately 5 million in the US) in relation to the number of cases of severe hepatotoxicity,[43] including death or liver transplantation, is good.[4] In contrast, in a survey of suspected drug-induced liver fatalities reported to the World Health Organization database, diclofenac was the only NSAID implicated among the top 20 causes.[57] A systematic review reported the prevalence of hospitalization as 22.4 per 100,000 patient-years of diclofenac exposure.[47]

Most patients with N-DILI caused by diclofenac are asymptomatic. Abnormal aminotransferases have been documented in approximately 15% of cases of chronic diclofenac use.[65] Elevation of aminotransferases greater than three times the upper limit of normal has been reported in 3.5% of cases.[48] An immunoallergic reaction characterized by fever, rash, and eosinophilia has been reported and associated with a clinical picture similar to that of autoimmune hepatitis with positive antinuclear antibodies.[66]

Symptomatic patients with hepatocellular jaundice (Hy's cases) are quite uncommon. In one series of 180 cases of diclofenac hepatotoxicity, 50% of the patients presented with jaundice and 8% of those patients died.[67] Documented risk factors for diclofenac hepatotoxicity include female gender, higher doses, prolonged duration of treatment, and OA.[68]

The type of hepatotoxicity caused by diclofenac is mainly hepatocellular, with idiosyncratic metabolic cause as the main mechanism of liver damage.[27] Mitochondrial injury, immunogenic adducts, toxic intermediates, and aberrant transport are other mechanisms of liver injury associated with diclofenac.[69] The aberrant metabolism by CYP2C9, with formation of adducts and immune responses or adduct antibodies, has also been described.[70] The increase in variant alleles for interleukin-10 and interleukin-4 in patients with diclofenac hepatotoxicity has been postulated as a T helper-2–mediated antibody response and associated disease susceptibility.[71] Genetic studies of the polymorphism of the genes encoding UGT2B7, CYP2C8, and ABCC2 have identified allelic variants that correlated with liver injury.[52] These genes are involved in the metabolism, conjugation, and excretion of diclofenac.

**Sulindac** Sulindac has been associated with 12.4% of cases of N-DILI and is considered the second most common NSAID associated with hepatotoxicity after diclofenac.[58] In another review of five population studies with more than 1 million patients on NSAIDs, sulindac was the only NSAID associated with a significant increase in liver injury.[59] Symptomatic liver injury is rare with approximately 5 cases in 100,000 prescriptions (0.1% of users). Fatality rate has been reported in 5% of cases but mostly secondary to generalized hypersensitivity reactions.[72] In the United States sulindac is available by prescription only. It is used mainly for management of pain in OA and other rheumatologic diseases. It has also been used in patients with familial adenomatous polyposis to decrease the number and size of colorectal adenomas.[73,74]

Clinical hepatotoxicity presents as allergic hepatitis with fever, nausea, vomiting, and abdominal pain within 8 weeks of starting the medication.[27] Analysis of 91 cases reported to the FDA found that two-thirds of cases had evidence of hypersensitivity, most of them were women, and the most common pattern of serum enzymes abnormalities was cholestatic followed by hepatocellular and mixed pattern. Five patients died but only one secondary to ALF.[72]

### Enolic acid derivatives (oxicams)

**Piroxicam** Piroxicam has an extended half-life up to 40 hours that allows administration once a day.[75] It is available by prescription only and is used for chronic arthritic pain. The hepatotoxicity associated with piroxicam has been estimated from 9 to 14 per 100,000 person-years of use.[59]

The spectrum of liver injury varies from mild abnormalities in serum enzymes to ALF with cholestatic jaundice and hepatic necrosis.[76–78] The pattern of liver damage is mainly cholestatic, but hepatocellular and mixed pattern have been described.[79,80] A component of hypersensitivity is seen in some patients that present fever, rash, and eosinophilia, although it is rare. The mechanism of injury is likely toxic metabolic. Recovery with normalization of serum enzymes usually takes weeks to several months.

### Selective Cox-2 inhibitors

The association of N-DILI with COX-2 inhibitors has been evaluated in a systematic review that found no increase in clinical liver injury with COX inhibitors.[81] A population study from Taiwan that included 4519 patients hospitalized with acute hepatitis secondary to NSAIDs revealed a similar risk of liver injury with celecoxib and other NSAIDs, although this has not been reported previously in other population-based studies.[44]

ALT abnormalities were reported in 2% of patients taking rofecoxib and 3% with high-doses of lumiracoxib[81]; both of these drugs have been withdrawn from the market. Rofecoxib was withdrawn because of increased risk of thrombotic cardiovascular events. Lumiracoxib was never approved for use in the United States and was withdrawn in Europe and Australia because of severe hepatotoxicity with several cases of ALF.[31,32]

**Celecoxib** Celecoxib is the only selective COX-2 inhibitor approved in the United States. The rate of ALT greater than three $\times$ ULN in celecoxib users has been calculated in a systematic review as 0.4% (N = 12,750) celecoxib-treated persons compared with 0.29% (N = 4084) in subjects using placebo.[48] This was similar to a combined analysis of 14 controlled trials of celecoxib (celecoxib 0.4%, N = 6376; placebo 0.5%, N = 1864).[82] No cases of clinical hepatitis were described. A pooled analysis of 41 randomized control trials found similar rates of ALT greater than five $\times$ ULN in patients taking celecoxib (1.1%) and placebo (0.9%); no clinical cases of hepatitis among 24,933 celecoxib users was reported.[83]

Case reports of severe cholestatic jaundice with ALF requiring transplantation have been published.[84] Previously, in approximately 50,000 liver transplant cases reported to the United Network for Organ Sharing from 1990 to 2002, 270 were associated with ALF secondary to DILI (0.5%); one case was related to bromfenac and one to naproxen but no cases were associated with celecoxib.[4] Other cases of clinical liver injury with hepatocellular and mixed pattern have been reported.[85]

### Salicylates

**Acetylsalicylic acid (aspirin)** The mechanism of action as with other NSAIDs is inhibition of COX-1 and COX-2 with decrease in proinflammatory prostaglandins. Aspirin is an irreversible noncompetitive COX-1 inhibitor that has been associated with gastrointestinal side effects, such as peptic ulcer disease and bleeding. It is one of the first and most commonly used analgesic and antipyretics and higher doses have been used in some rheumatologic diseases. The hepatotoxicity of aspirin is dose dependent. Most cases are usually asymptomatic. With higher doses there is mild elevation of serum ALT levels and mild elevations of bilirubin and AP. Severe hepatotoxicity with encephalopathy and coagulopathy has been seen with very high aspirin doses from 2 to 3 mg daily and salicylate levels greater than 25 mg/dL.[86] Hypersensitivity reactions are rare. The mechanism of hepatotoxicity has been characteristically secondary to mitochondrial dysfunction.

A unique form described with aspirin is Reye syndrome, initially reported in children receiving aspirin and later associated with interaction with concomitant viral illness (influenza, varicella).[40] ALF with severe encephalopathy and significant increase in serum aminotransferases with minimal or moderate serum bilirubin abnormalities was the typical presentation with evidence of fatty degeneration of the liver. Restrictions in the use of aspirin in children and teenagers decreased dramatically the number of cases of Reye syndrome.[87]

### SUMMARY

The mechanism of hepatotoxicity associated with NSAIDs is mainly idiosyncratic (with the exception of aspirin). The incidence of severe NSAIDs hepatotoxicity is very low with significant morbidity and mortality in cases of ALF. The surveillance and monitoring after approval of new medications and NSAIDs is extremely important to detect severe cases of hepatotoxicity because preapproval clinical trials may not be able to detect severe cases of hepatotoxicity because of the low incidence of idiosyncratic reactions. Among currently approved NSAIDs the safety profile for severe hepatotoxicity is equivalent with some evidence of cross-reactivity among some NSAIDs. A higher incidence of DILI has been described with diclofenac and sulindac. A genetic predisposition to develop DILI has been found with diclofenac and lumiracoxib. Pharmacogenomic studies are a promising way to evaluate individuals or populations with predisposition to DILI. The use of NSAIDs in patients with coexisting liver or renal disease and those taking other potential hepatotoxic medications must be avoided because this could increase the potential for severe hepatotoxicity.

## REFERENCES

1. Lee WM, Squires RH Jr, Nyberg SL, et al. Acute liver failure: summary of a workshop. Hepatology 2008;47(4):1401–15.
2. Navarro VJ, Senior JR. Drug-related hepatotoxicity. N Engl J Med 2006;354(7): 731–9.
3. Bjornsson E, Jerlstad P, Bergqvist A, et al. Fulminant drug-induced hepatic failure leading to death or liver transplantation in Sweden. Scand J Gastroenterol 2005;40(9):1095–101.
4. Russo MW, Galanko JA, Shrestha R, et al. Liver transplantation for acute liver failure from drug induced liver injury in the United States. Liver Transpl 2004; 10(8):1018–23.
5. Andrade RJ, Lucena MI, Fernandez MC, et al. Drug-induced liver injury: an analysis of 461 incidences submitted to the Spanish registry over a 10-year period. Gastroenterology 2005;129(2):512–21.
6. Chalasani N, Fontana RJ, Bonkovsky HL, et al. Causes, clinical features, and outcomes from a prospective study of drug-induced liver injury in the United States. Gastroenterology 2008;135(6):1924–34.
7. Sgro C, Clinard F, Ouazir K, et al. Incidence of drug-induced hepatic injuries: a French population-based study. Hepatology 2002;36(2):451–5.
8. Carey EJ, Vargas HE, Douglas DD, et al. Inpatient admissions for drug-induced liver injury: results from a single center. Dig Dis Sci 2008;53(7):1977–82.
9. Aithal GP, Watkins PB, Andrade RJ, et al. Case definition and phenotype standardization in drug-induced liver injury. Clin Pharmacol Ther 2011;89(6):806–15.
10. Zimmerman H. Drug-induced liver disease. In: Hepatotoxicity. The adverse effects of drugs and other chemicals on the liver. 1st edition. New York: Appleton-Century-Crofts; 1978. p. 353.
11. Reuben A. Hy's law. Hepatology 2004;39(2):574–8.
12. Senior JR. How can 'Hy's law' help the clinician? Pharmacoepidemiol Drug Saf 2006;15(4):235–9.
13. Bjornsson E, Olsson R. Outcome and prognostic markers in severe drug-induced liver disease. Hepatology 2005;42(2):481–9.
14. Temple R. Hy's law: predicting serious hepatotoxicity. Pharmacoepidemiol Drug Saf 2006;15(4):241–3.
15. Danan G, Benichou C. Causality assessment of adverse reactions to drugs–I. A novel method based on the conclusions of international consensus meetings: application to drug-induced liver injuries. J Clin Epidemiol 1993;46(11): 1323–30.

16. Suzuki A, Andrade RJ, Bjornsson E, et al. Drugs associated with hepatotoxicity and their reporting frequency of liver adverse events in vigibase: unified list based on international collaborative work. Drug Saf 2010;33(6):503–22.

17. Hunter EB, Johnston PE, Tanner G, et al. Bromfenac (Duract)-associated hepatic failure requiring liver transplantation. Am J Gastroenterol 1999;94(8): 2299–301.

18. Rabkin JM, Smith MJ, Orloff SL, et al. Fatal fulminant hepatitis associated with bromfenac use. Ann Pharmacother 1999;33(9):945–7.

19. Moses PL, Schroeder B, Alkhatib O, et al. Severe hepatotoxicity associated with bromfenac sodium. Am J Gastroenterol 1999;94(5):1393–6.

20. Fontana RJ, McCashland TM, Benner KG, et al. Acute liver failure associated with prolonged use of bromfenac leading to liver transplantation. The Acute Liver Failure Study Group. Liver Transpl Surg 1999;5(6):480–4.

21. Goldkind L, Laine L. A systematic review of NSAIDs withdrawn from the market due to hepatotoxicity: lessons learned from the bromfenac experience. Pharmacoepidemiol Drug Saf 2006;15(4):213–20.

22. Kaplowitz N. Idiosyncratic drug hepatotoxicity. Nat Rev Drug Discov 2005;4(6): 489–99.

23. Lee WM. Drug-induced hepatotoxicity. N Engl J Med 2003;349(5):474–85.

24. Kaplowitz N. Avoiding hepatic injury from drugs. Gastroenterology 1999;117(4): 759.

25. Duthie A, Nicholls A, Freeth M, et al. Fatal cholestatic jaundice in elderly patients taking benoxaprofen. Br Med J (Clin Res Ed) 1982;285(6334):62.

26. Taggart HM, Alderdice JM. Fatal cholestatic jaundice in elderly patients taking benoxaprofen. Br Med J (Clin Res Ed) 1982;284(6326):1372.

27. Lewis JH. Nonsteroidal anti-inflammatory drugs and leukotriene receptor antagonists: pathology and clinical presentation of hepatotoxicity. In: Kaplowitz N, DeLeve LD, editors. Drug-induced liver disease. 2nd edition. New York: Informa Healthcare USA; 2007. p. 439–64.

28. Chitturi S, Farrell GC. Identifying who is at risk of drug-induced liver injury: is human leukocyte antigen specificity the key? Hepatology 2011;53(1): 358–62.

29. Farkouh ME, Kirshner H, Harrington RA, et al. Comparison of lumiracoxib with naproxen and ibuprofen in the Therapeutic Arthritis Research and Gastrointestinal Event Trial (TARGET), cardiovascular outcomes: randomised controlled trial. Lancet 2004;364(9435):675–84.

30. Schnitzer TJ, Burmester GR, Mysler E, et al. Comparison of lumiracoxib with naproxen and ibuprofen in the Therapeutic Arthritis Research and Gastrointestinal Event Trial (TARGET), reduction in ulcer complications: randomised controlled trial. Lancet 2004;364(9435):665–74.

31. Chitturi S, Farrell GC. Lessons from Lumiracoxib: are cyclooxygenase-2 inhibitors less hepatotoxic than non-selective non-steroidal anti-inflammatory drugs? J Gastroenterol Hepatol 2012;27(6):993–4.

32. Pillans PI, Ghiculescu RA, Lampe G, et al. Severe acute liver injury associated with lumiracoxib. J Gastroenterol Hepatol 2012;27(6):1102–5.

33. Singer JB, Lewitzky S, Leroy E, et al. A genome-wide study identifies HLA alleles associated with lumiracoxib-related liver injury. Nature 2010;42(8):711–4.

34. Russmann S, Jetter A, Kullak-Ublick GA. Pharmacogenetics of drug-induced liver injury. Hepatology 2010;52(2):748–61.

35. Riley TR 3rd, Smith JP. Ibuprofen-induced hepatotoxicity in patients with chronic hepatitis C: a case series. Am J Gastroenterol 1998;93(9):1563–5.

36. Bessone F, Colombato L, Fassio E, et al. The spectrum of nimesulide-induced-hepatotoxicity. An overview. Antiinflamm Antiallergy Agents Med Chem 2010; 9(4):355–65.
37. Walker SL, Kennedy F, Niamh N, et al. Nimesulide associated fulminant hepatic failure. Pharmacoepidemiol Drug Saf 2008;17(11):1108–12.
38. Venegoni M, Da Cas R, Menniti-Ippolito F, et al. Effects of the European restrictive actions concerning nimesulide prescription: a simulation study on hepatopathies and gastrointestinal bleedings in Italy. Ann Ist Super Sanita 2010; 46(2):153–7.
39. Traversa G, Bianchi C, Da Cas R, et al. Cohort study of hepatotoxicity associated with nimesulide and other non-steroidal anti-inflammatory drugs. BMJ 2003;327(7405):18–22.
40. Rainsford KD. Members of the Consensus Report Group on N. Nimesulide: a multifactorial approach to inflammation and pain: scientific and clinical consensus. Curr Med Res Opin 2006;22(6):1161–70.
41. European Medicines Agency concludes review of systemic nimesulide-containing medicines. 2011. Available at: http://www.ema.europa.eu/ema/index.jsp?curl= pages/medicines/human/referrals/Nimesulide/human_referral_000275.jsp&mid= WC0b01ac0580024e99&murl=menus/regulations/regulations.jsp.
42. Bessone F. Non-steroidal anti-inflammatory drugs: what is the actual risk of liver damage? World J Gastroenterol 2010;16(45):5651–61.
43. Laine L, Goldkind L, Curtis SP, et al. How common is diclofenac-associated liver injury? Analysis of 17,289 arthritis patients in a long-term prospective clinical trial. Am J Gastroenterol 2009;104(2):356–62.
44. Lee CH, Wang JD, Chen PC. Increased risk of hospitalization for acute hepatitis in patients with previous exposure to NSAIDs. Pharmacoepidemiol Drug Saf 2010;19(7):708–14.
45. Sanchez-Matienzo D, Arana A, Castellsague J, et al. Hepatic disorders in patients treated with COX-2 selective inhibitors or nonselective NSAIDs: a case/noncase analysis of spontaneous reports. Clin Ther 2006;28(8):1123–32.
46. Lapeyre-Mestre M, de Castro AM, Bareille MP, et al. Non-steroidal antiinflammatory drug-related hepatic damage in France and Spain: analysis from national spontaneous reporting systems. Fundam Clin Pharmacol 2006;20(4):391–5.
47. Rubenstein JH, Laine L. Systematic review: the hepatotoxicity of nonsteroidal anti-inflammatory drugs. Aliment Pharmacol Ther 2004;20(4):373–80.
48. Rostom A, Goldkind L, Laine L. Nonsteroidal anti-inflammatory drugs and hepatic toxicity: a systematic review of randomized controlled trials in arthritis patients. Clin Gastroenterol Hepatol 2005;3(5):489–98.
49. Garcia Rodriguez LA, Williams R, Derby LE, et al. Acute liver injury associated with nonsteroidal anti-inflammatory drugs and the role of risk factors. Arch Intern Med 1994;154(3):311–6.
50. Chalasani N, Bjornsson E. Risk factors for idiosyncratic drug-induced liver injury. Gastroenterology 2010;138(7):2246–59.
51. Licata A, Calvaruso V, Cappello M, et al. Clinical course and outcomes of drug-induced liver injury: nimesulide as the first implicated medication. Dig Liver Dis 2010;42(2):143–8.
52. Daly AK, Aithal GP, Leathart JB, et al. Genetic susceptibility to diclofenac-induced hepatotoxicity: contribution of UGT2B7, CYP2C8, and ABCC2 genotypes. Gastroenterology 2007;132(1):272–81.
53. Zimmerman HJ. Update of hepatotoxicity due to classes of drugs in common clinical use: nonsteroidal drugs, antiinflammatory drugs, antibiotics,

antihypertensives, and cardiac and psychotropic agents. Semin Liver Dis 1990;10(4):322–8.

54. Alam I, Ferrell LD, Bass NM. Vanishing bile duct syndrome temporally associated with ibuprofen use. Am J Gastroenterol 1996;91(8):1626–30.

55. Srivastava M, Perez-Atayde A, Jonas MM. Drug-associated acute-onset vanishing bile duct and Stevens-Johnson syndromes in a child. Gastroenterology 1998;115(3):743–6.

56. Andrade RJ, Lucena MI, Garcia-Cortes M, et al. Chronic hepatitis C, ibuprofen, and liver damage. Am J Gastroenterol 2002;97(7):1854–5.

57. Bjornsson E, Olsson R. Suspected drug-induced liver fatalities reported to the WHO database. Dig Liver Dis 2006;38(1):33–8.

58. Agundez JA, Lucena MI, Martinez C, et al. Assessment of nonsteroidal antiinflammatory drug-induced hepatotoxicity. Expert Opin Drug Metab Toxicol 2011;7(7):817–28.

59. Walker AM. Quantitative studies of the risk of serious hepatic injury in persons using nonsteroidal antiinflammatory drugs. Arthritis Rheum 1997;40(2): 201–8.

60. Manoukian AV, Carson JL. Nonsteroidal anti-inflammatory drug-induced hepatic disorders. Incidence and prevention. Drug Saf 1996;15(1):64–71.

61. Andrejak M, Davion T, Gineston JL, et al. Cross hepatotoxicity between nonsteroidal anti-inflammatory drugs. Br Med J (Clin Res Ed) 1987;295(6591): 180–1.

62. Demirag MD, Ozenirler S, Goker B, et al. Idiosyncratic toxic hepatitis secondary to single dose of naproxen. Acta Gastroenterol Belg 2007;70(2):247–8.

63. Fredell EW, Strand LJ. Naproxen overdose. JAMA 1977;238(9):938.

64. Arellano FM, Yood MU, Wentworth CE, et al. Use of cyclo-oxygenase 2 inhibitors (COX-2) and prescription non-steroidal anti-inflammatory drugs (NSAIDS) in UK and USA populations. Implications for COX-2 cardiovascular profile. Pharmacoepidemiol Drug Saf 2006;15(12):861–72.

65. Zimmerman H. Drugs used to treat rheumatic and musculospastic disease. In: Zimmerman H, editor. Hepatotoxicity: the adverse effects of drugs and other chemicals on the liver. 2nd edition. Philadelphia: Lippincott Williams & Williams; 1999. p. 599–602.

66. Scully LJ, Clarke D, Barr RJ. Diclofenac induced hepatitis: 3 cases with features of autoimmune chronic active hepatitis. Dig Dis Sci 1993;38(4):744–51.

67. Banks AT, Zimmerman HJ, Ishak KG, et al. Diclofenac-associated hepatotoxicity: analysis of 180 cases reported to the Food-and-Drug-Administration as adverse reactions. Hepatology 1995;22(3):820–7.

68. de Abajo FJ, Montero D, Madurga M, et al. Acute and clinically relevant drug-induced liver injury: a population based case-control study. Br J Clin Pharmacol 2004;58(1):71–80.

69. Boelsterli UA. Diclofenac-induced liver injury: a paradigm of idiosyncratic drug toxicity. Toxicol Appl Pharmacol 2003;192(3):307–22.

70. Aithal GP, Ramsay L, Daly AK, et al. Hepatic adducts, circulating antibodies, and cytokine polymorphisms in patients with diclofenac hepatotoxicity. Hepatology 2004;39(5):1430–40.

71. Aithal GP. Diclofenac-induced liver injury: a paradigm of idiosyncratic drug toxicity. Expert Opin Drug Saf 2004;3(6):519–23.

72. Tarazi EM, Harter JG, Zimmerman HJ, et al. Sulindac-associated hepatic injury: analysis of 91 cases reported to the Food and Drug Administration. Gastroenterology 1993;104(2):569–74.

73. Giardiello FM, Hamilton SR, Krush AJ, et al. Treatment of colonic and rectal adenomas with sulindac in familial adenomatous polyposis. N Engl J Med 1993; 328(18):1313–6.
74. Guldenschuh I, Hurlimann R, Muller A, et al. Relationship between APC genotype, polyp distribution, and oral sulindac treatment in the colon and rectum of patients with familial adenomatous polyposis: reply. Dis Colon Rectum 2001;44(8):1098–9.
75. Brogden RN, Heel RC, Speight TM, et al. Piroxicam: a review of its pharmacological properties and therapeutic efficacy. Drugs 1981;22(3):165–87.
76. Lee SM, O'Brien CJ, Williams R, et al. Subacute hepatic necrosis induced by piroxicam. Br Med J (Clin Res Ed) 1986;293(6546):540–1.
77. Planas R, De Leon R, Quer JC, et al. Fatal submassive necrosis of the liver associated with piroxicam. Am J Gastroenterol 1990;85(4):468–70.
78. Paterson D, Kerlin P, Walker N, et al. Piroxicam induced submassive necrosis of the liver. Gut 1992;33(10):1436–8.
79. Hepps KS, Maliha GM, Estrada R, et al. Severe cholestatic jaundice associated with piroxicam. Gastroenterology 1991;101(6):1737–40.
80. Caballeria E, Masso RM, Arago JV, et al. Piroxicam hepatotoxicity. Am J Gastroenterol 1990;85(7):898–9.
81. Laine L, White WB, Rostom A, et al. COX-2 selective inhibitors in the treatment of osteoarthritis. Semin Arthritis Rheum 2008;38(3):165–87.
82. Maddrey WC, Maurath CJ, Verburg KM, et al. The hepatic safety and tolerability of the novel cyclooxygenase-2 inhibitor celecoxib. Am J Ther 2000;7(3):153–8.
83. Soni P, Shell B, Cawkwell G, et al. The hepatic safety and tolerability of the cyclooxygenase-2 selective NSAID celecoxib: pooled analysis of 41 randomized controlled trials. Curr Med Res Opin 2009;25(8):1841–51.
84. El Hajj II, Malik SM, Alwakeel HR, et al. Celecoxib-induced cholestatic liver failure requiring orthotopic liver transplantation. World J Gastroenterol 2009;15(31): 3937–9.
85. Nachimuthu S, Volfinzon L, Gopal L. Acute hepatocellular and cholestatic injury in a patient taking celecoxib. Postgrad Med J 2001;77(910):548–50.
86. Zimmerman HJ. Effects of aspirin and acetaminophen on the liver. Arch Intern Med 1981;141(3 Spec No):333–42.
87. Belay ED, Bresee JS, Holman RC, et al. Reye's syndrome in the United States from 1981 through 1997. N Engl J Med 1999;340(18):1377–82.

# Antiretroviral and Anti–Hepatitis C Virus Direct-Acting Antiviral-Related Hepatotoxicity

Hyosun Han, MD, Ritu Agarwal, MD, Valerie Martel-Laferriere, MD, Douglas T. Dieterich, MD*

## KEYWORDS

• HIV • HCV • Coinfection • ARV • DAAs • Hepatotoxicity • Drug-induced liver injury

## KEY POINTS

- The most common side effect of antiretroviral therapy in patients with HIV is liver injury.
- Antiretroviral-related hepatotoxicity includes hepatic steatosis, unconjugated hyperbilirubinemia, nodular regenerative hyperplasia, and transaminitis.
- Drug–drug interactions between antiretrovirals and anti–hepatitis C virus (HCV) therapy require dose adjustments depending on the class of drugs.
- First-generation HCV direct-acting antivirals have not been shown to adversely affect the liver in both patients monoinfected with HCV and those coinfected with HIV/HCV.

## ANTIRETROVIRAL-ASSOCIATED LIVER DISEASE

Antiretroviral therapy has become the cornerstone of treatment of patients with human immunodeficiency virus (HIV), and has reduced the rates of morbidity and mortality. However, side effects, including nephrotoxicity, cardiovascular disease, neuropsychiatric disease, and drug-related liver injury, can limit their use.[1,2,3]

Liver injury is one of the most common adverse effects of HIV treatment. Antiretroviral-related liver injury can range from asymptomatic elevations in transaminases (aspartate aminotransferase/alanine aminotransferase [ALT/AST]) to severe liver decompensation and death. Most antiretroviral-related liver injury cases are asymptomatic and resolve once the medication is withdrawn. Severe hepatotoxicity

Financial Disclosures: Dr Dieterich has received honoraria from and provided consulting for Merck & Co., Inc., Vertex Pharmaceuticals, Gilead Sciences, Inc., Boehringer Ingelheim GmbH, Idenix Pharmaceuticals, Bristol-Myers Squibb, and Tobira Therapeutics, Inc. Dr Martel-Laferriere was funded by the 2012 Grant of the CHUM Foundation.
Department of Medicine, Division of Liver Diseases, Icahn School of Medicine at Mount Sinai, 1468 Madison Avenue, Annenberg 21-42, New York, NY 10029, USA
* Corresponding author. Icahn School of Medicine at Mount Sinai, 1468 Madison Avenue, Box 1123, Room 11-70, New York, NY 10029.
E-mail address: douglas.dieterich@mountsinai.org

occurs in 5% to 10% of people with HIV in the first 12 months after initiation of anti-retroviral therapy.[4] Risk factors include coinfection with chronic viral hepatitis, abnormal baseline serum transaminases, alcohol consumption, drug use, opportunistic infections, and diabetes.[5]

The definition of antiretroviral-associated hepatotoxicity has not been consistent throughout clinical studies. The AIDS Clinical Trial Group defines hepatotoxicity as a change relative to pretreatment normal baseline ALT or AST: grade 0 (<1.25 times the upper limit of normal [ULN]), grade 1/mild (1.25–2.60 times the ULN), grade 2/moderate (2.5–5.0 times the ULN), grade 3 severe (5.1–10.0 times the ULN), and grade 4/life-threatening (>10 times the ULN) toxicity. Patients with elevated pretreatment ALT or AST values, such as those with viral hepatitis, follow this guideline, which may skew the interpretation of drug-induced liver injury.[6]

### Nucleoside Reverse Transcriptase Inhibitors

The nucleoside reverse transcriptase inhibitors (NRTIs) can be associated with liver toxicity. They have been reported to cause fatal lactic acidosis, nonalcoholic fatty liver disease, and noncirrhotic portal hypertension (NCPH). Liver injury is more common with stavudine, zalcitabine, and didanosine than other NRTIs, such as abacavir, zidovudine, lamivudine, and tenofovir.[7]

Mitochondrial toxicity is the cause of NRTI-associated hepatic steatosis and lactic acidosis. The mechanism is that NRTIs inhibit mitochondrial DNA (mtDNA) polymerase gamma. This enzyme is essential for mitochondrial DNA replication. The inhibition of mtDNA synthesis becomes clinically significant when an organ's energy threshold is not met by the affected mitochondria's energy-producing capacity.[8]

#### Lactic acidosis

Inhibiting mtDNA synthesis causes hyperlactatemia. The common presenting clinical symptoms can be nonspecific and include nausea, vomiting, abdominal pain, weight loss, malaise, and dyspnea. Mild hyperlactemia is defined as serum serum lactate of 2.1–5 mmol/L, serious hyperlactemia is serum lactate >5 mmol/L, lactic acidosis is serious hyperlactemia and bicarbonate >20 mmol/L.[9]

Clinically significant lactic acidosis is rare, occurring at an incidence of 0.013% to 2.5%.[8,10] Lactate levels can be used for monitoring and management of NRTI toxicity. Current practice suggests measuring lactate only in patients presenting with one of the following: extreme fatigue, sudden weight loss, abdominal pain, unexplained nausea and vomiting, or dyspnea. If the patient has mild hyperlactatemia, changing the NRTI or providing supportive treatment is recommended. In patients who present with serious hyperlactatemia (a serum lactate level of 5 mmol/L or greater), NRTIs should be discontinued and supportive treatment should be initiated. Routine measurement of lactate in asymptomatic patients is controversial and may lead to unnecessary treatment alterations.[11]

#### Hepatic steatosis

Although hepatosteatosis is rare, hepatotoxicity as measured by elevations in hepatic transaminases occurs at a rate of 5% to 15% in patients with HIV treated with NRTIs. Patients typically remain asymptomatic during the transaminitis, which is reversible after the medication is discontinued. Hepatosteatosis can present with hepatomegaly, nausea, ascites, edema, dyspnea, myopathy, and encephalopathy.[12] Liver histology may show microvesicular and/or macrovesicular steatosis with little necrosis and no inflammation.

*Noncirrhotic portal hypertension*
NCPH is an uncommon condition reported to be associated with long-term antiretroviral use and chronic HIV infection. Its prevalence has been reported to be 1%. It manifests as portal hypertension, including esophageal varices, life-threatening gastrointestinal bleeding, ascites, and splenomegaly. Liver function is typically preserved and liver enzymes are often only mildly elevated. Histologic findings are very heterogeneous and include nodular regenerative hyperplasia, hepatoportal sclerosis, periportal fibrosis, and obliterative portal venopathy, but not cirrhosis. Didanosine use has been most associated with NCPH. Management includes stopping the medication, variceal screening, and treatment.[13,14,15,16,17] Platelet counts less than 100,000 per microliter in a patient on NRTIs should be a signal to refer for variceal screening. Variceal bleeding can be the first presentation in 30% to 40% of patients, and the mortality from variceal bleeding is 30%.[18,19]

### Non-Nucleoside Reverse Transcriptase Inhibitors

Vast data have been published on the occurrence of non-nucleoside reverse transcriptase inhibitor (NNRTI)–associated liver injury. Two commonly used first-generation NNRTIs are efavirenz and nevirapine. Both medications undergo hepatic clearance and are associated with liver injury. The data show that the frequency of liver injury is higher with nevirapine than with efavirenz. The frequency of drug-induced liver injury in patients taking efavirenz ranges from 1% to 8%, whereas in patients treated with nevirapine, it ranges from 4% to 18%.

Patients with any preexisting liver disease, such as hepatitis C virus (HCV), are likely to have more serious disease. Coinfection with hepatitis B virus and coadministration with HIV protease inhibitors (PIs) are other risk factors.[20] Underlying liver diseases such as HCV can impair metabolite clearance and result in liver injury from any drug cleared by the liver.

A retrospective study conducted by the manufacturer of nevirapine, Boehringer Ingelheim GmbH (Ingelheim, Germany), found that the risk of rash-associated hepatotoxicity was significantly greater in women with a baseline CD4 count greater than 250 cells/mL (11.0% compared with 0.9% among women with baseline CD4 count <250 cells/mL). These findings led the U.S. Food and Drug Administration to issue a black box warning regarding using nevirapine to treat women with CD4 counts greater than 250 cells/mL and men with CD4 counts greater than 450 cells/mL, unless the benefits clearly outweigh the risks.[8]

Two types of hepatotoxicity can occur with NNRTI treatment. One is hypersensitivity reactions and the other is toxic hepatitis. Hypersensitivity can occur quickly after initiating therapy, either within a few days or in less than 12 weeks. Along with elevated transaminases, patients can present with constitutional symptoms, including skin rash, eosinophilia, lymphadenopathy, interstitial nephritis, and pneumonia.

Hypersensitivity events occur more frequently with nevirapine than with efavirenz. Female sex and high CD4 counts have also been associated with a higher rate of nevirapine-induced hypersensitivity. A genetic component is also believed to be related to nevirapine-related hypersensitivity. Those with DRB1*0101 histocompatibility antigen and a baseline percentage more than 25% of CD4 cells/mm$^3$ are more susceptible.[21] Intrinsic liver toxicity occurs later than hypersensitivity reactions, typically more than 12 weeks after initiating therapy.

Nevirapine-related hepatotoxicity may be dose-dependent. Small sample size studies have suggested that patients with higher trough levels of nevirapine have been associated with increased ALT levels. In a study of 70 patients infected with HIV, those with normal ALT levels had median trough levels of 5.2 µg/mL, whereas patients with increased ALT had higher trough levels (median, 6.25 µg/mL). Larger sample size studies, however, have not confirmed this finding.[22]

The Non-Nucleoside Reverse Transcriptase Inhibitor Response Study conducted in Zambia, Thailand, and Kenya prospectively evaluated treatment-naïve women initiating nevirapine. After initiating nevirapine-based antiretroviral therapy, severe hepatotoxicity occurred in 41 (5%) women, and rash-associated hepatotoxicity occurred in 27 (3%) women. In a multivariate logistic regression model, severe hepatotoxicity and rash-associated hepatotoxicity were both associated with baseline abnormal (grade 1) ALT or AST elevations, but not with a baseline CD4 cell count greater than 250 cells/mL. The authors concluded that among women taking nevirapine-based antiretroviral therapy, severe hepatotoxicity and rash-associated hepatotoxicity were predicted by abnormal baseline ALT or AST levels, not by CD4 counts greater than 250 cells/mL. Therefore, treatment monitoring should focus on transaminase testing.[23]

Transaminases should be monitored early in treatment. In a study defining 306 patients initiating nevirapine treatment, 8 developed acute hepatitis in a median of 24 days, and transaminases peaked at 28 days. Withdrawal of the medication led to rapid resolution of transaminases and symptoms. The study was not able to define a specific risk factor.[8]

High baseline ALT levels, advanced fibrosis, and prolonged antiretroviral experience before starting therapy with an NNRTIs have been associated with the development of severe nevirapine-induced liver toxicity.

### Protease inhibitors

All PIs used for the treatment for HIV have been associated with drug-induced hepatitis. More than 50% of patients develop asymptomatic mild elevation of transaminases.[7] A total of 10% to 20% of patients on PI therapy were reported to develop severe hepatotoxicity, with transaminase levels surpassing 5 times the ULN.[24]

Patients taking indinavir and atazanavir commonly experience unconjugated hyperbilirubinemia. The clinical presentation is similar to that of Gilbert syndrome, the most common inherited form of unconjugated hyperbilirubinemia. Both medications inhibit uridine 5'-diphospho-glucuronosyltransferase, the enzyme required for bilirubin glucuronidation. Although hyperbilirubinemia can commonly occur, it is rarely clinically significant enough to require treatment cessation. The UGT1A1*28 gene variant has been associated with hyperbilirubinemia, requiring atazanavir to be discontinued.[25]

Tipranavir is a nonpeptidic PI. It has low oral bioavailability and requires boosting with ritonavir. Tipranavir/ritonavir is a potent combination treatment for patients with PI-resistant infections. However, fatal hepatotoxicity has been reported for this combination. In a safety data analysis from the Randomized Evaluation of Strategic Intervention in multi-drug reSistant patients with Tipranavir (RESIST) trial, 6% of patients treated with tipranavir exhibited grade 3 or 4 elevations in aminotransferases versus 2% of patients in the other treatment arms. Risk was increased in patients with concomitant HCV infection and elevated baseline transaminases.[26] Tipranavir labeling states that the medication should not be given to patients with Child-Pugh class B or C cirrhosis.[27]

### CCR5 antagonists

Maraviroc is the first CCR5 antagonist approved for treatment-naïve and treatment-experienced patients. Concern was expressed about hepatotoxicity associated with CCR5 antagonists when severe cases were reported after use of alparivoc.[28] Maraviroc has a black box warning concerning hepatotoxicity based on possible class effects.

*Integrase inhibitors*
This class of antiretroviral therapy inhibits HIV integrase from inserting viral genome into cellular DNA. Raltegravir and elvitegravir are the 2 currently available integrase inhibitors. Hepatotoxicity has not been reported as a significant side effect of these medications.

*Fusion inhibitor*
Enfuvirtide prevents viral entry into a target cell. Hepatotoxicity has not been reported as a significant side effect.

## HEPATOTOXICITY OF ANTIRETROVIRAL THERAPY IN PATIENTS COINFECTED WITH HIV AND HCV

The prevalence of coinfection with HCV among persons with HIV is 30% to 50%.[29] This rate is high because of shared methods of transmission for both HCV and HIV. The progression of liver fibrosis to cirrhosis is accelerated in coinfected patients.[30,31,32,33] A recent meta-analysis showed that patients with coinfection not taking antiretrovirals have a relative risk (RR) of 2.49 for developing cirrhosis.[34] The RR of cirrhosis was lower (1.72) among coinfected patients on HIV treatment, but still significant even after accounting for the use of antiretroviral therapy. Furthermore, liver transplantation is not the answer for coinfected patients, given that HCV reinfection of the allograft is universal and progression to cirrhosis is further accelerated in coinfected patients who have undergone transplant. Recent studies indicate that survival rates posttransplantation remain low, at approximately a 50% 5-year survival rate.[35] The treatment of both HIV and chronic HCV is critical for improving the survival of coinfected individuals. However, treatment with antiretroviral therapy in combination with traditional HCV treatment is laden with the risk of further liver injury and drug–drug interactions (DDIs). With the advent of new direct-acting antivirals (DAAs), the concern intensifies, especially given the unknown side effects and unforeseen risks associated with these therapies.

The treatment of chronic HCV should be considered early in coinfected patients, because studies have shown that HCV enhances the risk of liver enzyme elevations in patients taking antiretrovirals.[36,37] This finding is thought to stem from lower activity of the cytochrome P450, which predisposes to drug overexposure necessitating dose adjustments.[38] Antiretrovirals requiring dose adjustments or that should be avoided in patients with cirrhosis with moderate to severe hepatic impairment (Child-Turcotte-Pugh class B and C) include nevirapine, amprenavir, atazanavir, fosamprenavir, indinavir, and tipranavir (**Tables 1** and **2**). Additionally, successful treatment of HCV is believed to improve tolerance of antiretrovirals.[39]

Sustained virologic response (SVR) is not easy to achieve in this subgroup of patients. Coinfected patients are less likely to achieve an SVR after pegylated interferon α (pegIFN)/ribavirin therapy than those infected with only HCV. The rate of SVR is approximately 30% and 70% for HCV genotypes 1/4 and 2/3, respectively.[40,41,42] The APRICOT trial showed similar SVR rates of 29% in coinfected patients with genotype 1, and 62% in those with genotype 2/3. If an SVR is achieved, however, regression of liver fibrosis and improved survival occur.[43,44,45,46]

DDIs are important to consider when treating HIV-infected patients with pegIFN and ribavirin. Among the NRTIs, emtricitabine, lamivudine, and tenofovir are safe. The combination of didanosine and ribavirin has been associated with an increased risk of lactic acidosis and pancreatitis via mitochondrial toxicity.[47,48,49] Additionally, zidovudine and ribavirin increase the risk of anemia.[47] Although safe, abacavir may reduce the efficacy of ribavirin. Drug-induced liver injury from non-nucleosides has long been

**Table 1**
**Antiretroviral medications and hepatic adverse effects**

| Class of Antiretroviral | Hepatic Adverse Effects |
|---|---|
| Nucleoside reverse transcriptase inhibitors | Steatosis, noncirrhotic portal hypertension, lactic acidosis |
| Non-nucleoside reverse transcriptase inhibitors | Risk with nevirapine is greater than risk with efavirenz<br>Hypersensitivity and toxic hepatitis |
| Protease inhibitors | Mild asymptomatic increase in transaminases<br>Indinavir and atazanavir: indirect hyperbilirubinemia<br>Tipranavir/Ritonavir: contraindicated in Child-Pugh class B or C cirrhosis |
| CCR5 antagonists | Maraviroc: hepatotoxicity associated with same class medication aplaviroc |
| Integrase inhibitors | None |
| Fusion inhibitors | None |

*Adapted from* US Department of Health and Human Services. Guidelines for the use of antiretroviral agents in HIV-1-infected adults and adolescents. Available at: aidsinfo.nih.gov/guidelines. Accessed March 3, 2013.

established, but they can still be used in combination with pegIFN and ribavirin.[50] In rare cases, etravirine has been described to cause hepatic failure. HIV PIs, integrase inhibitors, entry inhibitors, and CCR5 inhibitors seem to be safe in combination with pegIFN and ribavirin (see **Table 2**).

In the long-term, hepatotoxicity of antiretrovirals may enhance liver fibrogenesis through several mechanisms, such as metabolic abnormalities associated with their use.[51,52] Risk of direct drug injury, however, has declined significantly when using the most recently approved antiretroviral agents, such as raltegravir, maraviroc, etravirine, atazanavir, and darunavir.[53] The impact of antiretrovirals on coinfection may be significant and life-threatening. The improvement in the immune status, however, is associated with reduced liver damage induced by HCV, preventing end-stage liver disease complications and improving survival.[54,55,56]

### Why Are Coinfected Patients Being Treated?

Few coinfected patients have undergone treatment for HCV, either because many have not been eligible for treatment or because the perceived potential benefit was low. With the approval of first-generation DAAs, telaprevir and boceprevir, and many new DAAs on the horizon, more patients will be offered safe, tolerable, and successful treatment. Coinfected patients may also be eligible for off-label treatment.[57,58] New phase III trials are underway in coinfected patients, and preliminary results from phase II trials show negligible hepatotoxicity and efficacy equal to that seen in patients monoinfected with HCV.

The Adult AIDS Clinical Trials Group is studying additional drug interactions in coinfected patients. Preliminary data show promising results, but many questions remain. Data support the use of DAAs in patients with high CD4 T-cell counts who are not taking antiretroviral agents or those on select antiretroviral regimens with no DDIs.

### Interactions with Antiretrovirals

Drug interactions between DAAs and antiretroviral treatments are an important concern when considering triple regimens in coinfected patients.[50] The potential

**Table 2**
Interactions of antiretroviral medications, anti-HCV therapy, and first-generation direct-acting antivirals

| Class | Antiretroviral | Pegylated Interferon α/Ribavirin | First-Generation Direct-Acting Antivirals (Telaprevir) | First-Generation Direct-Acting Antivirals (Boceprevir) |
|---|---|---|---|---|
| Non-nucleoside reverse transcriptase inhibitor | Nevirapine | Dose-adjust | | Do not coadminister |
| | Etravirine | Hepatic failure | Safe | |
| | Rilpivirine | | Safe | Do not coadminister |
| | Delavirdine | | | Do not coadminister |
| | Efavirenz | | Safe but increase dosing | Do not coadminister |
| Nucleoside reverse transcriptase inhibitors (NRTI) | Emtricitabine | Safe | | Safe |
| | Lamivudine | | | Safe |
| | Tenofovir | | Telaprevir increases tenofovir 30% | Safe |
| | Didanosine | Lactic acidosis Pancreatitis | | |
| | Zidovudine | Anemia | | |
| | Abacavir | Safe, reduces ribavirin efficacy | | Safe |
| NtRTI/NRTI | Tenofovir/emtricitabine | | Safe | Safe |
| Protease inhibitor | Amprenavir | Safe | Reduces telaprevir efficacy | |
| | Indinavir | Dose-adjust | | |
| | Tipranavir | Dose-adjust | | |
| | Atazanavir | Dose-adjust | | |
| | Fosamprenavir | | 20% reduction of Telaprevir Telaprevir increases fosamprenavir by 47% | |
| | Ritonavir-boosted | | | Do not coadminister |
| CCR5 antagonists | | Safe | | |
| Integrase inhibitors | Raltegravir | Safe | Safe | Safe |
| Fusion inhibitors | | Safe | | |

interactions between first-generation DAAs and antiretrovirals are not completely characterized. More importantly, some interactions that would cause hepatotoxicity are unknown. Reports from some clinical trials are emerging on hepatotoxicity, specifically mitochondrial toxicity, associated with the use of new-generation DAAs, namely IDX184 (2-C-methylguanosine monophosphate prodrugs) and BMS-986094 (nucleotide polymerase inhibitors), which have led to the suspension of both trials. In the phase IIb Quantum study, one treatment arm was discontinued when abnormal liver function tests were noted with the use of PSI-938 (nucleotide analog) alone or in combination with PSI-7977.[59]

Telaprevir is a substrate and inhibitor of CYP 3A4 and the transporter P-glycoprotein. The recommended dose is 750 mg every 8 hours, except when used in combination with efavirenz, wherein the dose should be increased to 1125 mg every 8 hours.[60] All HIV PIs significantly reduce plasma levels of telaprevir. Atazanavir has a more limited interaction, with only a 20% reduction in area under the curve (AUC) of telaprevir. Efavirenz also moderately decreases the AUC by 20%. Telaprevir increases exposure to tenofovir by 30% in the AUC, and fosamprenavir by 47%. Telaprevir can be safely used in coinfected patients taking tenofovir/emtricitabine, atazanavir/ritonavir, efavirenz (with a higher dose of telaprevir), and raltegrevir.[60] Rilpivirine and etravirine have also been studied and are safe (see **Table 2**).[61,62]

Boceprevir inhibits both CYP3A4 and CYP3A5, but it is mainly metabolized by the enzyme aldoketoreductase.[63] No adjustments were needed when boceprevir was coadministered with tenofovir. Boceprevir cannot be coadministered with efavirenz. Similar to telaprevir, boceprevir has no significant interaction with raltegravir.[64] Data support the safe use of boceprevir in combination with abacavir, lamivudine, tenofovir, and emtricitabine plus raltegravir, but not efavirenz or other NNRTIs.[65] Boceprevir should not be given with ritonavir-boosted HIV PIs because of decreased AUC and minimum concentration, and the theoretical risk of HIV virologic breakthrough (see **Table 2**).[66]

### What Is New on the Horizon?

One of the new NS5B polymerase inhibitors, sofosbuvir (GS-7977), requires no dose adjustments when coadministered with antiretroviral agents in healthy volunteers.[67] In other phase III clinical trials, simeprevir (TMC435), an NS3/4A PI, when administered with pegIFN/ribavirin, exhibited rare instances of hyperbilirubinemia.[68] Daclatasvir (BMS-790052), an NS5A inhibitor, and faldaprevir (BI 201335), a second-generation NS3/4A PI, when used in combination with antiretrovirals, require dose adjustments.[69,70] A recent trial concluded that darunavir/ritonavir increases faldaprevir exposure, whereas efavirenz decreases it. Therefore, faldaprevir at the lower dose (120 mg) is recommended in combination with darunavir/ritonavir and at the higher dose (240 mg) if taken with efavirenz.[71] Moreover, when coadministered with atazanavir/ritonavir, the daclatasvir AUC was 110% higher and maximum concentration (Cmax) was 35% higher, whereas the AUC was 32% lower and the Cmax 67% lower when administered with efavirenz.[69] When daclatasvir is coadministered with efavirenz, the higher dose of 90 mg once daily is recommended, whereas 60 mg is recommended when used alone, and 30 mg when combined with atazanavir/ritonavir (**Table 3**).

The new DAAs used to treat coinfection seem as efficacious as those used for treating monoinfection, although no direct comparisons have been made.[58,72] Adverse events also are similar. DDIs are driving the protocols, and will drive the market when approved. Because liver disease is the leading cause of morbidity and mortality among coinfected persons, the safety of all new anti-HCV agents and their interactions with antiretrovirals remains a top priority.

**Table 3**
**Interactions between antiretrovirals with new-generation direct-acting antivirals**

| Class | Antiretroviral | NS5A Polymerase Inhibitors (Daclatasvir) | NS5B Polymerase Inhibitors (Sofosbuvir) | NS3/4A Protease Inhibitors (Faldaprevir) |
|---|---|---|---|---|
| Non-nucleoside reverse transcriptase inhibitor | Efavirenz | Decreases daclatasvir | Safe | Decreases faldaprevir |
| Protease inhibitor | Darunavir/ritonavir | | Safe | Increases faldaprevir |
| | Atazanavir/ritonavir | Increases daclatasvir | | |

## BRIEF SUMMARY

Hepatotoxicity is the most common side effect of antiretroviral medications in HIV. Antiretroviral-related liver injury can range from asymptomatic elevations in transaminases (ALT/AST) and NCPH to severe liver decompensation and death. Risk factors include coinfection with chronic viral hepatitis (particularly HCV), abnormal baseline serum transaminases, alcohol consumption, drug use, opportunistic infections, and diabetes. NRTIs, NNRTIs, and PIs are the most common culprits in liver injury. NRTIs cause fatty liver disease and lactic acidosis via mitochondrial toxicity, whereas liver injury from NNRTIs manifests as hypersensitivity or toxic hepatitis. PIs such as indinavir and atazanavir can induce unconjugated hyperbilirubinemia, whereas tipranavir has been associated with elevated aminotransferases, rarely leading to fatal hepatitis when combined with ribavirin. CCR5 antagonists, integrase inhibitors, and fusion inhibitors have not been shown to cause liver injury.

DDIs between DAA agents for HCV and some antiretroviral medications used to treat HIV are common, but are often modest and can be managed with dose adjustments when treating people with coinfection. Dose adjustments are made when combining ribavirin with zidovudine. Ribavirin should never be used with didanosine. Additionally, the new HIV and HCV drugs have limited DDIs. One of the first-generation DAAs, telaprevir, requires upward dose adjustment when combined with efavirenz. Boceprevir cannot be administered with specific NNRTIs and ritonavir-boosted HIV PIs because of concern for HIV breakthrough. Liver injury does not occur with the first-generation DAAs; however, emerging reports from clinical trials show some hepatotoxicity with the use of some of the new generation DAAs, namely IDX184 (2-C-methylguanosine monophosphate prodrugs), BMS-094 (nucleotide polymerase inhibitors), and PSI-938 (nucleotide analog), which resulted in their suspension. Simeprevir, on the other hand, causes a slight increase in unconjugated bilirubin, but no evidence of increase in transaminases. Other new-generation DAAs, such as daclatasvir and faldaprevir, require dose adjustments in combination with other antiretrovirals, but have proven to be safe in ongoing studies.

## REFERENCES

1. Calza L. Renal toxicity associated with antiretroviral therapy. HIV Clin Trials 2012;13(4):189–211.
2. Gibellini D, Borderi M, Clò A, et al. Antiretroviral molecules and cardiovascular diseases. New Microbiol 2012;35(4):359–75.

3. Gazzard B, Balkin A, Hill A. Analysis of neuropsychiatric adverse events during clinical trials of efavirnenz in antiretroviral-naïve patients: a systematic review. AIDS Rev 2010;12(2):67–75.
4. Akhtar M, Mathieson K, Arey B, et al. Hepatic histopathology and clinical characteristics associated with antiretroviral therapy in HIV patients without viral hepatitis. Eur J Gastroenterol Hepatol 2008;20(12):1194–204.
5. Dieterich D. Managing antiretroviral associated liver disease. J Acquir Immune Defic Syndr 2003;34:S34–9.
6. AIDS Clinical Trials Group. Table of grading severity of adult adverse experiences. Rockville (MD): Division of AIDS, National Institute of Allergy and Infectious Diseases; 1996.
7. Kontorinis N, Dieterich D. Hepatotoxicity of antiretroviral therapy. AIDS Rev 2003;5:36–43.
8. de Maat MM, ter Heine R, van Gorp EC, et al. Case series of acute hepatitis in a non-selected group of HIV-infected patients on nevirapine-containing antiretroviral treatment. AIDS 2003;17(15):2209–14.
9. Brinkman K. Hyperlactemia and hepatic steatosis as features of mitochondrial toxicity of nucleoside analogue reverse transcriptase inhibitors. Clin Infect Dis 2000;31:167–9.
10. Dagan T, Sable C, Bray J, et al. Mitochondrial dysfunction and antiretroviral nucleoside analog toxicities: what is the evidence? Mitochondrion 2002;1: 397–412.
11. Brinkman K. Management of hyperlactatemia: no need for routine lactate measurements. AIDS 2001;15:795.
12. Bleeker-Rovers CP, Kadir SW, van Leusen R, et al. Hepatic steatosis and lactic acidosis caused by stavudine in an HIV-infected patient. Neth J Med 2000; 57(5):190–3.
13. Puoti M, Moioli MC, Travi G, et al. The burden of liver disease in human immunodeficiency virus-infected patients. Semin Liver Dis 2012;32(2):103–13.
14. Chang HM, Tsai HC, Lee SS, et al. Noncirrhotic portal hypertension associated with didanosine: a case report and literature review. J Infect Dis 2012;65(1):61–5.
15. Kovari H, Weber R. Influence of antiretroviral therapy on liver disease. Curr Opin HIV AIDS 2011;6(4):272–7.
16. Vispo E, Morello J, Rodriguez-Novoa S, et al. Noncirrhotic portal hypertension in HIV infection. Curr Opin Infect Dis 2011;24(1):12–8.
17. Cesari M, Schiavini M, Marchetti G, et al. Noncirrhotic portal hypertension in HIV-infected patients: a case control evaluation and review of the literature. AIDS 2010;24(11):697–703.
18. Parikh N, Kushner T, Martel-Laferriere V, et al. Noncirrhotic portal hypertension in HIV-infected patients: a case control study. Gastroenterology 2012;142(5): S945–6.
19. Rivero A. Liver toxicity induced by non-nucleoside reverse transcriptase inhibitors. J Antimicrob Chemother 2007;59(3):342–6.
20. Sulkowski M, Thomas D, Mehta S, et al. Hepatotoxicity associated with nevirapine or efavirenz-containing antiretroviral therapy: role of hepatitis C and B infections. Hepatology 2002;35:182–9.
21. Martin AM, Nolan D, James I, et al. Predisposition to nevirapine hypersensitivity associated with HLA-DRB1*0101 and abrogated by low CD4 T-cell counts. AIDS 2005;19(1):97–9.
22. Gonzalez de Requena D, Nunez M, Jimenez-Nacher I, et al. Liver toxicity caused by nevirapine. AIDS 2002;16:290–1.

23. Peters PJ, Stringer J, McConnell MS, et al. Nevirapine-associated hepatotoxicity was not predicted by CD4 count≥250 cells/μL among women in Zambia, Thailand and Kenya. HIV Med 2010;11(10):650.

24. Sulkowski MS, Thomas D, Chaisson R. Hepatotoxicity associated with antiretroviral therapy in adults infected with HIV and the role of Hepatitis C or B virus infection. JAMA 2000;283:74–80.

25. Ribaudo HJ, Daar ES, Tierney C, et al. Impact of UGT1A1 Gilbert variant on discontinuation of ritonavir boosted atazanavir in AIDS Clinical Trials Group Study A5202. J Infect Dis 2013;207:420–5.

26. Streeck H, Rockstroh J. Review of tipranavir in the treatment of drug-resistant HIV. Ther Clin Risk Manag 2007;3(4):641–51.

27. US Department of Health and Human Services. Guidelines for the use of antiretroviral agents in HIV-1-infected adults and adolescents. Available at: aidsinfo.nih.gov/guidelines. Accessed March 3, 2013.

28. Nichols WG, Steel WM, Bonny T, et al. Hepatotoxicity observed in clinical trials of Aplaviroc (GW873140). Antimicrob Agents Chemother 2008;52(3):858–65.

29. Chang CY, Schiano TD. Review article: drug hepatotoxicity. Aliment Pharmacol Ther 2007;25(10):1135–51.

30. Eyster M, Diamonstone L, Lien J, et al. Natural history of hepatitis C virus infection in multitransfused hemophiliacs: effect of coinfection with human immunodeficiency virus. The Multicenter Hemophilia Cohort Study. J Acquir Immune Defic Syndr 1993;6(6):602–10.

31. Soto B, Sanchez-Quijano A, Rodrigo L, et al. Human immunodeficiency virus infection modifies the natural history of chronic parenterally-acquired hepatitis C with an unusually rapid progression to cirrhosis. J Hepatol 1997;26(1):1–5.

32. Benhamou Y, Bochet M, Di Martino V, et al. Liver fibrosis progression in human immunodeficiency virus and hepatitis C virus coinfected patients. The Multivirc Group. Hepatology 1999;30(4):1054–8.

33. Martin-Carbonero L, Benhamou Y, Puoti M, et al. Incidence and predictors of severe liver fibrosis in human immunodeficiency virus-infected patients with chronic hepatitis C: a European collaborative study. Clin Infect Dis 2004;38(1):128–33.

34. Thein HH, Yi Q, Dore GJ, et al. Natural history of hepatitis C virus infection in HIV-infected individuals and the impact of HIV in the era of highly active antiretroviral therapy: a meta-analysis. AIDS 2008;22(15):1979–91.

35. Tan-Tam CC, Frassetto LA, Stock PG. Liver and kidney transplantation in HIV-infected patients. AIDS Rev 2009;11(4):190–204.

36. Soriano V, Puoti M, Garcia-Gasco P, et al. Antiretroviral drugs and liver injury. AIDS 2008;22(1):1–13.

37. Nunez M. Clinical syndromes and consequences of antiretroviral-related hepatotoxicity. Hepatology 2010;52(3):1143–55.

38. Mariné-Barjoan E, Saint-Paul M, Pradier C, et al. Impact of antiretroviral treatment on progression of hepatic fibrosis in HIV/hepatitis C virus co-infected patients. AIDS 2004;18(16):2163–70.

39. Labarga P, Soriano V, Vispo E, et al. Hepatotoxicity of antiretroviral drugs is reduced after successful treatment of chronic hepatitis C in HIV-infected patients. J Infect Dis 2007;196(5):670–6.

40. Soriano V, Puoti M, Sulkowski M, et al. Care of patients coinfected with HIV and hepatitis C virus: 2007 updated recommendations from the HCV-HIV International Panel. AIDS 2007;21(9):1073–89.

41. Medrano J, Resino S, Vispo E, et al. Hepatitis C virus (HCV) treatment uptake and changes in the prevalence of HCV genotypes in HIV/HCV-coinfected patients. J Viral Hepat 2011;18(5):325–30.

42. Poveda E, Vispo E, Barreiro P, et al. Predicted effect of direct acting antivirals in the current HIV-HCV-coinfected population in Spain. Antivir Ther 2012;17(3): 571–5.

43. Barreiro P, Labarga P, Martín-Carbonero L, et al. Sustained virological response following HCV therapy is associated with non-progression of liver fibrosis in HCV/HIV-coinfected patients. Antivir Ther 2006;11(7):869–77.

44. Soriano V, Labarga P, Ruiz-Sancho A, et al. Regression of liver fibrosis in hepatitis C virus/HIV-co-infected patients after treatment with pegylated interferon plus ribavirin. AIDS 2006;20(17):2225–7.

45. Soriano V, Maida I, Núñez M, et al. Long-term follow-up of HIV-infected patients with chronic hepatitis C virus infection treated with interferon-based therapies. Antivir Ther 2004;9(6):987–92.

46. Berenguer J, Alvarez-Pellicer J, Martín P, et al. Sustained virological response to interferon plus ribavirin reduces liver-related complications and mortality in patients coinfected with human immunodeficiency virus and hepatitis C virus. Hepatology 2009;50(2):407–13.

47. Guidelines for the use of antiretroviral agents in HIV-1-infected adults and adolescents. Available at: aidsinfo.nih.gov/guidelines. Accessed February 23, 2013.

48. Mauss S, Valenti W, DePamphilis J, et al. Risk factors for hepatic decompensation in patients with HIV/HCV coinfection and liver cirrhosis during interferon-based therapy. AIDS 2004;18(13):F21–25.

49. Bani-Sadr F, Carrat F, Pol S, et al. Risk factors for symptomatic mitochondrial toxicity in HIV/hepatitis C virus-coinfected patients during interferon plus ribavirin-based therapy. J Acquir Immune Defic Syndr 2005;40(1):47–52.

50. Barreiro P, Vispo E, Labarga P, et al. Management and treatment of chronic hepatitis C in HIV patients. Semin Liver Dis 2012;32(2):138–46.

51. Blanco F, Barreiro P, Ryan P, et al. Risk factors for advanced liver fibrosis in HIV-infected individuals: role of antiretroviral drugs and insulin resistance. J Viral Hepat 2011;18(1):11–6.

52. Ingiliz P, Valantin M, Duvivier C, et al. Liver damage underlying unexplained transaminase elevation in human immunodeficiency virus-1 mono-infected patients on antiretroviral therapy. Hepatology 2009;49(2):436–42.

53. Vispo E, Mena A, Maida I, et al. Hepatic safety profile of raltegravir in HIV-infected patients with chronic hepatitis C. J Antimicrob Chemother 2010;65(3): 543–7.

54. Pineda J, Aguilar-Guisado M, Rivero A, et al. Natural history of compensated hepatitis C virus-related cirrhosis in HIV-infected patients. Clin Infect Dis 2009;49(8):1274–82.

55. Sulkowski M, Mast E, Seeff L, et al. Hepatitis C virus infection as an opportunistic disease in persons infected with human immunodeficiency virus. Clin Infect Dis 2000;30(Suppl 1):S77–84.

56. Qurishi N, Kreuzberg C, Lüchters G, et al. Effect of antiretroviral therapy on liver-related mortality in patients with HIV and hepatitis C virus coinfection. Lancet 2003;362(9397):1708–13.

57. Victrelis (boceprevir) [2011]. Available at: http://www.merck.com/product/usa/pi_circulars/v/victrelis/victrelis_pi.pdf. Accessed February 26, 2013.

58. Incivek (telaprevir) [2011]. Available at: http://pi.vrtx.com/files/uspi_telaprevir.pdf. Accessed February 26, 2013.

59. Xu K. Pharmasset's PSI938 discontinued; impact on other nukes in hepatitis C? Wm Blair & Co Analyst Equity Research Report. Available at: www.natap.org/2011/HCV/121711_02.htm. Accessed March 26, 2013.
60. Dieterich D, Soriano V, Shermann K, et al. Telaprevir in combination with peginterferon alfa-2a/ribavirin in HCV/HIV co-infected patients: SVR12 interim analysis. Presented at the19th Conference on Retrovirus and Opportunistic Infections. Seattle, March 5–8, 2012. Abstract 46.
61. Van Heeswijk R, Vandevoorde A, Boogaerts G, et al. Pharmacokinetic interactions between ARV agents and the investigational HCV protease inhibitor TVR in healthy volunteers. Presented at the 18th Conference on Retroviruses and Opportunistic Infections. Boston, February 27–March 2, 2011. Abstract 119.
62. Van Heeswijk R, Gard V, Boogaerts G, et al. The pharmacokinetic interaction between telaprevir and raltegravir in healthy volunteers. Presented at the 51st Interscience Conference on Antimicrobial Agents and Chemotherapy. Chicago, September 17–20, 2011. Abstract A1–1738a.
63. Ghosal A, Yuan Y, Tong W, et al. Characterization of human liver enzymes involved in the biotransformation of boceprevir, a hepatitis C virus protease inhibitor. Drug Metab Dispos 2011;39(3):510–21.
64. de Kanter CT, Blonk MI, Colbers AP, et al. Influence of the HCV Protease Inhibitor Boceprevir on the Pharmacokinetics of the HIV Integrase Inhibitor Raltegravir. Presented at the 19th Conference on Retroviruses and Opportunistic Infections; Seattle, March 6, 2012. Abstract 772LB.
65. Kassera C, Hughes E, Treitel M, et al. Clinical pharmacology of boceprevir: metabolism, excretion, and drug-drug interactions. Presented at the 18th Conference on Retroviruses and Opportunistic Infections. Boston, February 27–March 2, 2011. Abstract 118.
66. Hulskotte EG, Feng HP, Xuan F, et al. Pharmacokinetic Interaction between the HCV protease inhibitor boceprevir and ritonavir-boosted HIV-1 protease inhibitors atazanavir, lopinavir, and darunavir. Presented at the 19th Conference on Retroviruses and Opportunistic Infections. Seattle, March 5–8, 2011. Abstract 47.
67. Kirby B, Mathias A, Rossi S, et al. No clinically significant pharmacokinetic drug interactions between sofosbuvir (GS-7977) and HIV antiretrovirals atripla, rilpivirine, darunavir/ritonavir, or raltegravir in healthy volunteers. Presented at the 63rd Annual Meeting of the American Association for the Study of Liver Diseases. Boston, November 9–13, 2012. Abstract 1877.
68. Douglas DJ, Rockstroh K, Orkin C, et al. Simeprevir (TMC435) with peginterferon/ribavirin in patients co-infected with chronic genotype-1 HCV and HIV-1: week-24 interim analysis of the TMC435-C212 study. Presented at the 20th Conference on Retroviruses and Opportunistic Infections. Atlanta, March 3–6, 2013. Oral abstract 154LB.
69. Bifano M, Hwang C, Oosterhuis B, et al. Assessment of HIV ARV Drug Interactions with the HCV NS5A Replication Complex Inhibitor BMS-790052 Demonstrates a Pharmacokinetic Profile which Supports Co-administration with Tenofovir Disoproxil Fumarate, Efavirenz, and Atazanavir/ritonavir. Presented at the 19th Conference on Retroviruses and Opportunistic Infections. Seattle, March 5–8, 2012. Abstract 618.
70. Dieterich D, Soriano V, Nelson M, et al. STARTVerso 4: high rates of early virologic response in HCV genotype 1/HIV-co-infected patients treated with faldaprevir plus pegIFN and RBV. Presented at the 20th Conference on Retroviruses and Opportunistic Infections. Atlanta, March 3–6, 2013. Oral abstract 40LB.

71. Sabo JP, Kort J, Haschke M, et al. Pharmacokinetic interactions of darunavir/ritonavir, efavirenz, and tenofovir with the HCV protease inhibitor faldaprevir in healthy volunteers. Presented at the 20th Conference on Retroviruses and Opportunistic Infections. Atlanta, March 3–6, 2013. Oral abstract 35.
72. Sulkowski M, Pol S, Cooper C, et al. Boceprevir plus peginterferon/ribavirin for the treatment of HCV/HIV co-infected patients. Presented at the 19th Conference on Retroviruses and Opportunistic Infections. Seattle, March 5–8, 2011. Abstract 47.

# Chemotherapy-Induced Hepatotoxicity

Ameet V. Thatishetty, MD[a], Nicholas Agresti, MD[a],
Christopher B. O'Brien, MD, AGAF, FRCMI[b],*

## KEYWORDS

- Cancer • Chemotherapy • Liver • Hepatotoxicity • Drugs

## KEY POINTS

- Most hepatotoxicity secondary to chemotherapy is idiosyncratic.
- Preexisting abnormal liver function has been shown to increase the risk of hepatotoxicity, especially patients with chronic hepatitis B.
- Alterations in the patterns of abnormal liver test are helpful to characterize the type of presentation, but not the extent of damage.
- Presentations include hepatocellular injury, cholestasis, hepatic sinusoidal obstruction syndrome, and progressive liver fibrosis.
- Outcomes can range from asymptomatic liver function test abnormalities, which resolve spontaneously, to cirrhosis, despite discontinuation of the chemotherapeutic agent.

## INTRODUCTION

The newer chemotherapy agents have revolutionized the treatment options for a wide variety of cancers. Most hepatotoxicity from chemotherapeutic drugs is idiosyncratic. Alterations in the patterns of abnormal liver test can be used to determine changes in synthetic function, cellular injury, duct injury, or cholestasis, but not the extent of damage.[1]

### Liver Toxicity Criteria

The US National Cancer Institute (NCI) (**Table 1**) and the World Health Organization (WHO) have developed specific adverse event criteria for those undergoing chemotherapy.[2,3] The US NCI categories range from no adverse event (0), mild (1), moderate (2), severe (3), life-threatening (4), and death (5), but these are not specific to hepatotoxicity. The WHO classification grades (1–5) are specific to hepatotoxicity, but are

Commercial relationships: None.
[a] Department of Medicine, Memorial Health, University Medical Center, 4700 Waters Avenue, Savannah, GA 31403, USA; [b] Division of Liver and GI Transplantation, University of Miami School of Medicine, 1500 Northwest 12th Avenue, Suite 1101, Miami, FL 33136, USA
* Corresponding author.
*E-mail address:* cobrien@med.miami.edu

Clin Liver Dis 17 (2013) 671–686
http://dx.doi.org/10.1016/j.cld.2013.07.010
1089-3261/13/$ – see front matter © 2013 Elsevier Inc. All rights reserved.

**liver.theclinics.com**

**Table 1**
NCI common terminology criteria for adverse events grading of hepatic toxicity

| | 0 | 1 | 2 | Grade 3 | 4 | 5 |
|---|---|---|---|---|---|---|
| Alkaline phosphatase | WNL | >ULN to 2.5 × ULN | >2.5 to 5 × ULN | >5 to 20 × ULN | >20 × ULN | — |
| Bilirubin | WNL | >ULN to 1.5 × ULN | >1.5 to 3 × ULN | >3 to 10 × ULN | >10 × ULN | — |
| GGT (γ-glutamyl transpeptidase) | WNL | >ULN to 2.5 × ULN | >2.5 to 5 × ULN | >5 to 20 × ULN | >20 × ULN | — |
| Liver failure (clinical) | Normal | — | — | Asterixis; mild encephalopathy; limiting self-care ADL | Moderate to severe encephalopathy; coma; life-threatening consequences | Death |
| Portal hypertension | Normal | — | Decreased portal vein flow | Reversal/retrograde portal vein flow associated with varices or ascites | Life-threatening consequences; urgent operative intervention needed | Death |
| ALT | WNL | >ULN to 3 × ULN | >3 to 5 × ULN | >5 to 20 × ULN | >20 × ULN | — |
| AST | WNL | >ULN to 3 × ULN | >3 to 5 × ULN | >5 to 20 × ULN | >20 × ULN | — |

*Abbreviations:* ADL, activities of daily living; ALT, alanine aminotransferase; AST, aspartate aminotransferase; ULN, upper limit of normal; WNL, within normal limits.

*Adapted from* US Department of Health and Human Services; National Institutes of Health; National Cancer Institute. Common Terminology Criteria for Adverse Events (CTCAE). NIH Publication No. 09-5410.

poor predictors of severity of injury, because most are reversible, with the exception of sinusoidal obstruction syndrome.

## Mechanism of Injury and Risk Factors

Hepatotoxicity from chemotherapy occurs most often from an unpredictable or idiosyncratic reaction. Therefore, the incidence is rare, unrelated to the dose of the drug, unpredictable, typically noted 1 to 4 weeks after drug dosing, and more common after multiple exposures. Often, hepatotoxicity is not caused by the drug itself, but by a metabolite that acts as a hapten, binding to cell proteins, which induces the immunologic damage.[4] However, the adverse effects of these agents on the liver are also modified by preexisting liver disease, genetic sensitivity to chemotherapy, and whether the tumor is in the liver itself. This injury may be reversible or permanent depending on the genetic variability, age, sex, and hepatic adaptation of the patient. Increased age, female sex, and specific social habits such as tobacco and alcohol ingestion can increase the risk of toxicity.[5] Some familial clusters have been studied, with individuals having as high as a 25% likelihood of developing a drug reaction.[6] This unique genetic variability to specific drugs depends on the expression of the cytochrome pathway and immune response to medications.

## Clinical Presentation

The clinical presentations (**Table 2**) of those with hepatotoxicity vary from asymptomatic, increase of liver chemistries, overt cholestatic hepatitis, progression to fibrosis and cirrhosis, malignant transformation, sinusoidal obstruction, and fulminant hepatic failure.[7] Hepatic sinusoidal obstruction is caused by nonthrombotic obliteration of small intrahepatic veins and occurs in those undergoing stem cell transplantations.[8] The proposed mechanisms related to increase in age are decrease in blood flow, decrease in clearance, and lower levels of albumin, leading to an increase in unbound drugs.[9] The combination of chemotherapeutic agents in conjunction with radiation potentially causes augmented toxicity.

## SPECIFIC DRUGS
### Antimetabolites

Their mechanism of action is to affect both DNA and RNA synthesis and lead to apoptosis of cells. These drugs have variable hepatotoxic potential and because most are metabolized by the liver, they require dose adjustments in patients with hepatic dysfunction.

### Azathioprine (Imuran)
Azathioprine is a derivative of 6-mercaptopurine (6-MP). Azathioprine was developed to decrease the rate of inactivation of 6-MP by S-methylation by xanthine oxidase to thiourate. A study performed in 1974 examined 29 patients treated with azathioprine for psoriatic arthritis. Liver biopsies on 20 of these patients before and 6 months after starting treatment showed mild portal fibrosis and mild cholestasis, and follow-up biopsies at 24 months were within normal limits.[10] When compared with 6-MP, its effects are less frequent and less dose dependent.

### Capecitabine (Xeloda)
Capecitabine is a prodrug converted in the intestine into the active metabolite fluorouracil (5-FU). According to the product information, an increased serum bilirubin level occurred in 48% of patients with colorectal cancer in clinical trials. The changes were fully reversible. In contrast to 5-FU, the pharmacology of capecitabine is not

**Table 2**
Chemotherapeutic hepatotoxic histologic presentation patterns

| Drug | Hepatitis | Cholestasis | Biliary Stricture | Steatosis | Veno-Occlusive Disease |
|---|---|---|---|---|---|
| Asparaginase | Common | | | Common | |
| Axitinib | Common | | | | |
| Azathioprine | | Rare | | | Rare |
| Bendamustine | | | | | |
| Bleomycin | | | | | |
| Bortezomib | | | | | |
| Bosutinib | Common | | | | |
| Busulfan | | Rare | | | |
| Cabazitaxel | Rare | | | | |
| Capecitabine | | Common | | | |
| Carboplatin | | Rare | | | Rare |
| Carmustine | Common | | | | |
| Chlorambucil | | Rare | | | |
| Cisplatin | | Rare | | Rare | |
| Crizotinib | Common | | | | |
| Cyclophosphamide | Rare | | | | |
| Cytarabine | | | Common intravenously | | |
| Dacarbazine | | | | | Rare |
| Dactinomycin | Rare | | | | Rare |
| Docetaxel | | | | | |
| Doxorubicin | Rare | Rare | | | Rare |
| Erlotinib | Common | | | | |
| Etoposide | Rare | Rare | | | |
| Everolimus | | | | | |
| Floxuridine | Common | Significant | | | |
| Fluorouracil | Rare | | | | |
| Gefitinib | Rare | | | | |
| Gemcitabine | Rare | Rare | | | |
| Hydroxyurea | Rare | | | | |
| Ifosfamide | Rare | | | | |
| Imatinib | Common | | | | |
| Interferon α | Rare | | | | |
| Ipilimumab | Rare | | | | |
| Irinotecan | | | | Rare | Rare |
| Ixabepilone | | | | | |
| Lapatinib | Rare | | | | |
| Lomustine | Common | | | | |
| Melphalan | Rare | | | | |
| Mercaptopurine | | | | | Rare |
| Methotrexate | Common intravenously | | | | |

(continued on next page)

| Table 2 (continued) | | | | | |
|---|---|---|---|---|---|
| Drug | Hepatitis | Cholestasis | Biliary Stricture | Steatosis | Veno-Occlusive Disease |
| Mitomycin | Rare | | | | Rare |
| Mitoxantrone | Rare | | | | |
| Nitrogen mustard | | | | | |
| Oxaliplatin | | | | Rare | Rare |
| Paclitaxel | | Rare | | | |
| Pazopanib | Common | | | | |
| Ponatinib | Common | | | | |
| Procarbazine | Rare | | | | |
| Regorafenib | Rare | | | | |
| Sorafenib | Rare | Rare | | | |
| Streptozocin | | | | | |
| Sunitinib | Rare | | | | |
| Temozolomide | | | | | |
| Thioguanine | | | | | Rare |
| Trastuzumab | Rare | | | | |
| Vandetanib | Common | | | | |
| Vemurafenib | Common | | | | |
| Vinblastine | | | | | Rare |
| Vincristine | Rare | | | | |

significantly affected by hepatic dysfunction, therefore, dose reduction is not recommended.[11]

### Cytarabine/cytosine arabinoside (Cytosar-U; Depocyt)
Cytarabine combines a cytosine base with an arabinose sugar instead of deoxyribose, leading to cell death. This drug is the most important antimetabolite used in the treatment of acute myelogenous leukemia and non-Hodgkin lymphoma.[12] In recent studies, there have been transient increases in aminotransferase levels secondary to high-dose cytarabine; progression to cholestasis is rare.[13] The hepatotoxic effects of cytarabine are usually reversible, and the dose should be reduced in those with underlying liver diseases.

### 5-FU (Efudex)
5-FU is currently used in the treatment of gastrointestinal and head and neck as well as lung and bladder tumors. Even although the liver plays a key role in its catabolism, 5-FU has not been reported to cause liver damage when given orally, and only rare reports of possible hepatotoxicity have been noted when the drug is given intravenously.[14] 5-FU has been implicated with other agents such as oxaliplatin or irinotecan, leading to hepatotoxicity in 1 report.[15] A pattern of hepatic vascular injury is noted in patients receiving combinations of 5-FU and leucovorin with oxaliplatin or irinotecan for neoadjuvant therapy before the resection of colorectal cancer liver metastases.[16]

### Fluorodeoxyuridine (5-FUdR)
Unlike 5-FU, the metabolite fluorodeoxyuridine does cause hepatotoxicity, and guidelines have been established for dose reduction.[17] The development of irreversible biliary strictures is seen in variable numbers, but could present in as many as 25%

of patients. The strictures are permanent without intervention and are one of the serious liver toxicity issues.[18] A hepatitis pattern with this drug is also common, and in 1 report ranged from 40% to 100%.[19]

### Gemcitabine (Gemzar)

Gemcitabine is used in clinical practice for the treatment of lung, pancreatic, bladder, and breast carcinoma. It is a cytosine analogue that shows cell cycle–dependent and S-phase–specific cytotoxicity.[20] Increased levels of transaminases are commonly seen, with rapid reversal, and precautions should be taken in those with preexisting liver disease.[21] Gemcitabine is commonly used with other chemotherapeutic agents such as platinum derivatives with split dosing, causing systemic side effects in 20% of patients.

### 6-MP (Purinethol)

6-MP is a purine analogue, and both hepatocellular and cholestasis patterns have been observed in patients whose daily dose is more than 2 mg/kg.[22] Allopurinol can lead to additional toxicity with 6-MP by blocking the enzyme xanthine oxidase. The hepatocellular injury pattern usually occurs more than 30 days after treatment initiation with increase of bilirubin level up to 7 mg/dL.[23] Hepatotoxicity from 6-MP is felt to be an idiosyncratic reaction because the re-challenge did not decrease the latent period and systemic manifestations of hypersensitivity.

### Thioguanine/tioguan/thioguanine/6-thioguanine (Lanvis)

6-Thioguanine is a purine analogue similar to 6-MP, except that it may be administered concurrently with allopurinol without reduction in dosage, unlike 6-MP and azathioprine. The risk of veno-occlusive disease is serious and frequently irreversible and may be dose dependent based on 1 study.[24]

### Methotrexate (Trexall; Rheumatrex)

Methotrexate (MTX) is an inhibitor of dihydrofolate reductase, with an effect on folate requiring reactions in biosynthesis of thymidylate and purines. In low doses, MTX is excreted mainly unchanged in the urine, whereas in high doses (such as are used to treat osteosarcoma, and central nervous system [CNS] lymphoma), it is partially metabolized by the liver to 7-hydroxymethotrexate. MTX in high doses usually causes increase in transaminase levels in 60% to 80% of patients. However, in those undergoing treatment of long-term diseases, such as rheumatoid arthritis, it can lead to fibrosis and cirrhosis.[25] In patients who take daily oral MTX, fibrosis or cirrhosis is reported to develop more than twice as frequently as in those who take the drug intermittently by parenteral route.[26]

### Alkylating Agents

Alkylating agents function by adding an alkyl group to the guanine base of DNA. Overall, the alkylating agents are seldom implicated as hepatotoxins and can be given in the setting of altered liver function with relative safety. In clinical practice, dose reduction is usually not necessary, with the exception of cyclophosphamide and ifosfamide.

### Busulfan (Myleran; Busulfex)

Busulfan is the only drug of the alkylsulfonate class, rarely used for the myeloproliferative disorders because of its narrow therapeutic index. The mechanism of action of this drug lies in the cross-links produced between guanine-adenine intrastrand, which cannot be repaired by cell proofreading, leading to cell death.[27] Overall, busulfan rarely causes hepatic dysfunction, but there have been a few case reports of cholestatic hepatitis.[28]

#### Cyclophosphamide (Endoxan; Cytoxan; Neosar; Procytox; Revimmune)

The liver cytochrome P450 system converts cyclophosphamide to 4-hydroxycyclophosphamide to its intermediaries which are picked up by rapidly dividing cells and cleaved into compounds that are highly toxic.[29] Few cases of increased hepatic enzymes have been attributed to cyclophosphamide and it is believed that the reaction like most others is idiosyncratic.[30] When used to treat vasculitis, cyclophosphamide has been associated with liver damage when it was given after a course of azathioprine.[31]

#### Chlorambucil (Leukeran)

Chlorambucil was used to treat chronic lymphocytic leukemia, but has been replaced by fludarabine in young patients.[32] A variety of controversial reports, ranging from nonspecific findings to cholestasis, were published in the late 1950s and early 1960s.[33] This drug should be considered a rare cause of cholestatic hepatoxicity.

#### Ifosfamide (Ifex; Mitoxana)

Despite being metabolized by the liver, ifosfamide is rarely known to cause hepatotoxicity. Ifosfamide is mostly given in combination with other chemotherapy; its role in causing increase of aminotransferase levels is not clear.[34]

#### Melphalan (Alkeran)

This drug was first used in the treatment of melanoma and is currently used for multiple myeloma, bone marrow transplants, and ovarian cancer.[35] This drug has a short half-life, is rapidly hydrolyzed in plasma and is excreted in the urine. It may cause transient increase in liver function tests, especially in those undergoing bone marrow transplant using higher dosages.[36]

### Antitumor Antibiotics

Anthracycline antibiotics function by intercalating into DNA and are commonly used in the treatment of a wide range of cancers, including carcinoma, hematologic malignancies, and soft tissue sarcomas.

#### Actinomycin D/Dactinomycin (Cosmegen)

Actinomycin D was the first antibiotic known to have antitumor properties.[37] This drug binds to the double-helical DNA and blocks the transcription of DNA by RNA polymerase. The common side effects are hematopoietic in nature but can cause transient increase in aminotransferase levels if a specific site has been irradiated. This finding suggests that radiation-induced hepatic toxicity prolongs excretion and increases toxicity. Hepatic veno-occlusive disease has also been reported.[38]

#### Bleomycin (Blenoxane)

The cytotoxic action of bleomycin results from its ability to cause fragmentation of DNA. The largest review of more than 1000 patients treated with bleomycin found that hepatic toxicity was rare and it could not be specifically attributed to bleomycin.[39]

#### Dacarbazine (DTIZ; DTIC-Dome)

Dacarbazine functions as an alkylating agent after metabolic activation in the liver, leading to inhibition of RNA synthesis more than DNA. Cases of hepatovascular toxicity after receiving single-agent dicarbazine have been reported.[40] One such case was in a patient with melanoma with fatal hepatotoxicity after dicarbazine therapy. Autopsy revealed thrombosis in the hepatic veins and eosinophilic infiltrations around the vessels, suggesting an idiosyncratic hypersensitivity reaction, rather than endoluminal damage.[41]

### Doxorubicin (Adriamycin; Rubex) and daunorubicin (Cerubidine)

Both are produced by the bacterium *Streptomyces peucetius*. Drugs from this group, which includes epirubicin (Ellence) and idarubicin (Idamycin), seem similar in terms of their toxicity and metabolism. The mechanism of doxorubicin of action binds topoisomerase II, which normally relaxes the double helix and prevents its realignment.[42] Doxorubicin can cause an idiosyncratic reaction and potentially contribute to liver toxicity.[43] Impaired liver function delays excretion, increases accumulation of the drug in plasma and tissues, leading to systemic side effects like cardiomyopathy.[44]

### Mitomycin

Mitomycin is converted into an alkylating agent and works by inhibiting DNA synthesis.[45] This medication is rarely known to increase aminotransferase levels but has been reported in the literature for veno-occlusive disease at higher doses.[46]

### Nitrosureas

Nitrosureas as a class are lipophilic, enabling them to cross the blood-brain barrier and making them useful in treating CNS tumors. The potential hazard of this class of drugs is the depletion of hepatic stores of glutathione, which may increase the risk of oxidative injury from other sources like acetaminophen.[4]

### Carmustine (BiCNU) and lomustine (CeeNU)

Carmustine and lomustine have similar delayed onset of increase in aminotransferase levels with rare causes of fatalities. In 1 phase 2 study, hepatotoxicity occurred from 6 to 127 days after receiving treatment with carmustine.[47] Severe hepatotoxicity has been reported when carmustine was used in conjunction with etoposide (Etopophos)[48] as well as a combination of lomustine, procarbazine (Matulane), and vincristine (Oncovin).[49]

### Streptozotocin (STZ; Zanosar)

Streptozotocin was originally discovered as an antibiotic derived from *Streptomyces acromogenes*; it has a special affinity for β cells of the islets of Langerhans and is used in the treatment of pancreatic islet cell carcinoma and malignant carcinoid tumors. It has been reported to cause hepatotoxicity in as many as 67% of patients, most with rapid resolution after withdrawal of this agent.[50]

### Taxanes

### Paclitaxel (Abraxane; Taxol) and docetaxel (Taxotere)

These drugs belong to a new class of spindle inhibitors that function by binding to microtubules rather than tubulin dimers, inhibiting mitosis. Increases in aminotransferase levels are seen when these drugs interact with other drugs that are metabolized by cytochrome P450, including inhibitors and inducers of CYP3A4.[51] In particular, patients with liver dysfunction have decreased docetaxel clearance and are at increased risk for severe nonhepatic toxicity; hence a dose reduction is recommended.

### Cabazitaxel (Jevtana)

Cabazitaxel is a semisynthetic taxane that is metabolized by the liver. US Food and Drug Administration (FDA) guidelines suggest that this drug should not be given to patients with bilirubin levels greater than the upper limit of normal (ULN) or if either one of the aminotransferase levels is greater than 1.5 × ULN.

### Eribulin (Halaven)

Eribulin mesylate is a substrate derived from marine sponge. It is approved for metastatic breast cancer, sarcoma, and nonsmall cell carcinoma. Its mechanism of action is similar to other tubulin inhibitors.[1] Its exposure is increased in patients with mild and moderate hepatic dysfunction and should not be administered to anybody with Child-Pugh C disease.[52]

## Vinca Alkaloids

Vinca alkaloids are cytotoxic drugs that act on tubulin and microtubules derived from the periwinkle plant (*Catharanthus roseuso*).

### Vincristine (Oncovin) and vinorelbine (Navelbine)
A study revealed that alkaline phosphatase increases alone even when there was no evidence of liver dysfunction predicted delayed clearance of vincristine and may lead to increased neurotoxicity.[53] Abnormal liver function tests (LFTs) have been noticed after treatment with both vincristine and vinorelbine, and severe hepatotoxicity is reported in patients who received vincristine along with radiation therapy.[54]

## Topoisomerase Inhibitors

There are 2 topoisomerase I inhibitors available: irinotecan (Camptosar; Campto) and topotecan (Hycamtin). Irinotecan has been used in colorectal, cervical, and lung cancers.[55] It is metabolized in the intestine, plasma, and liver. Combinations of irinotecan and 5-FU have been used in patients with colorectal cancer before resection of liver metastasis and have been associated with steatosis and hepatic vascular injury.[56]

### Topotecan
Topotecan is used in ovarian cancer and myelodysplastic syndromes. Unlike irinotecan, topotecan is not extensively metabolized in liver and a significant portion is excreted in the urine. Mild and reversible increases in alkaline phosphatase and transaminase levels have been seen in 5% to 8% of patients.[57] Therefore topotecan may be safely used with bilirubin levels up to 10 mg/dL.

### Etoposide/VP-16 (Etopophos)
This drug is a topoisomerase II inhibitor, which is primarily excreted in bile. It is not known to be hepatotoxic, but 3 cases of severe hepatocellular necrosis after administration of standard doses have been reported.[58] Two cases of toxic hepatitis developed in approximately 3 weeks after high-dose etoposide treatment, but hepatitis resolved spontaneously over 12 weeks without any sequelae.

## Platinum Derivatives

### Carboplatin (Paraplatin)
Carboplatin is a cisplatin derivative. A case of carboplatin-induced liver failure was documented in an 18-year-old patient who was given high-dose carboplatin as part of leukemia treatment.[59] Another case of autopsy-documented hepatic sinusoidal obstruction syndrome has been reported in a patient who received high-dose carboplatin and etoposide along with multiple other medications, but the role of carboplatin could not be completely excluded.[60]

### Cisplatin (Platin)
Cisplatin occasionally has been associated with cholestasis or steatosis.[61] Mild increases in transaminase levels occur more frequently when given in higher doses.[62]

### Oxaliplatin (Eloxatin)
This drug is used more commonly in multidrug regimens, and reports of increased transaminase levels are frequent in this setting. Because this drug is excreted through the kidneys, there are some data to suggest that oxaliplatin can be safely given to

patients with underlying severe liver dysfunction caused by metastatic colorectal cancer.[63] However, this drug has also been linked to sinusoidal obstruction syndrome.[64]

### Kinase Inhibitors

#### Erlotinib (Tarceva) and Gefitinib (Iressa)

Both inhibit tyrosine kinase domain of the epidermal growth factor receptor. Hepatic dysfunction reduces clearance of erlotinib, which is metabolized by the P450 system in the liver.[65] There has been a case report of a patient with stage IV non–small cell lung cancer who died of fulminant hepatic failure as a result of treatment with erlotinib.[66] Gefitinib undergoes extensive hepatic metabolism. Rarely, it can cause abnormal alanine aminotransferase (ALT) and aspartate aminotransferase (AST) levels.[67]

#### Imatinib (Gleevec; Glivec)

Imatinib inhibits Bcr-Abl tyrosine kinase. It is used to treat chronic myelogenous leukemia, acute lymphocytic leukemia with the Philadelphia chromosome, and gastrointestinal stromal tumors. It too is metabolized by cytochrome P450 system. This drug has been shown to cause increases in serum LFTs in 15% to 20% of patients receiving the drug.[68] There has been 1 case report of a woman who received this drug and developed fatal acute liver failure.[69]

#### Pazopanib (Votrient)

Pazopanib is an oral agent that targets platelet-derived growth factor receptor, vascular endothelial growth factor (VEGF) receptor, and KIT tyrosine kinases. Pazopanib undergoes liver metabolism. Data suggest that some instances of isolated hyperbilirubinemia in pazopanib-treated patients are benign manifestations of Gilbert syndrome.[70] However, there have been reports of hepatoxicity in 18% of 977 patients receiving this drug as part of a clinical trial, with 2 deaths.[71]

#### Regorafenib (Stivarga)

Regorafenib is a novel receptor tyrosine kinase inhibitor. A review[72] reported a 2% risk of hepatic failure out of 132 patients. Manufacturer recommends checking LFTs every 2 weeks during the first 2 months of therapy.

#### Sorafenib (Nexavar)

The primary mode of action of sorafenib is mediated through inhibitory effects on tyrosine kinases associated with vascular endothelial growth and platelet-derived growth factor receptors. In a phase 1 study involving 44 patients, adverse hepatic effects, such as increased transaminase levels, occurred in 50% of the patients, increase of alkaline phosphatase level in 30% of patients and increased bilirubin level in 40%. Drug-related toxicity was less than grade 3 in all groups with doses up to 800 mg twice daily.[73] However, sorafenib has been associated with fatal liver failure.[74]

### Mammalian Target of Rapamycin Inhibitors

#### Everolimus (Zortress; Afinitor; Certican)

Everolimus is a macrolide inhibitor of the mammalian target of rapamycin (mTOR), which has antiproliferative and antiangiogenic properties. Everolimus is extensively metabolized in the liver via CYP3A4, and hence, exposure is increased in patients with hepatic dysfunction. Dose reduction is recommended for patients with cirrhosis.[75]

#### Temsirolimus (Torisel)

Temsirolimus and its active metabolite, sirolimus, are targeted inhibitors of mTOR kinase activity. This drug is mostly metabolized in liver to sirolimus and 4 other minor metabolites. FDA-approved labeling guidelines recommend that the drug should not be given to patients with serum bilirubin greater than 1.5 × ULN.

## Monoclonal Antibodies

### Bevacizumab (Avastin)
Bevacizumab is a recombinant humanized monoclonal IgG1 antibody targeted against VEGF. Data regarding hepatotoxicity are in combination with multiagent regimens using 5-FU/leucovorin and bevacizumab or 5-FU/leucovorin, irinotecan and bevacizumab, with hyperbilirubinemia in 7% and 1%, respectively.[76]

### Trastuzumab (Herclon; Herceptin)
An antibody-drug conjugate, trastuzumab has resulted in serious hepatotoxicity, including liver failure and death. A hepatocellular pattern of injury is the most commonly seen.[77] During clinical trials, 3 cases of nodular regenerative hyperplasia were identified on liver biopsies.

## Immunotherapy

### Pegylated interferon α
High-dose, recombinant α-interferon is used in the treatment of hairy cell leukemia, multiple myeloma, non-Hodgkin lymphomas, AIDS-related Kaposi sarcoma, and myeloproliferative disorders.[78] Its use is often accompanied by an increase in aminotransferase levels, which resolves with discontinuation of therapy. At high doses (>10 million units daily), hepatotoxicity may be dose limiting.[79]

### Interleukin 2
In a study conducted on 210 patients who received this drug, most patients were found to have increases in bilirubin, AST, AST, and alkaline phosphatase levels. These findings support the development of profound reversible cholestasis as the primary basis for the increased bilirubin level in these patients.[80] Interleukin 2 (IL-2) activates Kupffer cells and induces leukocyte and platelet adhesion to hepatic sinusoidal endothelium, with subsequent impaired sinusoidal perfusion and hypoxic damage, likely leading to cholestasis. A return to normal levels of bilirubin was noted within 5.6 days of stopping IL-2.[81]

## Miscellaneous Agents

### Arsenic trioxide
Severe hepatotoxicity occurred in 63.7% (7/11) of newly diagnosed patients with acute promyelocytic leukemia receiving a 10-mg daily intravenous infusion of arsenic trioxide; this was fatal in 2 of the cases. In the same study, 32% developed modest toxicity, which responded with symptomatic treatment.[82]

### Asparaginase (Elspar)
Hepatotoxicity is frequent with this drug.[83] The reason for hepatotoxicity is believed to be the depletion of asparagine, leading to abnormal protein synthesis, although it tends to be reversible. However, in another study, liver steatosis was found at autopsy in 42% to 87% of patients.[84] Asparaginase breaks down asparagine to aspartic acid and ammonia, and for this reason, hyperammonemia may be seen in patients.

### Bortezomib (Velcade)
Bortezomib is a reversible inhibitor of the chymotrypsinlike activity of the 26S proteasome and is used in the treatment of relapsed or refractory multiple myeloma. Bortezomib is metabolized by the liver. Its exposure is increased in patients with moderate

to severe hepatic impairment. In addition, there have been reports of portal vein thrombosis and hyperbilirubinemia.[85]

### Hydroxyurea (Hydrea; Droxia)

Hydroxyurea is an antimetabolite that selectively inhibits ribonucleoside diphosphate reductase, preventing the conversion of ribonucleotides to deoxyribonucleotides; halting the cell at the G1/S phase. Hepatotoxicity is unusual, although a case of hydroxyurea-induced self-limited hepatitis with an influenzalike reaction has been reported.[86]

### Procarbazine (Matulane; Natulan)

Originally synthesized as a potential monoamine oxidase inhibitor, procarbazine was later found to have antineoplastic effects on Hodgkin disease, non-Hodgkin lymphomas, melanoma, and small cell lung cancer. Hepatotoxicity is uncommon with procarbazine, but it has been associated with granulomatous hepatitis in 1 study.[87]

### REFERENCES

1. Lewis JH. Drug-induced liver disease. Med Clin North Am 2000;84(5):1275–311.
2. World Health Organization. Common terminology criteria for adverse events v3.0 (CTCAE). World Health Organization; 2006. Available at: http://ctep. cancer.gov/protocolDevelopment/electronic_applications/docs/ctcaev3.pdf. Accessed March 11, 2013.
3. National Cancer Institute. Cancer therapy evaluation program. National Cancer Institute; 2005. Available at: http://ctep.cancer.gov/protocolDevelopment/elec tronic_applications/docs/newadverse_2006.pdf. Accessed March 11, 2013.
4. King P, Perry MC. Hepatotoxicity of chemotherapy. Oncologist 2001;6: 162–76.
5. Hamilton M, Wolf JL, Rusk J, et al. Effects of smoking on the pharmacokinetics of erlotinib. Clin Cancer Res 2006;12:2166–71.
6. Farrell GC. Drug induced liver disease. J Hepatol 2000;32:77–88.
7. Zafrani ES, Leclercq B, Vernant JP, et al. Massive blastic infiltration of the liver: a cause of fulminant hepatic failure. Hepatology 1983;3:428–32.
8. Ceci G, Bella M, Melissari M, et al. Fatal hepatic vascular toxicity of DTIC. Is it really a rare event? Cancer 1988;61(10):1988–91.
9. Le Counter DG, Cogger VC, Markus AM, et al. Pseudocapillarization and asso-ciated energy limitation in the aged rat liver. Hepatology 2001;33:537–43.
10. Duvier A, Munro A, Verboy J. Treatment of psoriasis with azathioprine. Br Med J 1974;1:49–51.
11. Twelves C, Glynne-Jones R. Effect of hepatic dysfunction due to liver metasta-ses on the pharmacokinetics of capecitabine and its metabolites. Clin Cancer Res 1999;5(7):1696.
12. Wang WS, Tzeng CH, Chiou TJ, et al. High-dose cytarabine and mitoxantrone as salvage therapy for refractory non-Hodgkin's lymphoma. Jpn J Clin Oncol 1997; 27(3):154–7.
13. Pizzuto J, Avilés A. Cytosine arabinoside induced liver damage: histopathologic demonstration. Med Pediatr Oncol 1983;11(4):287.
14. Bateman JR, Pugh RP, Cassidy FR, et al. 5-Fluorouracil given once weekly: com-parison of intravenous and oral administration. Cancer 1971;28:907–13.
15. Aloia T, Sebagh M, Plasse M, et al. Liver histology and surgical outcomes after preoperative chemotherapy with fluorouracil plus oxaliplatin in colorectal cancer liver metastases. J Clin Oncol 2006;24(31):4983.

16. Hubert C, Sempoux C, Horsmans Y, et al. Nodular regenerative hyperplasia: a deleterious consequence of chemotherapy for colorectal liver metastases? Liver Int 2007;27(7):938.

17. Zalcberg JR, Kemeny NE. Systemic or regional chemotherapy for liver metastases from colorectal cancer: has the wheel stopped spinning? Cancer J 2004; 10:271.

18. Doria MI, Shepard KV, Levin B, et al. Liver pathology following hepatic arterial infusion chemotherapy. Hepatic toxicity with FUDR. Cancer 1986;58:855–61.

19. Chang AE, Schneider PD, Sugarbaker PH, et al. A prospective randomized trial of regional versus systemic continuous 5-FudR chemotherapy in the treatment of colorectal liver metastases. Ann Surg 1987;206:685–93.

20. Cerqueira PA, Fernandes MJ. Understanding ribonucleotide reductase inactivation by gemcitabine. Chemistry 2007;13(30):8507–15.

21. Aapro MS, Martin C, Hatty S. Gemcitabine–a safety review. Anticancer Drugs 1998;9(3):191.

22. Adamson PC, Zimm S, Ragab AH, et al. A phase II trial of continuous-infusion 6-mercaptopurine for childhood solid tumors. Cancer Chemother Pharmacol 1990;26:343–4.

23. Present DH, Meltzer SJ, Krumholtz MP, et al. 6-Mercaptopurine in the management of inflammatory bowel disease: short- and long-term toxicity. Ann Intern Med 1989;111:641–9.

24. Oancea I, Png CW, Das I, et al. A novel mouse model of veno-occlusive disease provides strategies to prevent thioguanine-induced hepatic toxicity. Gut 2013; 62(4):594–605.

25. Podurgiel BJ, McGill DB, Ludwig J, et al. Liver injury associated with methotrexate therapy for psoriasis. Mayo Clin Proc 1973;48:787–92.

26. Palmer HM. Hepatotoxicity of methotrexate in the treatment of psoriasis. Practitioner 1973;263:324–8.

27. Karstens A, Kramer I. Chemical and physical stability of diluted busulfan infusion solutions. EJHP Science 2007;13:40–7.

28. Morris LE, Guthrie TH. Busulfan induced hepatitis. Am J Gastroenterol 1988;83: 682–3.

29. Snyder LS, Heigh RL, Anderson ML. Cyclophosphamide induced hepatotoxicity in a patient with Wegener's granulomatosis. Mayo Clin Proc 1993;68: 1203–4.

30. Goldberg JW, Lidsky MD. Cyclophosphamide associated hepatotoxicity. South Med J 1985;78:222–3.

31. Bacon AM, Rosenberg SA. Cyclophosphamide hepatotoxicity in a patient with systemic lupus erythematosus. Ann Intern Med 1982;97:62–6.

32. Rai KR, Peterson BL, Appelbaum FR, et al. Fludarabine compared with chlorambucil as primary therapy for chronic lymphocytic leukemia. N Engl J Med 2000; 343(24):1750–7.

33. Amromin GD, Delman RM, Shanbran E. Liver damage after chemotherapy for leukemia and lymphoma. Gastroenterology 1962;42:401–10.

34. Bruhl P, Gunther U, Hoefer-Janker H, et al. Results obtained with fractionated ifosfamide massive-dose treatment in generalized malignant tumors. Int J Clin Pharmacol 1976;14:29–39.

35. Facon T, Mary JY, Hulin C, et al. Melphalan and prednisone plus thalidomide versus melphalan and prednisone alone or reduced-intensity autologous stem cell transplantation in elderly patients with multiple myeloma (IFM 99-06): a randomized trial. Lancet 2007;370(9594):1209–18.

36. Giralt S, Thall PF, Khouri I, et al. Melphalan and purine analog-containing preparative regimens: reduced-intensity conditioning for patients with hematologic malignancies undergoing allogeneic progenitor cell transplantation. Blood 2001; 97(3):631.

37. Waksman SA, Woodruff HB. Bacteriostatic and bacteriocidal substances produced by soil actinomycetes. Proc Soc Exp Biol 1940;45:609–14.

38. Ludwig R, Weirich A, Abel U, et al. Hepatotoxicity in patients treated according to the nephroblastoma trial and study SIOP-9/GPOH. Med Pediatr Oncol 1999; 33:462–9.

39. Blum RH, Carter SK, Agre K. A clinical review of bleomycin. A new antineoplastic agent. Cancer 1973;31:903–14.

40. Erichsen C, Jönsson PE. Veno-occlusive liver disease after dacarbazine therapy (DTIC) for melanoma. J Surg Oncol 1984;27(4):268.

41. McClay E, Lusch CJ, Mastrangelo MJ. Allergy-induced hepatic toxicity associated with dacarbazine. Cancer Treat Rep 1987;71(2):219.

42. Frederick CA, Williams LD, Ughetto G, et al. Structural comparison of anticancer drug-DNA complexes: adriamycin and daunomycin. Biochemistry 1990;29(10): 2538–49.

43. Avilés A, Herrera J, Ramos E, et al. Hepatic injury during doxorubicin therapy. Arch Pathol Lab Med 1984;108(11):912.

44. Brenner DE, Wiernik PE, Wesley M, et al. Acute doxorubicin toxicity. Relationship to pretreatment liver function, response, and pharmacokinetics in patients with acute non-lymphocytic leukemia. Cancer 1984;53:1042–8.

45. Dorr RT, Bowden GT, Alberts DS, et al. Interaction of mitomycin C with mammalian DNA detected by alkaline elution. Cancer Res 1985;45:3510–6.

46. Lazarus HM, Gottfried MR, Herzig RH, et al. Veno-occlusive disease of the liver after high-dose mitomycin C therapy and autologous bone marrow transplantation. Cancer 1982;49(9):1789.

47. De Vita VT, Carbone PP, Owens AH, et al. Clinical trials with 1,3-bis (2-chloroethyl)-nitrosourea, NSC-409962. Cancer Res 1965;25:1876–81.

48. Wolff SN. High-dose carmustine and high-dose etoposide: a treatment regimen resulting in enhanced hepatic toxicity. Cancer Treat Rep 1986;70:1464–5.

49. Postma TJ, van Groeningen CJ, Witjes RJ, et al. Neurotoxicity of combination chemotherapy with procarbazine, CCNU [lomustine] and vincristine (PCV) for recurrent glioma. J Neurooncol 1998;38(1):69–75.

50. Broder LE, Carter SK. Pancreatic islet cell carcinoma II: results of therapy with streptozotocin in 52 patients. Ann Intern Med 1973;79:108–18.

51. Hirth J, Watkins PB, Strawderman M, et al. The effect of an individual's cytochrome CYP3A4 activity on docetaxel clearance. Clin Cancer Res 2000;6(4):1255.

52. Witteveen P, Marchetti S, Mergui-Roelvink M, et al. Eribulin mesylate pharmacokinetics in patients with hepatic impairment [abstract # 2582]. J Clin Oncol 2010; 28:224s.

53. Desai ZR, Van den Berg HW, Bridges JM, et al. Can severe vincristine neurotoxicity be prevented? Cancer Chemother Pharmacol 1982;8(2):211.

54. Hohneker JA. A summary of vinorelbine (Navelbine) safety data from North American clinical trials. Semin Oncol 1994;21(5 Suppl 10):42.

55. Saltz LB, Douillard JY, Pirotta N, et al. Irinotecan plus fluorouracil/leucovorin for metastatic colorectal cancer, a new survival standard. Oncologist 2001;6:81–91.

56. Felix FG, Ritter J, Goodwin JW, et al. Effect of steatohepatitis associated with irinotecan or oxaliplatin pretreatment on respectability of hepatic colorectal metastases. J Am Coll Surg 2000;205:845–53.

57. Creemers GJ, Lund B, Verweijt J. Topoisomersase I inhibitors: topotecan and iri-notecan. Cancer Treat Rev 1994;20:73–96.
58. Tran A, Housset C, Boboc B, et al. Etoposide (VP 16-213) induced hepatitis. Report of three cases following standard-dose treatments. J Hepatol 1991; 12(1):36.
59. Hruban RH, Sternberg SS, Meyers P, et al. Fatal thrombocytopenia and liver fail-ure associated with carboplatin therapy. Cancer Invest 1991;9(3):263.
60. Christian MC. Two toxicities associated with carboplatin use: A. gross hematuria B. hepatic veno-occlusive disease. Bethesda (MD): Department of Health & Human Services bulletin, National Institutes of Health, National Cancer Institute; 1989.
61. Cavalli F, Tschopp L, Sonntag RW, et al. A case of liver toxicity following cis-dichlorodiammineplatinum(II) treatment. Cancer Treat Rep 1978;62(12):2125.
62. Pollera CF, Ameglio F, Nardi M, et al. Cisplatin-induced hepatic toxicity. J Clin Oncol 1987;5(2):318.
63. Fakih MG. 5-fluorouracil leucovorin and oxaliplatin (FOLFOX) in the treatment of metastatic colon cancer with severe liver dysfunction. Oncology 2004; 67(3–4):222.
64. Rubbia-Brandt L, Audard V, Sartoretti P, et al. Severe hepatic sinusoidal obstruc-tion associated with oxaliplatin-based chemotherapy in patients with metastatic colorectal cancer. Ann Oncol 2004;15:460–6.
65. Miller AA, Murry DJ, Owzar K, et al. Phase I and pharmacokinetic study of erlo-tinib for solid tumors in patients with hepatic or renal dysfunction. J Clin Oncol 2007;25(21):3055.
66. Liu W, Makrauer FL, Qamar AA, et al. Fulminant hepatic failure secondary to er-lotinib. Clin Gastroenterol Hepatol 2007;5(8):91.
67. Iressa (gefitinib) [package insert]. Macclesfield (United Kingdom): AstraZe-neca; 2004.
68. Gleevac (imatinib mesylate) [package insert]. East Hanover (NJ): Novartis Pharma; 2001.
69. Cross TJ, Bagot C, Portmann B, et al. Imatinib mesylate as a cause of acute liver failure. Am J Hematol 2006;81(3):189.
70. Xu CF, Reck BH, Xue Z, et al. Pazopanib-induced hyperbilirubinemia is associ-ated with Gilbert's syndrome UGT1A1 polymorphism. Br J Cancer 2010;102(9): 1371.
71. Teo YL, Ho HK, Chan A. Risk of tyrosine kinase inhibitors-induced hepatotox-icity in cancer patients: a meta-analysis. Cancer Treat Rev 2013;39(2): 199–206.
72. George DD, Peter R, Yoon-Koo K, et al. Efficacy and safety of regorafenib for advanced gastrointestinal stromal tumours after failure of imatinib and sunitinib (GRID): an international, multicentre, randomised, placebo-controlled, phase 3 trial. Lancet 2013;381(9863):295–302.
73. Awada A, Hendlisz T, Gil T, et al. A Phase I safety and pharmacokinetics of BAY 43-9006 administered for 21 days on/7 days off in patients with advanced, re-fractory solid tumors. Br J Cancer 1992;92:1855–61.
74. Fairfax B, Pratap S, Roberts I, et al. Fatal case of sorafenib-associated idiosyn-cratic hepatotoxicity in the adjuvant treatment of a patient with renal cell carci-noma. BMC Cancer 2012;11:590.
75. Amarapurkar DN. Prescribing medications in patients with decompensated liver cirrhosis. Int J Hepatol 2011;2011:519526. http://dx.doi.org/10.4061/2011/519526.

76. Avastin [package insert]. South San Francisco (CA): Genentech; 2004.
77. Susan D, Basak O, Honig A, et al. HER2-targeted therapy in breast cancer: a systematic review of neoadjuvant trials. Cancer Treat Rev 2013;39(6):622–31.
78. Quesada J, Hersh EM, Manning J, et al. Treatment of hairy cell leukemia with recombinant alpha interferon. Blood 1985;68:493–7.
79. Quesada JR, Talpaz M, Rios A, et al. Clinical toxicity of interferons in cancer patients. J Clin Oncol 1986;4:234–43.
80. Nakagawa K, Miller FN, Simds DE, et al. Mechanisms of interleukin-2 induced hepatic toxicity. Cancer Res 1996;56:507–10.
81. Fisher B, Keenan AM, Garra BS, et al. Interleukin-2 induces profound reversible cholestasis: a detailed analysis in treated cancer patients. J Clin Oncol 1989;7: 1852–62.
82. Niu C, Yan H, Yu T, et al. Studies on treatment of acute promyelocytic leukemia with arsenic trioxide: remission induction, follow-up, and molecular monitoring in 11 newly diagnosed and 47 relapsed acute promyelocytic leukemia patients. Blood 1999;94:3315–24.
83. Avramis VI, Panosyan EH. Pharmacokinetic/pharmacodynamic relationships of asparaginase formulations: the past, the present and recommendations for the future. Clin Pharmacokinet 2005;44(4):367–93.
84. Haskell CM, Canellos GP, Leventhal BG, et al. Lasparaginase: therapeutic and toxic effects in patients with neoplastic disease. N Engl J Med 1969;281: 1028–34.
85. Velcade (bortezomib) [package insert]. Cambridge (MA): Millennium Pharmaceuticals; 2003.
86. Heddle R, Calvert AF. Hydroxyurea induced hepatitis. Med J Aust 1980;1(3): 121.
87. McMaster KR 3rd, Hennigar GR. Drug-induced granulomatous hepatitis. Lab Invest 1981;44(1):61.

# Drug-Induced Liver Injury from Antiepileptic Drugs

Jennifer S. Au, MD[a], Paul J. Pockros, MD[b],*

## KEYWORDS

- Antiepileptic drugs • Drug-induced liver injury • Hepatotoxicity

## KEY POINTS

- The mechanism of action for DILI in antiepileptic drugs is varied and includes immune-mediated, direct cytotoxic, or idiosyncratic reactions.
- Valproic acid is a common cause of hepatotoxicity with demonstrated transient transaminase elevations in 10% to 15% of patients. However, fatal cases occur in only 1 per 10,000 patients.
- Chronic mild liver enzyme elevations are relatively common with longstanding phenytoin (PHT) therapy with an estimated incidence of 10% to 25%. However, severe hepatic injury from PHT is idiosyncratic and rare.
- Severe hepatotoxicity due to carbamazepine is idiosyncratic with risk factors for more severe liver injury including younger age, longer duration of therapy and absence of signs of hypersensitivity.
- Elevations in transaminases occur in less than 1% of patients on lamotrigine and severe hepatotoxicity is rare.
- In approximately 9% of patients on phenobarbital, hepatotoxicity is seen in the form of the reactive metabolic syndrome and accompanied by fever, rash, eosinophilia, and lymphadenopathy.
- A subsequent retrospective cohort study of the United Network for Organ Sharing database from 1987 through 2006 identified 661 patients diagnosed with drug-induced acute liver failure, accounting for 12% of all transplants for acute liver failure in that time period.

## BACKGROUND

Drug-induced liver injury (DILI) is a potential complication of innumerable medications. Most cases of DILI do not occur in a predictable, dose-dependent manner. This often leads to delayed recognition of a drug's hepatotoxic potential until after its release into

[a] Division of Gastroenterology/Hepatology, Scripps Clinic, and Scripps Translational Science Institute, 10666 North Torrey Pines Road, La Jolla, CA 92037, USA; [b] Division of Gastroenterology/Hepatology, Liver Disease Center, Scripps Clinic, and Scripps Translational Science Institute, 10666 North Torrey Pines Road, La Jolla, CA 92037, USA
* Corresponding author.
*E-mail address:* Pockros.Paul@scrippshealth.org

Clin Liver Dis 17 (2013) 687–697
http://dx.doi.org/10.1016/j.cld.2013.07.011
1089-3261/13/$ – see front matter © 2013 Elsevier Inc. All rights reserved.
**liver.theclinics.com**

the market and exposure in many thousands of patients. The mechanisms of action for DILI in antiepileptic drugs (AEDs) are varied and include immune-mediated, direct cytotoxic, or idiosyncratic reactions. The estimated occurrence of DILI is 1 in 10,000 to 100,000 patients. However, the rates are likely higher because many cases of DILI go unrecognized owing to lack of reporting or missed diagnosis.[1]

Epilepsy is one of the most common neurologic diseases, affecting approximately 20 million Americans and 3% of the population worldwide. The term epilepsy actually refers to a group of syndromes characterized by a predisposition to recurrent unprovoked seizures. The different types of epilepsy are classified by the clinical features of the seizures, the presence of neurologic abnormalities, and the electroencephalographic results. Onset is typically in infants and the elderly or because of brain injury.[2]

AEDs are a class of medications that were first introduced in 1857 with the use of potassium bromide to treat women with "hysterical epilepsy connected with the menstrual period." This was followed by the introduction of phenobarbital (PB) in 1912, phenytoin (PHT) in 1938, and, subsequently, primidone, ethosuximide, carbamazepine (CBZ), and valproic acid (VPA), the first generation of antiepileptics.[3] Since then, many more AEDs have been introduced, with 15 new AEDs released between 1990 and 2011.[4] AEDs do not cure epilepsy. They are used to control seizure activity and, therefore, are typically long-term (or lifetime) medications. Even with AED use, approximately 20% of patients continue to have seizure activity.[5] Many AEDs have been implicated in cases of DILI (**Table 1**). This article reviews the AEDs most commonly associated with DILI.

## VPA

VPA is a chiral, short-chain, branched fatty acid with a structure different from other AEDs and a mechanism of action that is not clearly understood. Its antiepileptic properties were first discovered in 1962 and it was approved for use as an AED by the US Food and Drug Administration (FDA) in 1978. Proposed mechanisms include the inhibition of voltage-gated sodium channels,[6] increased gamma aminobutyric acid (GABA) neurotransmission,[7] attenuation of N-methyl-d-aspartate (NMDA) receptor–mediated neural excitation,[8] and reduced aspartate neurotransmission resulting in reduced neuronal excitation (**Table 2**).[9]

VPA is widely used in the treatment of partial and generalized seizures, migraine, and cluster headaches, as well as bipolar disorder.[10] It is 80% to 90% protein bound and is primarily metabolized by the liver. The drug is primarily metabolized by glucuronidation and beta oxidation. However, it is also metabolized by cytochrome P450 through a process known as omega oxidation. Omega oxidation increases when the P450 system is induced by other medications and results in the production of 4-en-VPA. This metabolite has been implicated in most VPA-induced hepatotoxicity as altering fatty acid metabolism through the inhibition of beta oxidation. VPA therapy also results in carnitine, coenzyme A, and free radical scavenging enzyme depletion, which may further hepatic injury.[6,11]

Retrospective studies have demonstrated transient transaminase elevations in 10% to 15% of patients, and hyperbilirubinemia in up to 44% of patients on VPA.[12] Less commonly, elevations in alkaline phosphatase (ALP) and gamma-glutamyltransferase (GGT) have been reported. In patients whose hepatic function tests become elevated, therapy can be continued as long as the elevations are less than three times the upper limit of normal. In some patients, a normalization of liver function tests (LFTs) occurs, likely because of adaptation.

**Table 1**
**Uses and routes of metabolism of AEDs commonly implicated in DILI**

| Antiepileptic Drug | Primary Route of Metabolism | Clinical Use |
|---|---|---|
| Valproic acid | Hepatic | Complex partial seizures<br>Simple and complex absence seizures<br>Generalized tonic-clonic seizures<br>Migraine headache prophylaxis<br>Cluster headaches<br>Mania associated with bipolar disorder |
| Phenytoin | Hepatic | Generalized tonic-clonic seizures<br>Complex partial seizures<br>Prevention of seizures after neurosurgery and<br>   following traumatic brain injury<br>Status epilepticus |
| Carbamazepine | Hepatic | Generalized tonic-clonic seizures<br>Partial seizures<br>Mixed seizure patterns<br>Trigeminal neuralgia<br>Glossopharyngeal neuralgia<br>Mania associated with bipolar I disorder |
| Lamotrigine | Hepatic | Partial seizures<br>Primary generalized tonic-clonic seizures<br>Medically refractory epilepsy in children<br>Lennox-Gastaut syndrome<br>Maintenance treatment of bipolar I disorder |
| Phenobarbital | Hepatic | Generalized tonic-clonic seizures<br>Status epilepticus<br>Partial seizures<br>Sedative or hypnotic |
| Felbamate | Hepatic | Not a first-line medication<br>Medically refractory partial and generalized seizures<br>Lennox-Gastaut syndrome |

Hyperammonemia in the setting of VPA use and normal LFTs has also been described. In a literature review, the prevalence of hyperammonemia, defined as a level more than two times the upper limit of normal, ranged from 70% to 100% in prospective studies. However, no relationship between elevated ammonia and clinical symptoms was defined.[13] Multiple case reports and series exist in neurologic and psychiatric literature and define valproate-induced hyperammonemic encephalopathy. It is described as a clinically rare occurrence in which patients experience confusion, typically seen around the time of initiation of VPA therapy, but it may be seen months into treatment. The encephalopathy typically resolves with the cessation of VPA treatment.[14,15]

VPA hepatotoxicity is rare, idiosyncratic, and commonly occurs within the first 3 months of use. The most common presenting symptoms include lethargy, vomiting, and seizure exacerbation.[16–18] In a series of three retrospective studies by Dreifuss and colleagues, the experience of hepatic fatalities from VPA therapy in the United States was examined from 1978 to 1993.[17,19,20] The first study, 1978 to 1982, revealed that children younger than 2 years, those treated with multiple anticonvulsants, and patients with developmental delay, neurologic disorders, and congenital abnormalities were at highest risk for hepatic fatalities. The overall fatality rate was 1 per 10,000 patients; in children younger 2 years, it was approximately 1 per 500. Most cases occurred within the first 90 days of therapy and LFTs were not reflective of ongoing hepatic injury.[17]

In the subsequent reports, a decreased frequency of hepatic complications was noted, as well as a decreased use of VPA in patients previously deemed at high risk for complications of therapy.[19,20] Patients with inborn errors of metabolism were also recognized at high risk for developing hepatic complications. VPA toxicity in young children was frequently misdiagnosed as Alpers disease.[17,19,20]

Koenig and colleagues[18] performed a questionnaire-based survey of German physicians on their experience with VPA hepatotoxicity from 1994 to 2003. Thirty-one cases of nonfatal and nine cases of fatal hepatotoxicity were reported. Corroborating the results of Dreifuss and colleagues in the United States, patients on multiple AEDs, those with inborn errors of metabolism, and those with psychomotor retardation were at highest risk for hepatotoxicity. In those patients with nonfatal disease, early identification of VPA-related hepatotoxicity, cessation of the medication, and intravenous carnitine supplementation were thought to contribute to recovery.

Schmid and colleagues[21] performed a pharmacovigilance study examining cases of VPA hepatotoxicity reported to the German Federal Institute for Drugs and Medical Devices between 1993 and 2009. Hepatotoxicity was higher in patients on multiple AEDS, as well as in those on concomitant benzodiazepine or antipsychotic therapy. However, the use of multiple medications did not increase the rate of fatalities. Pathologic injury was examined in 23 cases of fatal VPA hepatotoxicity in the United States by Zimmerman and Ishak.[22] Microvesicular steatosis was found in 80% of cases and most were accompanied by centrizonal necrosis or cirrhosis. The pathologic features are frequently indistinguishable from those of acute fatty liver of pregnancy.[23]

The treatment of VPA hepatotoxicity is typically withdrawal of VPA. Because carnitine is an amino acid that is essential in the metabolism of fatty acids, it has been hypothesized that VPA hepatotoxicity and hyperammonemia are due in part to carnitine deficiency. This theory has prompted the use of carnitine as a treatment of VPA hepatotoxicity. In review articles, carnitine has been reported to increase the rate of elimination of ammonia in some patients with encephalopathy.[24]

**Table 2**
**Patterns of liver injury induced by AEDs**

| Antiepileptic Drug | Pathologic Findings |
| --- | --- |
| Valproic acid | Microvesicular steatosis<br>Centrizonal necrosis<br>Cirrhosis |
| Phenytoin | Reactive metabolite syndrome |
| Carbamazepine | Granulomatous hepatitis<br>Vanishing bile duct syndrome<br>Immunoallergic hepatitis<br>Hepatic necrosis |
| Lamotrigine | Acute hepatic necrosis<br>Focal hepatitis with mild portal inflammation |
| Phenobarbitol | Granulomatous hepatitis<br>Hepatic necrosis |
| Felbamate | Acute hepatic necrosis |

## PHT

PHT was first synthesized in 1908; however, was not available for use as an AED until 1938. It was the first AED to be assessed by preclinical studies rather than clinical observation and was the first nonsedating AED.[25] PHT is now one of the most commonly used medications to treat generalized tonic-clonic seizures and status epilepticus.[26] The liver metabolizes 95% of the medication and less than 5% is excreted by the kidneys.[27] PHT is metabolized by cytochrome P450 to arene oxides, which are processed by the enzyme epoxide hydrolase. Reductions in epoxide hydrolase levels result in an elevated level of arene oxides. Arene oxides are reactive electrophilic compounds that can result in protein binding leading to cell death, mutations, and tumor formation. They can also act as haptens leading to secondary immune phenomena and hepatotoxicity.[28]

Chronic mild liver enzyme elevations are relatively common with longstanding PHT therapy with an estimated incidence of 10% to 25%. However, severe hepatic injury from PHT is idiosyncratic and rare. Most patients who experience elevations in LFTs with PHT therapy later have normalization of their LFTs because of adaptation.[29] GGT elevations are seen in 50% to 90% of patients on PHT. ALP elevations can also be seen, but are less common. The most common pattern of liver injury is cholestatic or mixed, although hepatocellular injury can occur. The incidence of clinically significant hepatotoxicity has been estimated at 1 in 10,000 to 150,000.[30]

Liver biopsies of patients with transaminase elevations have revealed hepatocyte swelling without necrosis, inflammation, fibrosis, or disturbance in hepatic architecture.[29] More than 70% of hepatotoxic reactions from PHT occur as part of reactive metabolite syndrome (RMS).[31]

RMS, also known as anticonvulsant hypersensitivity syndrome or pseudomononucleosis syndrome, is characterized by fever, rash, eosinophilia, and internal organ involvement seen with the use of a variety of anticonvulsants, including PB, CBZ, and lamotrigine. The frequency is estimated at 10 to 100 per 100,000 patients exposed. Symptoms typically occur 1 to 8 weeks after initiation of the AED. Hepatic abnormalities are seen in approximately 50% of those who develop RMS, typically with abnormal LFTs, but can also manifest with severe hepatitis.[32] Risk factors for developing RMS include earlier reactions to PHT, CBZ, or PB; first-degree relatives who have experienced RMS; and African descent.[33]

Toxicity because of drug overdose infrequently results in hepatic and renal toxicity. Given the hepatic metabolism and renal excretion of the medications, impairment of liver or kidney function can elevate PHT levels. Total serum levels greater than 80 μm are associated with clinically relevant toxicity. Typically, toxicity from overdose primarily affects the central nervous system and results in neurotoxicity.[34]

The risk of PHT hepatotoxicity is equal in males and females and typically seen within 6 weeks of initiation of therapy. The most common symptoms, other than those associated with RMS, include nausea and fatigue. Most hepatotoxicity is acute and reversible with prompt discontinuation of PHT. However, cases of irreversible, fatal hepatotoxicity, as well as chronic liver injury, have been described. Patients who experience RMS typically have recurrent hepatotoxicity when rechallenged with PHT.

Fatal reactions have been reported among patients who have symptomatic hepatotoxicity, with mortality rates between 10% and 40%. Patients deemed at highest risk for fatal hepatotoxicity are those with hepatic necrosis on liver biopsy and/or a hepatocellular pattern of injury.[29]

When hepatotoxicity does not improve with medication withdrawal, treatment with activated charcoal and the molecular adsorbents recirculating system (MARS) have been used with success. MARS is used as a therapy because PHT is 90% albumin bound. MARS is a blood purification system that uses an albumin filter. The albumin concentration within the filter is significantly higher than plasma concentrations. This results in the preferential binding of PHT to albumin within the filter when a patient is placed on MARS and the PHT is subsequently removed within a charcoal column.[35] Hemodialysis cannot remove PHT. However, in patients with renal failure, uremic toxins are thought to displace PHT from albumin, resulting in increased free drug levels. Hemodialysis with a high-flux cellulose membrane can serve to decrease levels of uremic toxins and lower free PHT levels.[36]

## CBZ

CBZ was first synthesized in the late 1950s. It is chemically related to tricyclic antidepressants; however, its mechanism of action is thought to be similar to PHT. CBZ was first approved by the FDA in 1964 for the treatment of trigeminal neuralgia and in 1974 as an AED. It is currently approved for use in the treatment of partial and secondarily generalized tonic-clonic seizures, as well as bipolar disorder.[4] Its off-label uses include treatment of borderline personality disorder and aggression in those with acquired brain injury.

CBZ is primarily metabolized by cytochrome P450 in the liver through epoxidation, hydroxylation, and, to a lesser extent, conjugation.[37] Reactive metabolites that are formed can lead to hepatotoxicity through direct injury or immune-related mechanisms.[38] The most important metabolite is 10, 11-CBZ epoxide, which is pharmacologically active and implicated in the development of hepatotoxicity.[39] Other chemically reactive metabolites, such as 3-OH CBZ, are thought to be important in CBZ hepatotoxicity through the production of reactive oxygen species resulting in mitochondrial dysfunction, suppression of glutathione expression, and alteration of oxidative stress markers.[40]

Hypersensitivity to CBZ is noted in up to 10% of patients. This commonly results in a rash and can progress to fevers, eosinophilia, and, rarely, Stevens-Johnson syndrome and toxic epidermal necrolysis.[41] Studies show hypersensitivity reactions are associated with major histocompatibility complex haplotype tumor necrosis factor (TNF)2-DR3-DQ2 and HLA-B*1502.[42,43] Hepatic adverse reactions make up approximately 10% of all CBZ adverse events.[44]

Asymptomatic elevations in LFTs are seen in up to 61% of patients and are commonly transient.[45] The most common laboratory abnormality is an elevated GGT. LFT abnormalities typically develop within 2 months of initiation of CBZ therapy, with a median of 5 weeks.[31]

Severe hepatotoxicity is idiosyncratic and can manifest with a variety of hepatic pathologic conditions. Risk factors for more severe liver injury or death include younger age, longer duration of therapy, and absence of signs of hypersensitivity. Prognosis has improved with the prompt recognition of CBZ-induced hepatotoxicity and discontinuation of drug use. Overall mortality rates have been recently estimated at 17%.[31]

Ductopenia, hepatic necrosis, granulomatous hepatitis, and immunoallergic hepatitis are known pathologic manifestations of CBZ hepatotoxicity. Vanishing bile duct syndrome is a rare complication of CBZ therapy. It is often seen with elevated GGT or ALP levels and characterized by loss of small bile ducts and development of jaundice and hepatic impairment. Owing to its rare occurrence, little is known about risk factors associated with vanishing bile duct syndrome. Cases described have included patients on long-standing CBZ therapy, as well as those recently initiated to CBZ therapy.[46,47] In some case reports, CBZ therapy clinically manifests with jaundice and cholangitis and liver biopsies reveal noncaseating granulomatous hepatitis, which typically resolves with drug discontinuation.[48,49]

A common manifestation of hepatic injury is RMS, also seen with PHT use. Hepatic adverse events have been reported to constitute 10% of all hypersensitivity reactions.[43] Approximately 30% of patients with DILI from CBZ were found to have features of hypersensitivity, namely peripheral or hepatic eosinophilia. The pattern of liver injury can be cholestatic or hepatocellular. In case reports, hepatocellular injury has shown worse outcomes, often demonstrating hepatic necrosis on biopsy and leading to death or liver transplantation.[31]

## LAMOTRIGINE

Lamotrigine belongs to the phenyltriazine class of medications. It was approved for use as an AED in 1994. It is used in the treatment of partial and generalized seizures, either as a single agent or in conjunction with other AEDs, and for resistant epilepsy.[50] In children, it is effective in partial, absence, and atonic seizures.[51]

Lamotrigine blocks voltage-sensitive sodium channels, thereby inhibiting the release of excitatory neurotransmitters, including glutamate and aspartate, which have been associated with epilepsy. It is primarily metabolized by the liver and, in a similar fashion to CBZ and PHT, is metabolized to an arene oxide, which is known to cause hepatotoxicity via RMS.[52] The most common side effects of the medication are cutaneous. They occur in approximately 10% of patients and they are often accompanied by fever and eosinophilia, indicating an immune-mediated toxicity.

Elevations in transaminases occur in less than 1% of patients on lamotrigine. Hepatotoxicity is rare, idiosyncratic, and typically exhibits a hepatocellular pattern of injury. The onset of hepatic injury is typically within 1 month of lamotrigine initiation. Case reports of acute hepatic failure have been described. Patients who developed hepatic failure were typically on multiple medications, including other AEDs, as well as non-AEDs.

Cases of hepatotoxicity have also been noted in patients who had a rapid titration of the medication, those who were in status epilepticus, and in children. Acute hepatic failure has been associated with disseminated intravascular coagulation, rhabdomyolysis, hyperthermia, and rash. Acute hepatic necrosis or focal hepatitis and mild portal inflammation were seen on liver biopsy. In most cases, hepatotoxicity resolved with discontinuation of lamotrigine; however, cases of fatal hepatic necrosis have been described.[53–60]

## PB

PB is a barbiturate derivative first discovered to have antiepileptic properties in 1912. Its antiepileptic properties were discovered when patients with epilepsy who were sedated with PB had fewer seizures than those given other sedating agents. Since then, it has been used as an AED and is effective in the treatment of partial and secondarily generalized tonic-clonic seizures, status epilepticus, and to prevent febrile seizures.[61] PB enhances the effects of GABA, therefore raising the seizure threshold.

PB is primarily metabolized by the liver and is a potent inducer of hepatic microsomal enzymes that can increase the metabolism of other medications. Prospective studies have suggested that long-term PB therapy results in elevated transaminase levels in less than 1% of patients. More commonly, elevations in ALP or GGT are seen and are asymptomatic and clinically insignificant. Liver injury is most commonly a mixed pattern, but may also be hepatocellular or cholestatic. Hepatotoxicity is a rare occurrence and typically severe and abrupt in onset. In approximately 9% of patients on PB, hepatotoxicity is seen in the form of RMS and accompanied by fever, rash, eosinophilia, and lymphadenopathy.[29] Liver biopsy often shows eosinophils and granulomatous inflammation; however, necrosis has also been described.[62] Hepatotoxicity is rapidly reversible with discontinuation of PB.

## FELBAMATE

Felbamate is a dicarbamate derivative that was approved for use as an AED by the FDA in 1993. It was approved for use in combination with other AEDs to treat refractory partial and generalized seizures. Since its approval, use has been severely limited due to the association of felbamate with acute liver failure (ALF) and aplastic anemia. It is now used to treat severe epilepsy refractory to other AEDs.[63]

Common medication side effects include nausea, dizziness, somnolence, and fatigue.[64] Hepatotoxicity is rare, idiosyncratic, and typically exhibits a hepatocellular pattern. There is an estimated occurrence of 1 in 18,500 to 20,000 patients exposed.[65] Despite the low frequency of hepatotoxicity, events are often severe and typically occur within 6 months of initiation of felbamate therapy. The mechanism by which toxicity is induced is unclear. Atropaldehyde, a reactive metabolite, has been implicated in causing both DILI and aplastic anemia.[66]

## OUTCOMES OF ALF FROM AED DILI

DILI is the leading cause of ALF in the adult and pediatric populations in the United States. Between 1998 and 2007, 31% of patients with nonacetaminophen-related, drug-induced ALF (DIALF) died and 41% underwent liver transplantation. Liver transplantation is the treatment of choice for patients with ALF who do not spontaneously recover.[67]

An analysis of the United Network for Organ Sharing (UNOS) liver transplant database, from 1990 until 2002, identified that 15% of all transplants for ALF were the result of DILI. In 96% of cases, a single drug was implicated. PHT and valproate were two of the top four most common prescription medications implicated in cases of ALF, each making up 7.3% of all cases. In comparison to patients undergoing transplantation for acetaminophen hepatotoxicity, those undergoing transplantation for AED-related ALF had significantly higher serum bilirubin and those with valproate toxicity had significantly lower creatinine. One-year graft and patient survival for all patients receiving a transplant for DILI were 77% and 71%, respectively.[68]

A subsequent retrospective cohort study of the UNOS database from 1987 through 2006 identified 661 patients diagnosed with DIALF, accounting for 12% of all transplants for ALF in that time period. Antiepileptic medications were the third leading class of drugs implicated in DIALF in adults, accounting for 7% of all cases. In the pediatric populations, AEDs accounted for 23% of cases and was the second leading cause of DIALF; VPA toxicity accounted for 73% of all cases.

Overall, the median age for patients undergoing transplantation because of DIALF was 36 years old. However, the median age of patients transplanted because of AED-induced DIALF was 22 years old. Those receiving a transplant for AED-induced DIALF had the highest mortality rate after liver transplantation. One-year survival after transplantation is only 27% for those younger than 18 years but 75% for patients older than 18 years, indicating a greater than 4-fold increased risk of death in children. The one-year survival rate for all patients receiving a transplant for DIALF was 76%. Patients undergoing a transplant for AED-induced DIALF also had higher rates of retransplantation. Retransplantation occurred in 24% of AED patients and only 4% to 9% of all other DIALF patients.[69]

## REFERENCES

1. Larry D. Epidemiology and individual susceptibility to adverse drug reaction affecting the liver. Semin Liver Dis 2002;22:145–55.
2. Chang BS, Lowenstein DH. Epilepsy. N Engl J Med 2003;349:1257–66.
3. Brodie MJ. Antiepileptic drug therapy the story so far. Seizure 2010;19(10): 650–5.
4. Bialer M. Chemical properties of antiepileptic drugs. Adv Drug Deliv Rev 2012; 64:887–95.
5. Engel J Jr. Surgery for seizures. N Engl J Med 1996;334:647–53.
6. Stahl SM. Anticonvulsants as mood stabilizers and adjuncts to antipsychotics: valproate, lamotrigine, carbamazepine, and oxcarbazepine and actions at voltage-gated sodium channels. J Clin Psychiatry 2004;65:738–9.
7. Loscher W. In vivo administration of valproate reduced the nerve terminal (synaptosomal) activity of GABA aminotransferase in discrete brain areas of rats. Neurosci Lett 1993;160:177–80.
8. Silva MF, Aires CC, Luis PB, et al. Valproic acid metabolism and its effects on mitochondrial fatty acid oxidation: a review. J Inherit Metab Dis 2008;31:205–16.
9. Morland C, Nordengen K, Gundersen V. Valproate causes reduction of the excitatory amino acid aspartate in nerve terminals. Neurosci Lett 2012;527:100–4.
10. Nalivaeva NN, Belyaev ND, Turner AJ. Sodium valproate: an old drug with new roles. Trends Pharmacol Sci 2009;30:509–14.
11. Baillie TA, Levy R. Metabolic fate of valproid acid in humans. In: Levy RH, Penry JK, editors. Idiosyncratic reactions to valproate. New York: Raven; 1991. p. 19–24.
12. Cotariu D, Zaidman JL. Valproic acid and the liver. Clin Chem 1988;34:890–7.
13. Chicharro AV, Marinis AJ, Kanner AM. The measurement of ammonia blood levels in patients taking valproic acid: looking for problems where they do not exist. Epilepsy Behav 2007;11:361–6.
14. Dealberto MJ. Valproate-induced hyperammonaemic encephalopathy: review of 14 cases in the psychiatric setting. Int Clin Psychopharmacol 2007;22:330–7.
15. Wadzinski J, Franks R, Roane D, et al. Valproate-associated hyperammonemic encephalopathy. J Am Board Fam Med 2007;20:499–502.
16. Willmore LJ. Clinical manifestations of valproate hepatotoxicity. In: Levy RH, Penry JK, editors. Idiosyncratic reactions to valproate. New York: Raven; 1991. p. 3–6.
17. Dreifuss FE, Santilli N, Langer DH, et al. Valproic acid hepatic fatalities: a retrospective review. Neurology 1987;37:379–85.
18. Koenig SA, Buesing D, Longin E, et al. Valproic acid-induced hepatopathy: nine new fatalities in Germany from 1994 to 2003. Epilepsia 2006;47:2027–31.
19. Dreifuss FE, Langer DH, Moline KA, et al. Valproic acid hepatic fatalities. II. US experience since 1984. Neurology 1989;39:201–7.
20. Bryant AE, Dreifuss FE. Valproic acid hepatic fatalities III US experience since 1986. Neurology 1996;46:465–9.
21. Schmid MM, Freudenmann RW, Keller F, et al. Non-fatal and fatal liver failure associated with valproic acid. Pharmacopsychiatry 2012;46:36–8.
22. Zimmerman HJ, Ishak KG. Valproate-induced hepatic Injury: analyses of 23 fatal cases. Hepatology 1982;2:591–7.

23. Pockros PJ, Esrason KT. Microvesicular fat diseases of the liver. In: Haubrich WS, Schaffner F, editors. Bockus gastroenterology. 5th edition. Philadelphia: W.B. Saunders Co; 1995. p. 2254–75.
24. Lheureux PE, Hantson P. Carnitine in the treatment of valproic acid-induced toxicity. Clin Toxicol 2009;47:101–11.
25. Porter RJ. Antiepileptic drugs:efficacy and inadequacy. In: Meldrum BS, Porter RJ, editors. New anticonvulsant drugs. 4th edition. London: John Libby; 1986. p. 3–15.
26. Walker M. Status epilepticus: an evidence based guide. BMJ 2005;331:673–7.
27. Bajpai M, Roskos LK, Shen DD, et al. Roles of cytochrome P4502C9 and cytochrome P4502C19 in the stereoselective metabolism of phenytoin to its major metabolite. Drug Metab Dispos 1996;24(12):1401–3.
28. Spielberg P, Gordon GB, Blake DA, et al. Predisposition to phenytoin hepatotoxicity assessed in vitro. N Engl J Med 1981;305:722–7.
29. Aiges HW, Daum F, Olson M, et al. The effects of phenobarbital and diphenylhydantoin on liver function and morphology. J Pediatr 1980;97:22–6.
30. Farrell OC. Drug-induced liver disease. London: Churchill Livingston; 1994.
31. Bjornsson E, Kalaitzakis E, Olsson R. The impact of eosinophilia and hepatic necrosis on prognosis in patients with drug-induced liver injury. Aliment Pharmacol Ther 2007;25:1411–21.
32. Knowles SR, Uetrecht J, Shear NH. Idiosyncratic drug reactions: the reactive metabolite syndromes. Lancet 2000;356:1587–91.
33. Vittorio CC, Muglia JJ. Anticonvulsant hypersensitivity syndrome. Arch Intern Med 1995;27:2285–90.
34. Chua HC, Venketasubramanian N, Tjia H, et al. Elimination of phenytoin in toxic overdose. Clin Neurol Neurosurg 2000;102:6–8.
35. Sen S, Ratnaraj N, Davies NA, et al. Treatment of phenytoin toxicity by molecular adsorbents recirculating system (MARS). Epilepsia 2003;44:265–7.
36. Frenchie D, Bastani B. Significant removal of phenytoin during high flux dialysis with cellulose triacetate dialyzer. Nephrol Dial Transplant 1998;13:817–8.
37. Bernus I, Dickinson RG, Hooper WD, et al. Dose-dependent metabolism of carbamazepine in humans. Epilepsy Res 1996;24:163–72.
38. Park BK, Kitteringham NR, Powell H, et al. Advances in molecular toxicology-towards understanding idiosyncratic drug toxicity. Toxicology 2000;153:39–60.
39. Leeder JS, Pirmohamed M. Anticonvulsant agents. In: Kaplowitz N, DeLeve LD, editors. Drug induced liver disease. New York: Marcel Decker, Inc; 2003. p. 425–46.
40. Lu W, Uetrecht JP. Peroxidase-mediated bioactivation of hydroxylated metabolites of carbamazepine and phenytoin. Drug Metab Dispos 2008;36:1624–36.
41. Rzany B, Correia O, Kelly JP, et al. Risk of Stevens-Johnson syndrome and toxic epidermal necrolysis during first weeks of antiepileptic therapy: a case-control study. Study group of the international case control study on severe cutaneous adverse reaction. Lancet 1999;353:2190–4.
42. Pirmohamed M, Lin K, Chadwick D, et al. TNF alpha promoter region gene polymorphisms in CBZ- hypersensitive patients. Neurology 2001;56:890–6.
43. Chung WH, Hung SI, Hong HS, et al. Medical genetics: a marker for Stevens-Johnson syndrome. Nature 2004;428:486.
44. Ashmark H, Wilholm B. Epidemiology of adverse reactions to carbamazepine as seen in a spontaneous reporting system. Acta Neurol Scand 1990;81:131–40.
45. Benedetti MS, Ruty B, Baltes E. Induction of endogenous pathways by antiepileptics and clinical implications. Fundam Clin Pharmacol 2005;19:511–29.

46. Forbes GM, Jeffrey GP, Shilkin KB, et al. Carbamazepine hepatotoxicity: another cause of the vanishing bile duct syndrome. Gastroenterology 1992;102:1385–8.

47. Ramos AM, Gayotto LC, Clemente CM, et al. Reversible vanishing bile duct syndrome induced by carbamazepine. Eur J Gastroenterol Hepatol 2002;14: 1019–22.

48. Mitchell MC, Boinott JK, Arregui A, et al. Granulomatous hepatitis associated with carbamazepine therapy. Am J Med 1981;71:733–5.

49. Levy M, Goodman MW, Van Dyne BJ, et al. Granulomatous hepatitis secondary to carbamazepine. Ann Intern Med 1981;95:64–5.

50. Brodie MJ. Lamotrigine. Lancet 1992;339:1397–400.

51. Besag FM, Wallace SJ, Dulac O, et al. Lamotrigine for the treatment of epilepsy in childhood. J Pediatr 1995;127:991–7.

52. Maggs JL, Naisbitt DJ, Tettey JN, et al. Metabolism of lamotrigine to a reactive arene oxide intermediate. Chem Res Toxicol 2000;13:1075–81.

53. Ouellet G, Tremblay L, Marleau D. Fulminant hepatitis induced by lamotrigine. South Med J 2009;102:82–4.

54. Fix OK, Peters MG, Davern TJ. Eosinophilic hepatitis caused by lamotrigine. Clin Gastroenterol Hepatol 2006;4:xxvi.

55. Fayad M, Choueiri R, Mikati M. Potential hepatotoxicity of lamotrigine. Pediatr Neurol 2000;22:49–52.

56. Sauve G, Bresson-Hadni S, Prost P, et al. Acute hepatitis after lamotrigine administration. Dig Dis Sci 2000;45:1874–7.

57. Overstreet K, Costaanza C, Behling C, et al. Fatal progressive hepatic necrosis associated with lamotrigine treatment: a case report and literature review. Dig Dis Sci 2002;47:1921–5.

58. Amante MF, Filippini AV, Cejas N, et al. Dress syndrome and fulminant hepatic failure induced by lamotrigine. Ann Hepatol 2009;8:75–7.

59. Su-Yin AN, Tai WW, Olson KR. Lamotrigine-associated reversible severe hepatitis: a case report. J Med Toxicol 2008;4:258–60.

60. Moeller KE, Wei L, Jewell AD, et al. Acute hepatotoxicity associated with lamotrigine. Am J Psychiatry 2008;165:539–40.

61. Kwan P, Brodie M. Phenobarbital for the treatment of epilepsy in the 21st century: a critical review. Epilepsia 2004;45:1141–9.

62. Shapiro PA, Antonioli DA, Peppercorn MA. Barbiturate-induced submassive hepatic necrosis. Am J Gastroenterol 1980;74:270–3.

63. Pellock JM, Brodie MJ. Felbamate: 1997 update. Epilepsia 1997;38:1261–4.

64. Li LM, Nashef L, Moriarty J, et al. Felbamate as add-on therapy. Eur Neurol 1996;36:146–8.

65. Pirmohamed M, Leeder SJ. Anticonvulsant agents. In: Kaplowitz N, DeLeve LD, editors. Drug-induced liver disease. 2nd edition. New York: Informa Healthcare USA; 2007. p. 485–506.

66. Dieckhaus CM, Thompson CD, Roller SG, et al. Mechanisms of idiosyncratic drug reactions: the case of felbamate. Chem Biol Interact 2002;142:99–117.

67. Lee WM, Squires RH Jr, Nyberg SL, et al. Acute liver failure: summary of a workshop. Hepatology 2008;47:1401–15.

68. Russo MW, Galanko JA, Shrestha R, et al. Liver transplantation for acute liver failure from drug induced liver injury in the United States. Liver Transpl 2004; 10:1018–23.

69. Mindikoglu AL, Magder LS, Regev A. Outcome of liver transplantation for drug-induced acute liver failure in the United States: analysis of the United Network for Organ Sharing Database. Liver Transpl 2009;15:719–29.

# Lipid-Lowering Agents and Hepatotoxicity

Michael Demyen, MD[a], Kawtar Alkhalloufi, MD[b],
Nikolaos T. Pyrsopoulos, MD, PhD, MBA[a,*]

KEYWORDS

- Lipid-lowering agents • Hepatotoxicity • Statins • Drug-induced liver injury

KEY POINTS

- Lipid-lowering therapy is increasingly being used in patients for a variety of diseases, the most important being the secondary prevention of cardiovascular disease.
- Many lipid-lowering drugs carry side effects that include elevations in hepatic function tests and liver toxicity.
- In many cases, these drugs are not prescribed or they are underprescribed because of fears of injury to the liver.
- This article attempts to review key trials with respect to the hepatotoxicity of these drugs.
- Recommendations are also provided with respect to the selection of low-risk patients and strategies to lower the risk of hepatotoxicity when prescribing these medications.

## INTRODUCTION

One of the main causes of death in industrialized countries is ischemic heart disease, accounting for approximately 1 out of every 6 deaths in the United States according to 2007 data.[1] Aggressive lipid management strategies have been successful in reducing risk of events in patients with coronary heart disease. Lowering low-density lipoprotein cholesterol (LDL-C) has shown to decrease cardiovascular morbidity and mortality in patients with coronary artery disease and at risk groups for ischemic heart disease. In addition, lowering of non HDL cholesterol is advocated in some circles for primary prevention of heart disease as well.[2]

Concern among primary care physicians and specialists for liver injury due to lipid lowering agents (**Table 1**) may prevent many patients from benefiting from these medications.[3] This article attempts to present the data regarding the risk of hepatotoxicity of these agents and provide strategies and patient selection criteria that will reduce the risk of these side effects.

Conflict of Interest: The authors have nothing to disclose.
[a] Rutgers New Jersey Medical School, Newark, New Jersey 07103, USA; [b] Howard University College of Medicine, Washington, DC 20059, USA
* Corresponding author.
E-mail address: npyrsopoulos@yahoo.com

Clin Liver Dis 17 (2013) 699–714
http://dx.doi.org/10.1016/j.cld.2013.07.016
1089-3261/13/$ – see front matter © 2013 Elsevier Inc. All rights reserved.

**Table 1**
**Lipid-lowering drug therapies, usual starting doses and dose ranges**

| Agent | Recommended Starting Daily Dose | Dose Range |
|---|---|---|
| Statins | | |
|   Lovastatin | 20 mg | 10–80 mg |
|   Pravastatin | 40 mg | 10–80 mg |
|   Simvastatin | 20–40 mg | 5–80 mg |
|   Fluvastatin | 40 mg | 20–80 mg |
|   Atorvastatin | 10–20 mg | 10–80 mg |
|   Rosuvastatin | 10 mg | 5–40 mg |
|   Pitavastatin | 2 mg | 2–4 mg |
| Fibrates | | |
|   Fenofibrate | 48–145 mg | 48–145 mg |
|   Gemfibrozil | 1200 mg | 1200 mg |
|   Fenofibric acid | 45–135 mg | 45–135 mg |
| Niacin | | |
|   Immediate release | 250 mg | 250–3000 mg |
|   Extended release | 500 mg | 50 mg 0–2000 mg |
| Bile acid sequestrants | | |
|   Cholestyramine | 8–16 g | 4–24 g |
|   Colestipol | 2 g | 2–16 g |
|   Colesevelam | 3.8 g | 3.8–4.5 g |
| Cholesterol absorption inhibitors | | |
|   Ezetimibe | 10 mg | 10 mg |
| Combination therapies (single pill) | | |
|   Ezetimibe/simvastatin | 10/20 mg | 10/10–10/80 mg |
|   Extended release | | |
|   Niacin/simvastatin | 500/20 mg | 500/20–1000/20 mg |

*Data from* Jellinger PS, Smith DA, Mehta AE, et al. American Association of Clinical Endocrinologists' guidelines for management of dyslipidemia and prevention of atherosclerosis. Endocr Pract 2012;18(Suppl 1):18.

## STATINS

Statins are competitive inhibitors of the 3-hydroxy-3-methylglutarylcoenzyme A (HMG-CoA) reductase enzyme and are efficient agents in reducing plasma cholesterol and LDL. The effects of the HMG-CoA reductase inhibitors are related to their capacity to reduce endogenous cholesterol synthesis by inhibiting the enzyme that converts HMG-CoA into mevalonic acid, a cholesterol precursor. Statins also increase plasma LDL uptake of hepatocytes by upregulation of these receptors because of the reduction in plasma concentrations (**Table 2**).[4]

The initial safety trials and postmarketing surveillance studies of statins consistently show that although a significant portion of patients may have elevated aminotransferases, these are usually mild. One of the most convincing articles to demonstrate this was the Greek Atorvastatin and Coronary Heart Disease Evaluation (GREACE) study, by Law and colleagues,[5] which attempted to assess the severity of these abnormalities in hepatic function tests in patients who are prescribed statin medication. The

**Table 2**
**Primary lipid-lowering drug classes and their metabolic effect**

| Drug Class | Metabolic Effect |
|---|---|
| HMG-CoA reductase inhibitors (statins: lovastatin, pravastatin, fluvastatin, simvastatin, atorvastatin, rosuvastatin, pitavastatin) | Primarily ↓ LDL-C 21%–55% by competitively inhibiting rate-limiting step of cholesterol synthesis in the liver<br>Effect on HDL-C is less pronounced (↑ 2%–10%) ↓ TG 6%–30% |
| Fibric acid derivatives (gemfibrozil, fenofibrate, fenofibric acid) | Primarily ↓ TG 20%–35%, ↑ HDL-C 6%–18% by stimulating lipoprotein lipase activity<br>Fenofibrate may ↓ TC and LDL-C 20%–25%<br>Lower VLDL-C and LDL-C; reciprocal increase in LDL-C transforms the profile into a less atherogenic form by shifting fewer LDL particles to larger size<br>Fenofibrate ↓ fibrinogen level |
| Niacin (nicotinic acid) | ↓ LDL-C 10%–25%, ↓ TG 20%–30%, ↑HDL-C 10%–35% by decreasing hepatic synthesis of LDL-C and VLDL-C<br>↓ Lipoprotein (a)<br>Transforms LDL-C to less atherogenic form by increasing particle size and thus decreasing particle number |
| Bile acid sequestrants (cholestyramine, colestipol, colesevelam hydrochloride) | Primarily ↓ LDL-C 15%–25% by binding bile acids at the intestinal level<br>Colesevelam ↓ glucose and hemoglobin A1c (∼0.5%) |
| Cholesterol absorption inhibitors (ezetimibe) | Primarily ↓ LDL-C 10%–18% by inhibiting intestinal absorption of cholesterol and decreasing delivery to the liver, ↓ Apo B 11%–16% |

*Abbreviations:* Apo B, apolipoprotein B; HDL-C, HDL cholesterol; TC, total cholesterol; TG, triglyceride; VLDL-C, very low-density lipoprotein cholesterol.
*Data from* Jellinger PS, Smith DA, Mehta AE, et al. American Association of Clinical Endocrinologists' guidelines for management of dyslipidemia and prevention of atherosclerosis. Endocr Pract 2012;18(Suppl 1):16–17.

study used Hy's law, which used serum bilirubin twice the upper limit of normal (ULN) or alanine aminotransferase (ALT) more than 3 times the ULN in patients without other liver dysfunction as a definition of serious drug-induced toxicity. In a placebo-matched control trial, 10- to 40-mg doses of simvastatin, lovastatin, fluvastatin, atorvastatin, and pravastatin were given to patients; hepatic function tests were compared. The incidence of an ALT elevation more than 3 times the ULN was 1.3% with the tested drugs and 1.1% to placebo, statistically insignificant (**Table 3**).[5]

Data from other trials seem to confirm this data. In one meta-analysis, 4 large trials, involving more than 48,000 patients, compared statins with placebo in patients and showed no difference in the frequency or degree of abnormal Hepatic Function Tests between the treatment and placebo groups. Moreover, if abnormal hepatic function tests were seen, these values tended to normalize, even with continuation of the same dose of statin.[6] Other studies have reported only an insignificant increase in ALT after statin administration.[7]

Perhaps the most striking endorsement for the safety of statins comes from the American Journal of Cardiology in 2006, which stated that after systematically

**Table 3**
Incidence rate of liver enzyme increase in participants of randomized controlled trials of statins

| Trials | Participants (N) | | Type of Statins | Duration (y) | Single Measure (%) | | 2 Consecutive Measures (%) | |
|---|---|---|---|---|---|---|---|---|
| | Statin | Placebo | | | Statin | Placebo | Statin | Placebo |
| HPS | 10,269 | 10,267 | Simvastatin | 5.3 | 0.4 | 0.3 | 0.1 | 0.0 |
| EXCEL | 6582 | 1663 | Lovastatin | 0.9 | 1.4 | 0.9 | 0.7 | 0.1 |
| ASCOT | 5168 | 5137 | Atorvastatin | 3.3 | — | — | — | — |
| LIPID | 4512 | 4502 | Pravastatin | 6.1 | 2.1 | 1.9 | — | — |
| AFCAPS/TexCAPS | 3304 | 3301 | Lovastatin | 5.2 | — | — | 0.5 | 0.3 |
| WOSCOPS | 3302 | 3293 | Pravastatin | 4.9 | 0.5 | 0.4 | — | — |
| PROSPER | 2891 | 2913 | Pravastatin | 3.2 | 0.0 | 0.0 | — | — |
| 4S | 2221 | 2223 | Simvastatin | 5.4 | 2.1 | 1.4 | 0.6 | 0.5 |
| CARE | 2081 | 2078 | Pravastatin | 5.0 | 3.2 | 3.5 | — | — |
| MIRACL | 1538 | 1548 | Atorvastatin | 0.3 | 2.5 | 0.6 | — | — |
| LIPS | 844 | 833 | Fluvastatin | 3.9 | — | — | 1.2 | 0.4 |

| Study | | | | | | | | |
|---|---|---|---|---|---|---|---|---|
| GREACE | 800 | 800 | Atorvastatin | 3.0 | — | — | — | 0.0 |
| PMSG | 530 | 535 | Pravastatin | 0.5 | 1.1 | 0.2 | 0.0 | 0.0 |
| ACAPS | 460 | 459 | Lovastatin | 3.0 | 1.3 | 1.3 | — | — |
| REGRESS | 450 | 434 | Pravastatin | 2.0 | 0.0 | 0.2 | 0.0 | 0.0 |
| FLARE | 409 | 425 | Fluvastatin | 0.8 | 1.7 | 0.7 | 0.0 | 0.0 |
| KAPS | 224 | 223 | Pravastatin | 3.0 | 1.8 | 1.3 | — | — |
| LRT | 203 | 201 | Lovastatin | 0.5 | 1.5 | 0.5 | — | — |
| MAAS | 193 | 188 | Simvastatin | 4.0 | 0.0 | 0.0 | — | — |
| Riegger et al[55] | 187 | 178 | Fluvastatin | 2.5 | 0.0 | 0.0 | — | — |
| LCAS | 157 | 164 | Fluvastatin | 0.9 | — | — | 1.3 | 0.1 |
| **Total** | **46,355** | **41,362** | — | — | — | — | — | — |
| Incidence per 1000 per person-year | 82,411 | 72,457 | — | — | 3.0 | 2.0 | 1.1 | 0.4 |

The liver enzyme increase is defined as more than 3 times the ULN or more than 120 U/L.

*Abbreviations:* **4S**, The Scandinavian Simvastatin Survival Study; ACAPS, Asymptomatic Carotid Artery Progression Study; AFCAPS/TexCAPS, Air Force/Texas Coronary Atherosclerosis Prevention Study; ASCOT, Anglo-Scandinavian Cardiac Outcomes Trial; CARE, Cholesterol and Recurrent Events; EXCEL, Expanded Clinical Evaluation of Lovastatin; FLARE, Fluvastatin Angioplasty Restenosis; GREACE, GREek Atorvastatin and Coronary-heart-disease Evaluation; HPS, Heart Protection Study; KAPS, Kuopio Atherosclerosis Prevention Study; LCAS, Lipoprotein and Coronary Atherosclerosis Study; LIPID, The Long-Term Intervention with Pravastatin in Ischaemic Disease; LIPS, Lescol Intervention Prevention Study; LRT, Lovastatin Restenosis; MAAS, Multicentre Anti-Atheroma Study; MIRACL, Myocardial Ischemia Reduction with Acute Cholesterol Lowering; PMSG, Pravastatin Multinational Study Group; PROSPER, The Prospective Study of Pravastatin in the Elderly at Risk; REGRESS, Regression growth evaluation statin study; WOSCOPS, West of Scotland Coronary Prevention Study.

*Adapted from* Law M, Rudnicka AR. Statin safety: a systematic review. Am J Cardiol 2006;97(8A):52C–60C; with permission.

reviewing cohort studies, randomized trials, voluntary notifications to national regulatory authorities, and published case reports, fewer hepatobiliary disorders were found in statin patients than in placebo patients.[8]

### Hepatotoxicity of Different Statins

The safety of statins with regard to hepatotoxicity seems to be a class-wide phenomenon, as evidenced by multiple trials. In the Expanded Clinical Evaluation of Lovastatin Study (EXCEL), a double-blinded, diet- and placebo-controlled trial, 6500 patients were randomized and followed for a median of 5 years. The number of patients who developed ALT elevations greater than 3 times the ULN did not differ between the lovastatin and the placebo group (18 [0.6%] vs 11 [0.3%]).[9]

In the Scandinavian Simvastatin Survival Study (4S), involving over 4000 subjects, the number of patients developing an ALT level greater than 3 times the ULN did not differ between the simvastatin and placebo groups (14 [0.7%] vs 12 [0.6%]).[10] In the Heart Protection Study, another simvastatin-placebo controlled trial with more than 20,000 patients monitored over 5 years, no evidence of hepatitis (defined as ALT of more than 4 ULN) was found in either group.[11]

Pravastatin also shows robust safety data. Pooled data from 3 large trials involving more than 19,000 patients that were randomized into drug versus placebo showed that marked ALT or aspartate aminotransferase (AST) elevations occurred with similarly low frequency in the pravastatin or placebo group (1.2%).[12–14]

Rosuvastatin was also shown to have a low incidence of hepatoxicity because a 2.5-year database survey of more than 10,000 patients did not show any cases of acute hepatitis.[15]

With atorvastatin, a review article looked at randomized trials, postmarketing analysis, and case reports and concluded that the drug is safe with respect to hepatotoxicity, especially if the dosage is kept less than 80 mg/d.[16]

In a meta-analysis of all statins, fluvastatin was the only statin found to have a significant difference versus placebo in liver test abnormalities (1.13% vs 0.29% with placebo [$P = .04$]). However, this was in a relatively small group of just more than 2000 patients in 2 small trials (**Box 1**).[7]

### Hydrophilicity

There was a suggestion in a meta-analysis that higher-intensity hydrophilic statin therapy (ie, rosuvastatin and pravastatin) may increase the risk of elevated

---

**Box 1**
**Percentages of aminotransferase increases in patients treated with placebo and different doses of statins**

| Stain | Placebo (%) | STATIN Dose (%) | | | |
|---|---|---|---|---|---|
| | | 10 mg | 20 mg | 40 mg | 80 mg |
| Lovastatin | 0.1 | — | 0.1 | 0.9 | 2.3 |
| Simvastatin | — | — | 0.7 | 0.9 | 2.3 |
| Pravastatin | 1.3 | — | — | 1.4 | — |
| Fluvastatin | 0.3 | — | 0.2 | 1.5 | 2.7 |
| Atorvastatin | — | 0.2 | 0.2 | 0.6 | 2.3 |

*Data from* De Denus S, Spinler SA, Miller K, et al. Statins and liver toxicity: a meta-analysis. Pharmacotherapy 2004;24:584–91; and *Adapted from* Bellosta S, Paoletti R, Corsini A. Safety of statins: focus on clinical pharmacokinetics and drug interactions. Circulation 2004;109(23 Suppl 1):III50–7, with permission.

aminotransferases (risk ratio [RR] 3.54 [95% confidence interval (CI), 1.83–6.85]) over higher-intensity lipophilic therapy (RR 1.58 [95% CI, 0.81–3.08]). However, this meta-analysis included only 9 trials, and pravastatin was the only hydrophilic statin evaluated. More data are needed before this relationship can be proven.[17]

### Statins Dose

There are many studies that demonstrate a dose-dependence risk of aminotransferase elevation in statins. In a 2007 meta-analysis of 9 trials involving multiple statin drugs, there was an increased risk of elevated aminotransferases in patients on high statin therapy when compared with low statin therapy (RR 3.1 [95% CI, 1.72–5.58]).[17] An article by Law and Rudnicka[8] further attempted to quantify the risk as approximately 2 per 1000 patient-years with high doses and 1 per 1000 patient-years with a low-dose regimen. Perhaps the most well-known dose-related risk of hepatic enzyme abnormalities is found in atorvastatin. In a retrospective analysis of data reported in 49 clinical trials, no differences were identified between low-dose atorvastatin (10 mg) versus placebo; however, elevated aminotransferases were significantly elevated in a higher (80 mg) dose of atorvastatin.[18]

It is important to note that the effectiveness of the statin on LDL does not relate in any meaningful way to the risk of liver toxicity. In a large prospective randomized trial of 23 treatment arms, the dose of therapy rather than the effectiveness in lowering LDL was a more important determinant of liver toxicity.[19] The results were similar to a pooled analysis of all statin new drug application data.[20]

### Hepatic Function Testing in Patients Taking Statins

There is no evidence that monitoring hepatic function tests while on treatment with statins reduces the rate of hepatotoxicity.[21] According to the US Food and Drug Administration (FDA), a baseline hepatic function tests should be done before starting statins except lovastatin, for which liver-function monitoring is no longer requested for asymptomatic patients without a history of liver disease. Although these warnings and considerations are required on package inserts, the clinical utility may not be warranted.

As so eloquently calculated in Bader's article in the *American Journal of Gastroenterology*, the estimated cost of routine liver function tests on patients prescribed statins in 2005 might approach $3 billion a year.[3] The number has almost certainly increased in the years after this as more patients are found to benefit from this class of drug.

The lack of data supporting routine testing does not imply, however, that patients on statins should not be monitored for liver damage. As pointed out in the article by Björnsson and colleagues,[22] most of the safety studies of statin drugs were severely

---

**Risk factors for adverse hepatotoxic effects of statins**

- High dose
- Recent addition of statin (within 3 months)
- Drug-drug interactions
- Advanced age and chronic illness
- Concomitant use of other lipid-lowering agents

*Adapted from* Bellosta S, Paoletti R, Corsini A. Safety of statins: focus on clinical pharmacokinetics and drug interactions. Circulation 2004;109(23 Suppl 1):III50–7.

underpowered to detect such a rare side effect as clinically significant statin hepato-toxicity. Although rare, the side effects, including liver failure, have been reported and should be investigated aggressively in symptomatic patients starting statins for the first time.

### Drug Interaction

Hepatotoxicity in statins is more common among patients receiving drugs that are metabolized by the cytochrome P450 enzyme systems (**Table 4**).[23] All statins undergo metabolism by cytochrome P450, with the exception of pravastatin, which is trans-formed enzymatically inside hepatocytes, and rosuvastatin, which is only minimally metabolized by cytochrome P450 2C9. In studies comparing the interaction profiles of pravastatin, simvastatin, and atorvastatin alone versus coadministration with cyto-chrome P450 3A4 inhibitors in healthy subjects, variable effects were reported with different statin preparations. The coadministration of pravastatin with verapamil or itraconazole does not seem to change its pharmacokinetics. However, verapamil increased simvastatin concentrations; itraconazole increased atorvastatin concentra-tions; and clarithromycin enhanced all 3 statin concentrations.[24] Additionally, there has been evidence that cyclosporine may interact with statins via mechanisms that are not exclusively CYP450 3A4 inhibitor related because increases in pravastatin bioavailability have been reported in the literature.[23] This interaction does not seem to affect the overall safety of administration, as was shown in the renal transplant patients receiving cyclosporine in the Assessment of Lescol in Renal Transplantation (ALERT) trial.[25]

### Statins in Patients with Chronic Liver Disease

#### Statin and chronic hepatitis C
Several large trials have shown the administration of statins is safe in patients with hepatitis C.[26] In a study by Khorashadi and colleagues,[27] 830 patients matched for body mass index were randomized into 3 groups: 166 patients who were hepatitis C positive on statin therapy, 332 patients who were hepatitis C negative on statin ther-apy, and 332 patients who were hepatitis C positive who did not receive statin treat-ment. Liver function tests were evaluated 1 year before therapy as well as 1 year after starting the trial. The results showed that all patients receiving statins had a higher inci-dence of mild to moderate increases in liver biochemistry values, but no difference in the frequency or severity of these increases existed between hepatitis C positive and

**Table 4**
**Summary of important drug-drug interactions with statin use**

| May Interact with Statins | Potentiated by Statin Therapy | Similar Side Effects to Statins |
|---|---|---|
| Macrolides | Digoxin | Fibrates |
| HIV protease inhibitors | Coumarin anticoagulants | Niacin |
| Azole antifungals | Oral contraceptives | |
| Diclofenac | | |
| Nefazodone | | |
| Calcium antagonists | | |
| Cyclosporine, tacrolimus | | |

*Abbreviation:* HIV, human immunodeficiency virus.
*Adapted from* Bellosta S, Paoletti R, Corsini A. Safety of statins: focus on clinical pharmacoki-netics and drug interactions. Circulation 2004;109(23 Suppl 1):III50–7.

negative patients on statin therapy. It was the nontreated group who had the highest incidence of severe increases in laboratory values. There were no significant differences in the discontinuation rates of patients taking statins, regardless of hepatitis C status. There is even evidence that the statins may possess antiviral properties, as a fluvastatin trial suggested in hepatitis C interferon treatment failures.[28]

### Statins in nonalcoholic steatohepatitis

Statins cannot only be used safely in patients with nonalcoholic fatty liver disease or nonalcoholic steatohepatitis (NASH), there are several trials that suggest statin use may improve or normalize aminotransferases in these patients.[29] Post hoc data from the GREACE trial sought to report the safety of statins in patients with NASH and ALT values that were more than 3 times the ULN versus a control. Serious increases of ALT were no different in each group, and ALT values in the statin group were improved in contrast to the control group. More strikingly, this resulted in an overall 68% risk reduction in cardiovascular events (including all-cause mortality and coronary heart disease mortality and morbidity) in patients taking statins over the control group.[30,31]

### Statins in cirrhosis and transplant

Low doses of statins can be used with careful monitoring in compensated cirrhosis, chronic liver disease, and partially obstructed liver disease. One of the best studies was performed by Lewis and colleagues,[32] which was a placebo-controlled trial with 80 mg of pravastatin in more than 300 well-compensated patients with chronic liver disease of all types. Some patients in the group had up to 5 times the normal limit of aminotransferase levels before the study started. Nevertheless, no significant ALT elevations were observed between the two groups, prompting the Liver Expert Panel to recommend that statin therapy not be contraindicated in patients with well-compensated liver disease.[33]

In patients with decompensated cirrhosis, the data support extreme caution with the use of statins because these patients may have severely impaired metabolic pathways. This finding was revealed in a study by Simonson and colleagues[34] in which concentrations of rosuvastatin were increased significantly in a Child-Pugh B cohort when compared with a Child-Pugh A patient population. Uncertainties in plasma concentration might increase the risk of severe hepatotoxicity in these patients.

After a liver transplant, patients must be monitored carefully when they are placed on statins mostly because of the effects of immunosuppressive agents. As noted earlier, these drugs are metabolized by the cytochrome P450 system and increase the risk of statin toxicity. Using pravastatin, which is not metabolized through this pathway, might mitigate these risks. In a controlled crossover study, 6 weeks of pravastatin or cerivastatin did not show significant effects in liver function and immunosuppression. However, the study was small and short-term, so more clinical evidence is likely needed.[35] As noted earlier though, care must be taken when combining pravastatin and cyclosporine because increased bioavailability was seen in these patients.[23]

In the future, statins may play a role in the treatment of patients with cirrhosis as one study suggests. In this trial, simvastatin decreased the hepatic venous pressure gradient and improved liver perfusion in patients with cirrhosis as compared with placebo.[36]

### Acute liver failure associated with statin use

The rate of statin-induced hepatic failure is exceedingly rare. Only 30 cases were reported to the FDA between 1987 and 2000. The rate of liver failure with statins use is estimated at about one case per million person-years of use.[5,33] The incidence is very similar to the rate of idiopathic acute liver failure in the general public, which in the United States ranges from 0.5 to 1.0 cases per million.[21]

In an article by Bjornsson and colleagues,[22] all 3 patients who suffered acute liver failure related to statin therapy experienced similar toxicity when rechallenged with the medication.

This finding reinforces the consensus opinion among hepatologists that "if a causal relationship between significant liver injury and statins therapy cannot be excluded, then re-initiation of statin therapy is not recommended."[33]

### Summary of the hepatotoxic effects of statins

Mild elevations of ALT (less than 3 times the ULN value) commonly occur in patients who are started on statin therapy; however, this rarely reflects true hepatotoxicity. Such elevations are usually transient, asymptomatic, and do not require interruption of therapy.

Lower doses of statins and lipophilic statin preparations might further reduce that risk. Care should be taken in reducing drug-drug interactions, especially in medications that use the cytochrome P450 3A4 pathway. Many patients with chronic liver disease, such as patients with chronic hepatitis C and patients with NASH, can safely take statins with little risk and possible hepatoprotective benefits. Patients with well-compensated NASH should be strongly considered for statin therapy because of their high cardiovascular risk.[33] On the other hand, statin hepatotoxicity should be monitored more carefully in patients with cirrhosis and in posttransplant patients, especially with patients on significant doses of immunosuppressive medication.

Routine monitoring of hepatic function tests in average-risk patients taking statins, although recommended in several package inserts, is not helpful in discovering serious hepatic events. Björnsson and colleagues[22] suggested a reasonable monitoring strategy whereby patients are counseled on the rare, serious risk of idiosyncratic statin-induced hepatitis; patients with signs and symptoms of this reaction are vigilantly monitored and treated.

Statins should be discontinued in patients having unexplained, persistent elevations of more than 3 times the ULN. Statins should not be restarted in these patients who have hepatotoxic reactions unless another cause for the laboratory abnormality is found. Acute liver failure associated with statins is rare but has been reported.

### EZETIMIBE

Ezetimibe was the first member of the lipid-lowering drugs that inhibit the uptake of dietary and biliary cholesterol. The FDA approved it in 2002 for hypercholesterolemia alone or in combination with statins. Ezetimibe inhibits the absorption of dietary and biliary cholesterol by blocking transport proteins, specifically the Niemann-Pick C1-Like 1 protein found in jejunal enterocytes.[37] Ezetimibe reduces the LDL level by 15% to 20%,[38] triglyceride (TG) levels by 5%, and increases the HDL level by 1% to 2% (see **Table 2**).[39] Ezetimibe is commonly combined with a statin and is marketed with simvastatin under the trade name Zetia.

Clinical safety trials of ezetimibe report the incidence of asymptomatic, reversible elevations in aminotransferase levels 3 or more times the ULN at 0.7%, which were similar to placebo.[40] There has been a single case report of a woman who developed a serious hepatocellular drug-induced liver disease after 4 months of therapy with 10 mg daily of ezetimibe, with withdrawal of the drug resulting in slow recovery.[41] To date, no cases of liver failure, liver transplantation, or death have been reported with ezetimibe.

Aminotransferase levels may be slightly higher with combination ezetimibe-simvastatin therapy compared with simvastatin alone,[42] although another trial involving atorvastatin monotherapy versus an atorvastatin-ezetimibe combination showed no significant difference in aminotransferase elevations.[43] In conclusion, ezetimibe monotherapy seems to be extremely safe with regard to aminotransferase elevations, and the value of monitoring liver function among patients receiving a statin-ezetimibe regimen (as stated on the package insert of Zetia [Merck & Co., Inc., Whitehouse Station, NJ, 2001]) should be similar to that of statin therapy alone.

## BILE ACID SEQUESTRANTS

As a class, bile acid sequestrants, by the nature of their mechanism, are poorly absorbed and so theoretically have little potential for hepatotoxicity. However, hepatic abnormalities are seen in patients that are administered these drugs.[44] Typical preparations (cholestyramine, colestipol, and colesevelam) bind bile acids in the intestine, preventing enterohepatic recirculation of cholesterol. As a result, the hepatic cholesterol content declines, stimulating the production of LDL receptors, which leads to increased LDL clearance and, thus, low LDL levels. In the Coronary Primary Prevention Trial, cholestyramine reduced the total cholesterol by 13%, LDL by 20%, and Coronary Heart Disease (CHD) events (fatal and nonfatal) by 19% (see **Table 2**). Higher AST levels were seen, on average, in patients on cholestyramine versus placebo in this trial, although this was only seen in the first year of therapy and no episodes of acute liver injury or serious adverse hepatic events were seen.[45] Similarly, in the Lovastatin Study Group III, ALT levels more than 2 times the ULN occurred in 9% of patients in the study.[46]

Colestipol has been shown to have a similar excellent safety record with regard to hepatic derangement; however, there is a case report of a patient with type IIa dyslipidemia who developed asymptomatic elevation of his liver enzymes 10 times the ULN after a 3-month treatment period. One week after discontinuing colestipol, serum aminotransferases decreased dramatically. Four weeks after colestipol was discontinued, all liver function tests were normal.[47]

Colesevelam has greater specificity for bile acids and, thus, has less drug interactions and gastrointestinal adverse effects as compared with cholestyramine and colestipol. In the best study looking at hepatic effects of colesevelam, 509 patients with type 2 diabetes were followed for a year in an open-label study. Only one patient had ALT of more than 3 times the ULN and 2 patients had AST of more than 3 times the ULN. These abnormalities resolved despite the fact that the drug was not stopped during the trial.[48]

In summary, these drugs seem to be extremely safe with regard to serious hepatotoxic events, although they do seem, in some cases, to raise aminotransferase levels. In nearly all cases, these elevations are mild and self-limited and, in cases of severe insult, resolve with the discontinuation of the drug.

## NIACIN

Niacin inhibits the lipolysis of TG by hormone-sensitive lipase, thereby decreasing hepatic TG synthesis. Niacin also reduces TG synthesis by inhibiting both the synthesis and esterification of fatty acids in the liver. Niacin reduces TG by 35% to 50% and LDL by 25% and increases the HDL level by 15% to 30% (see **Table 2**).

There are 3 different formulations of niacin: immediate release (IR) or crystalline, extended release (ER), and sustained released (SR), with absorption rates of 1 hour,

8 hours, and 12 hours, respectively. ER and SR preparations are given to reduce the rate of unwanted physical side effects, such as flushing.

IR niacin has been shown to have the least risk of hepatotoxicity, whereas ER and SR preparations seem to be more commonly associated with dose-dependent amino-transferase elevations.[49]

A comparative study indicated that approximately 50% of those receiving SR niacin experienced hepatotoxicity, especially with dosages of more than 2000 mg/d, compared with none in the IR niacin group.[50] The differences in hepatotoxicity among formulations are likely explained by 2 different metabolic pathways. Conjugation of niacin with glycine to form nicotinic acid is a low-affinity, high-capacity system, which leads to flushing. The second nonconjugative pathway involves multiple reactions that convert niacin to nicotinamide and is a high-affinity, low-capacity system with greater potential for hepatotoxicity. IR products will quickly saturate the nonconjugative pathway, with most of the drug being metabolized by conjugation, resulting in increased flushing and a low incidence of hepatotoxicity. Slowly absorbed preparations (SR niacin) are metabolized primarily by the high-affinity nonconjugative pathway, resulting in less flushing but increased hepatotoxicity.[49]

Thus, as is so often the case with niacin, the benefits of this drug must be weighed against the physical and metabolic side effects of the drug. Preparations of SR niacin less than 2 g/d might reduce the risk of hepatic events in these patients.

## FIBRATES

Currently, 5 fibrates are used clinically; 3 are available in the United States, 2 of which are found in generic formulations: gemfibrozil and fenofibrate. The FDA has not approved bezafibrate and ciprofibrate, which are available in Europe and elsewhere. The FDA has approved a new fenofibrate formulation known as fenofibric acid (Trilipix) with a specific indication for use with a statin in patients with mixed dyslipidemia.[51]

The pharmacologic actions of fibrates are mediated by their interaction with peroxisome proliferator-activated receptor alpha. Fibrates decrease TG levels by up to 50% and LDL by 15% to 20% and increases HDL by 15%. Most of the fibrates have potential antithrombotic effects, including the inhibition of coagulation and enhancement of fibrinolysis (see **Table 2**).

The effects of fibrate monotherapy on the liver have been discussed and succinctly summarized in Dr Zimmerman's[44] textbook on hepatotoxicity. Clofibrate is associated with several different adverse liver effects. The first is a 10% incidence of AST elevations, which may be partly caused by muscle injury. There have also been case reports of granulomatous cholestatic jaundice and anicteric hepatitis. Also, care should be taken in patients who are at risk for gallbladder disease because this may enhance the formation of stones or in patients with primary biliary cirrhosis in whom clofibrate may increase plasma cholesterol. As far as fenofibrate, elevated aminotransferases have been seen in up to 20% of patients, and several cases of cholestatic and chronic hepatitis have been reported. Gemfibrozil seems to have the least hepatic effects, although a low incidence of elevated aminotransferases have been reported as well as possible evidence of microvesicular steatosis.[44]

The most common use of fibrates today is in combination with other lipid-lowering agents, such as statins; in these preparations, an increased risk of myopathy and elevated aminotransferase levels have been observed, especially when a high dose of statin is used.[52] However, if the concomitant statin dose remains low to moderate, adverse events, including hepatotoxicity, generally remain low.[53] In case of transaminase elevations, levels normalized within weeks after the discontinuation of the drug treatment.[54]

## SUMMARY

In patients with hypercholesterolemia and heart disease, lipid-lowering agents have been shown to decrease cardiovascular events and extend lifespans. Nearly all lipid-lowering agents may cause an elevation in aminotransferases in patients. The risk of hepatotoxicity from lipid-lowering agents, however, is generally very low; this risk can be minimized using careful patient selection, attention to the type of drugs used, and knowledge of the potential for drug-drug interactions. Statins, in particular, seem to be extremely safe in most patients, including patients with chronic compensated liver disease. Special care must be taken in patients with evidence of decompensated disease and in patients who are on immunosuppressive medications after undergoing a transplant. Physicians must be vigilant for the signs and symptoms of serious statin-related idiosyncratic drug reaction; statins should never be restarted in these patients.

Ezetimibe seems to be extremely safe with regard to liver toxicity, but physicians should be aware that this drug might be combined with other lipid-lowering agents that may increase the risk of hepatic derangement.

Bile acid sequestrants are also considered very safe with respect to liver toxicity, although mild elevated aminotransferases may be experienced in a significant proportion of patients, which is almost always completely reversible.

Niacin doses of 2 g or more in the ER or higher doses in the SR are associated with higher rates of hepatotoxicity events and should be avoided if possible.

Fibrates, as a class, also have a low risk of elevated aminotransferases; however, this risk is increased when the medication is used in combination with statin therapy.

It seems that hepatic function testing does not need to be routinely performed except in patients that are at risk for hepatic injury, although clinicians should be wary of the small but serious risk of severe liver injury that has been reported with these medications. In general, mild elevations in aminotransferases less than 3 times the ULN should not merit discontinuation of therapy. In elevations greater than 3 times the ULN or in more ominous signs of liver damage, such as hepatomegaly, clinical evidence of jaundice, elevated direct bilirubin, or increased prothrombin time, the discontinuation of statin therapy should be seriously considered.[33]

As always, with any therapy, the overall benefit to patients must be considered when therapy is considered. Indeed, as originally stated in Ted Bader's editorial in the *Journal of Hepatology*, the benefits of lipid-lowering drugs, such as statin therapy, in patients with liver disease and cardiac risk factors may increase the overall lifespan more than any other therapy. In addition, this mortality benefit is accomplished with only minimal risk, especially when compared with the extremely risky therapies offered to many patients with liver disease, such as liver transplantation for patients with NASH or peg interferon–based triple therapy for hepatitis C.[51]

## REFERENCES

1. Jellinger PS, Smith DA, Mehta AE, et al. American Association of Clinical Endocrinologists' guidelines for management of dyslipidemia and prevention of atherosclerosis. Endocr Pract 2012;18(Suppl 1):1–78.
2. Smith SC Jr, Benjamin EJ, Bonow RO, et al. AHA/ACCF secondary prevention and risk reduction therapy for patients with coronary and other atherosclerotic vascular disease: 2011 update: a guideline from the American Heart Association and American College of Cardiology Foundation endorsed by the World Heart

Federation and the Preventive Cardiovascular Nurses Association. J Am Coll Cardiol 2011;58(23):2432–46.

3. Bader T. The myth of statin-induced hepatotoxicity. Am J Gastroenterol 2010; 105:978–80. http://dx.doi.org/10.1038/ajg.2010.102.

4. Hunninghake DB. HMG-CoA reductase inhibitors. Curr Opin Lipidol 1992;3: 22–8.

5. Law MR, Wald NJ, Rudnicka AR. Quantifying effect of statins on low density lipoprotein cholesterol, ischaemic heart disease, and stroke: systematic review and meta-analysis. BMJ 2003;326:1423.

6. Rzouq FS, Volk ML, Hatoum HH, et al. Hepatotoxicity fears contribute to under-utilization of statin medications by primary care physicians. Am J Med Sci 2010; 340:89–93.

7. De Denus S, Spinler SA, Miller K, et al. Statins and liver toxicity: a meta-analysis. Pharmacotherapy 2004;24:584–91.

8. Law M, Rudnicka AR. Statin safety: a systematic review. Am J Cardiol 2006; 97(8A):52C–60C.

9. Bradford RH, Shear CL, Chremos AN, et al. Expanded Clinical Evaluation of Lovastatin (EXCEL) study results. I. Efficacy in modifying plasma lipoproteins and adverse event profile in 8245 patients with moderate hypercholesterolemia. Arch Intern Med 1991;151(1):43–9.

10. Randomised trial of cholesterol lowering in 4444 patients with coronary heart disease: the Scandinavian Simvastatin Survival Study (4S). Lancet 1994; 344(8934):1383–9.

11. MRC/BHF Heart Protection Study Collaborative Group, Armitage J, Bowman L, Collins R, et al. Effects of simvastatin 40 mg daily on muscle and liver adverse effects in a 5-year randomized placebo-controlled trial in 20,536 high-risk people. BMC Clin Pharmacol 2009;9:6.

12. Shepherd J, Cobbe SM, Ford I, et al, for the West of Scotland Coronary Prevention Study Group (WOS). Prevention of coronary heart disease with pravastatin in men with hypercholesterolemia. N Engl J Med 1995;333:1301–7.

13. The Long-term Intervention with Pravastatin in Ischemic Disease Group (LIPID). Prevention of cardiovascular events and death with pravastatin in patients with coronary heart disease and a broad range of initial cholesterol levels. N Engl J Med 1998;339:1349–57.

14. Sacks FM, Pfeffer MA, Moye LA, et al, for the Cholesterol and Recurrent Events Trial Investigators (CARE). The effect of pravastatin on coronary events after myocardial infarction in patients with average cholesterol levels. N Engl J Med 1996;335:1001–9.

15. Garcia-Rodriguez LA, Masso-Gonzalez EL, Wallander MA, et al. The safety of rosuvastatin in comparison with other statins in over 100,000 statin users in UK primary care. Pharmacoepidemiol Drug Saf 2008;17:943–52.

16. Arca M. Atorvastatin: a safety and tolerability profile. Drugs 2007;67(Suppl 1): 63–9.

17. Dale KM, White CM, Henyan NN, et al. Impact of statin dosing intensity on transaminase and creatine kinase. Am J Med 2007;120(8):706–12.

18. Newman C, Tsai J, Szarek M, et al. Comparative safety of atorvastatin 80 mg versus 10 mg derived from analysis of 49 completed trials in 14,236 patients. Am J Cardiol 2006;97(1):61–7.

19. Alsheikh-Ali AA, Maddukuri PV, Han H, et al. Effect of the magnitude of lipid lowering on risk of elevated liver enzymes, rhabdomyolysis, and cancer: insights from large randomized statin trials. J Am Coll Cardiol 2007;50:409–18.

20. Jacobson TA. Statin safety: lessons from new drug applications for marketed statins. Am J Cardiol 2006;97(8A):44C–51C.
21. Tolman KG. Defining patient risks from expanded preventive therapies. Am J Cardiol 2000;85:15E–9E.
22. Björnsson E, Jacobsen EI, Kalaitzakis E. Hepatotoxicity associated with statins: reports of idiosyncratic liver injury post-marketing. J Hepatol 2012;56(2):374–80. http://dx.doi.org/10.1016/j.jhep.2011.07.023.
23. Bellosta S, Paoletti R, Corsini A. Safety of statins: focus on clinical pharmacokinetics and drug interactions. Circulation 2004;109(23 Suppl 1):III50–7.
24. Jacobson TA. Comparative pharmacokinetic interaction profiles of pravastatin, simvastatin, and atorvastatin when coadministered with cytochrome P450 inhibitors. Am J Cardiol 2004;94(9):1140–6.
25. Holdaas H, Fellström B, Jardine AG, et al. Effect of fluvastatin on cardiac outcomes in renal transplant recipients: a multicentre, randomised, placebo-controlled trial. Lancet 2003;361(9374):2024–31.
26. Madhoun MF, Bader T. Statins improve ALT values in chronic hepatitis C patients with abnormal values. Dig Dis Sci 2010;55:870–1.
27. Khorashadi S, Hasson NK, Cheung RC. Incidence of statin hepatotoxicity in patients with hepatitis C. Clin Gastroenterol Hepatol 2006;4(7):902–7 [quiz: 806].
28. Bader T, Fazili J, Madhoun M, et al. Fluvastatin inhibits hepatitis C replication in humans. Am J Gastroenterol 2008;103:1383–9.
29. Matalka MS, Ravnan MC, Deedwania PC. Is alternate daily dose of atorvastatin effective in treating patients with hyperlipidemia? The Alternate Day versus Daily Dosing of Atorvastatin Study (ADDAS). Am Heart J 2002;144:674–7.
30. Athyros VG, Tziomalos K, Gossios TD, et al. Safety and efficacy of long-term statin treatment for cardiovascular events in patients with coronary heart disease and abnormal liver tests in the Greek Atorvastatin and Coronary Heart Disease Evaluation (GREACE) study: a post hoc analysis. Lancet 2010;376:1916–22.
31. Bader T. Liver tests are irrelevant when prescribing statins. Lancet 2010;376:1882–3.
32. Lewis JH, Mortensen ME, Zweig S, et al. Efficacy and safety of high-dose pravastatin in hypercholesterolemic patients with well-compensated chronic liver disease: Results of a prospective, randomized, double-blind, placebo-controlled, multicenter trial. Hepatology 2007;46(5):1453–63.
33. Cohen D, Anania F, Chalasani N. An assessment of statin safety by hepatologists. Am J Cardiol 2006;97:C77–81.
34. Simonson SG, Martin PD, Mitchell P, et al. Pharmacokinetics and pharmacodynamics of rosuvastatin in subjects with hepatic impairment. Eur J Clin Pharmacol 2003;58(10):669–75.
35. Onofrei MD, Butler KL, Fuke DC, et al. Safety of statin therapy in patients with preexisting liver disease. Pharmacotherapy 2008;28(4):522–9.
36. Abraldes JG, Albillos A, Bañares R, et al. Simvastatin lowers portal pressure in patients with cirrhosis and portal hypertension: a randomized controlled trial. Gastroenterology 2009;136:1651–8.
37. Garcia-Calvo M, Lisnock J, Bull HG, et al. The target of ezetimibe is Niemann-Pick C1-Like 1 (NPC1L1). Proc Natl Acad Sci U S A 2005;102:8132–7.
38. Gagné C, Bays HE, Weiss SR, et al. Efficacy and safety of ezetimibe added to ongoing statin therapy for treatment of patients with primary hypercholesterolemia. Am J Cardiol 2002;90:1084–91.

39. Knopp RH, Dujovne CA, Le Beaut A, et al. Evaluation of the efficacy, safety, and tolerability of ezetimibe in primary hypercholesterolaemia: a pooled analysis from two controlled phase III clinical studies. Int J Clin Pract 2003;57:363–8.

40. Dujovne CA, Suresh R, McCrary Sisk C, et al. Safety and efficacy of ezetimibe monotherapy in 1624 primary hypercholesterolaemic patients for up to 2 years. Int J Clin Pract 2008;62:1332–6.

41. Castellote J, Ariza J, Rota R, et al. Xavier Xiol Serious drug-induced liver disease secondary to ezetimibe. World J Gastroenterol 2008;14(32):5098–9.

42. Goldman-Levine JD, Bohlman LG. Ezetimibe/simvastatin (Vytorin) for hypercholesterolemia. Am Fam Physician 2005;72:2081–2.

43. Conard S, Bays H, Leiter LA, et al. Ezetimibe added to atorvastatin compared with doubling the atorvastatin dose in patients at high risk for coronary heart disease with diabetes mellitus, metabolic syndrome or neither. Diabetes Obes Metab 2010;12:210–8.

44. Zimmerman HJ. Hepatotoxicity: the adverse effects of drugs and other chemicals on the liver. 2nd edition. Philadelphia: Lippincott; 1999. p. 660, 662.

45. The Lipid Research Clinics Coronary Primary Prevention Trial results. I. Reduction in incidence of coronary heart disease. JAMA 1984;251(3):351–64.

46. The Lovastatin Study Group III. A multicenter comparison of lovastatin and cholestyramine therapy for severe primary hypercholesterolemia. JAMA 1988; 260:359–66.

47. Sirmans SM, Beck JK, Banh HL, et al. Colestipol-induced hepatotoxicity. Pharmacotherapy 2001;21(4):513–6.

48. Goldfine AB, Fonseca VA, Jones MR, et al. Long-term safety and tolerability of colesevelam HCl in subjects with type 2 diabetes. Horm Metab Res 2010;42: 23–30.

49. Backes JM, Padley RJ, Moriarty PM. Important considerations for treatment with dietary supplement versus prescription niacin products. Postgrad Med 2011; 123:70–83.

50. Mckenney JM, Proctor JD, Harris S, et al. A comparison of the efficacy and toxic effects of sustained versus immediate release niacin in hypercholesterolemic patients. JAMA 1994;271:672–7.

51. Mohiuddin SM, Pepine CJ, Kelly MT, et al. Efficacy and safety of ABT-335 (fenofibric acid) in combination with simvastatin in patients with mixed dyslipidemia: a phase 3, randomized, controlled study. Am Heart J 2009;157(1):195–203.

52. Backes JM, Howard PA, Ruisinger JF, et al. Does simvastatin cause more myotoxicity compared with other statins? Ann Pharmacother 2009;43:2012–20.

53. Murdock DK, Murdock AK, Murdock RW, et al. Long-term safety and efficacy of combination gemfibrozil and HMG-CoA reductase inhibitors for the treatment of mixed lipid disorders. Am Heart J 1999;138:151–5.

54. Athyros VG, Papageorgiou AA, Hatzikonstandinou HA, et al. Safety and efficacy of long-term statin-fibrate combinations in patients with refractory familial combined hyperlipidemia. Am J Cardiol 1997;80:608–13.

55. Riegger G, Abletshauser C, Ludwig M, et al. The effect of fluvastatin on cardiac events in patients with symptomatic coronary artery disease during one year of treatment. Atherosclerosis 1999;144(1):263–70.

# Liver Injury Induced by Herbal Complementary and Alternative Medicine

Victor J. Navarro, MD[a],*, Leonard B. Seeff, MD[b]

## KEYWORDS

- Regulatory • Herbal • Dietary supplements • Hepatotoxicity • Causality assessment

## KEY POINTS

- Herbal and dietary supplements (HDSs) are being used with increasing frequency in American households. Several products and specific ingredients have been implicated in liver injury.
- The regulatory environment for HDSs is different than that for conventional medications; premarket testing for safety and efficacy is not required.
- The diagnosis of liver injury caused by an HDS is made as it is for drugs. However, the causality assessment process is confounded by the possibility of product adulteration and contamination, which may account for injury.
- Many different single herbal ingredients have been implicated in liver injury. However, multicomponent products are more likely to be implicated in liver injury, each with many ingredients making it difficult, if not impossible, to impugn any of them with certainty.

## INTRODUCTION

Before the emergence of pharmacology as a science and the proliferation of the pharmaceutical industry that fueled the development of chemical and biologic medications, indigenous peoples who suffered illnesses or injuries depended on unconventional means of treatment, some now referred to as alternative medicine. A local healer was often consulted and might conduct animal sacrifice, perform incantations, or apply specific forms of scarification, whereas other approaches considered included prayer, massage, acupuncture, body manipulations, and especially the use of herbal medications. The use of herbal medications was particularly prevalent in the Far East,

Disclaimer: Dr Seeff, The views expressed here are those solely of the author and not those of the U.S. Food and Drug Administration.
Disclosures: The authors have nothing to disclose.
Funding: Supported by NIDDK, NIH (7U01DK083027-06; PI: V.J. Navarro).
[a] Division of Hepatology, Einstein Healthcare Network, 5401 Old York Road, Klein Building, Suite 505, Philadelphia, PA 19141, USA; [b] The Hill Group, 6903 Rockledge Drive, Suite 540, Bethesda, MD 20817, USA
* Corresponding author.
E-mail address: navarrov@einstein.edu

dating back centuries. The herbals used came from the leaves, stems, roots, seeds, and berries of local plants and also from the barks of trees. Thought to have potential medicinal properties, they differed by geographic location, local weather conditions, the available local plants, and by soil characteristics and the elevation at which the plant was grown.

The original use of herbals consisted of applying the plant or leaf directly to the injured or painful body part, or the administration by mouth of an extract of the plant or a concoction made from boiling the plant. Without knowing the medicinal component, what was thought to be helpful was far from pure and may have been contaminated. Nevertheless, for centuries, the traditional use of herbals consisted of administering what was thought to be a single herbal ingredient or a mix of a small number of individual ingredients thought to have a complementary effect when used together, selected and mixed by an herbalist with long experience. As scientific measures became available, the supposed principal medicinal ingredient could be isolated, facilitating access to these single-ingredient products. The next step in more recent times has been for commercial interests to become involved by developing products containing multiple individual herbal ingredients. These mixtures have generally consisted of 10 or more separate constituents, each ingredient thought to have its own medicinal effect, but without necessarily having the complementary effect thought to be important by the experienced herbalist. Although many such commercially created herbal products are sold in established health care stores, as many or even more are advertised and sold via the Internet.

At present, many peoples in third world countries use single-ingredient herbals to treat illnesses, in part because of custom but also because of the lack of availability and high cost of Western commercial drugs.[1] In Western countries, even though there is easy access to pharmaceutically developed drugs, there has been a growing interest in herbal and dietary supplements (HDSs) used either in conjunction with standard medications (complementary medicine) or on their own (alternative medicine). The reasons are multiple, including the high cost of many drugs, but additionally the unpleasant or even serious side effects from some drugs, the disillusionment with general medical care, the wish to take personal control of one's health, the effort to increase well-being, and the belief in the effectiveness of herbal remedies. Moreover, there is the conviction that herbals are safe, having been used for centuries, and that conventional medical providers may not be well informed about these remedies.[2] Unlike peoples in less developed countries, westernized individuals are more likely to use products containing multiple ingredients, purchased either in health care stores or from the Internet, which they trust as sources of information.[3] Although early use focused largely on improving well-being, herbal products are now more commonly used for bodybuilding purposes and in the hope of promoting weight loss. Furthermore, they are used frequently to treat a wide variety of chronic diseases, including cancers, chronic pain, rheumatologic and cardiovascular diseases, diabetes, human immunodeficiency virus infection, and even liver diseases.[4–6] This pattern of use has raised concern because they have sometimes supplanted clearly effective treatments using standard medications with supposed medications that are less likely or even unlikely to be effective. Interactions with standard medical therapies is an additional concern,[7] the potential for which has recently been studied in patients being treated for cancer.[8]

## EPIDEMIOLOGY

Interest in and the level of use of HDS products seem to have increased in most Western countries, particularly in the United States. One of the earliest rigorous efforts to assess the frequency of use of herbals and vitamins in the United States took place in 1990 via a telephone survey.[9] Thirty-four percent of respondents disclosed the use of one or another form of complementary or alternative medicine (CAM), 2.5% admitting to a focus on herbals. A similar survey by the same researchers conducted 7 years later found an increase both in overall CAM use to 42% and in the use of herbals to 12.1%.[10] Data from the National Health and Nutrition Examination Surveys (NHANES) have been particularly revealing. Beginning with the NHANES I survey conducted between 1971 and 1974, when 23% of the studied population reported the use of vitamin supplements,[11] there has been a consistent increase in reported usage of HDS products in subsequent NHANES surveys,[12,13] reaching a figure of 52% of all respondents in the NHANES IV survey conducted between 1999 and 2000.[14] Similar increases have been identified in other national surveys, including the National Health Interview Survey (NHIS) involving the noninstitutionalized US civilian population, the frequency of admitted herbal use increasing from 9.6% to 19% in 2 successive surveys,[15,16] and a US Food and Drug Administration (FDA)–sponsored health and dietary survey conducted in 2002 finding that 73% of the screened population used supplements, half of which were herbals.[17]

Another indicator of the growing interest in the use of CAM practices in the United States is the extent of commerce attributed to purchasing products or in payment to CAM practitioners. One survey estimated that, in 1990, $14.6 million was spent on CAM therapies, increasing to an estimated $27 million in 1997,[10] whereas another analysis, conducted by the National Center for Complementary and Alternative Medicine, National Institutes of Health (NIH), concluded that the annual expenditure had increased to $33.9 million in 2007.[18] Most telling of all are data published by the American Botanical Council. This organization has been maintaining records of the estimated annual sales of herbs, noting that, in 1999, total sales were $4110 million, increasing each year thereafter, with the exception of 2002 and 2003, to reach an expenditure of $5200 million in 2010.[19] Equally informative are the data from an ongoing study supported by the National Institute of Diabetes and Digestive and Kidney Diseases, NIH. The Drug-Induced Liver Injury Network (DILIN) Study involves 8 academic centers in the United States charged with identifying cases of liver injury from either conventional pharmaceutical drugs or from herbal products.[20] In a preliminary report of the DILIN's experience between 2003 and 2011, 679 cases of drug-induced liver injury (DILI) were enrolled, of which 109 (16%) were attributed to HDS products. This group accounted for the second most common class of agents causing drug-related hepatotoxicity. Most of these agents consisted of commercial mixtures. Moreover, the data show that there has been an increase over time of the proportion of HDS DILI cases relative to the total number of all identified cases of drug injury, conventional and HDS related.[21]

## REGULATORY ENVIRONMENT

Perhaps the most common perception among the general public is that HDS products are safe and effective, which is presumably valid for vitamin supplements but may not be so for all herbal products. This perception may result from their accessibility, easy-to-read labeling, and effective marketing. However, the regulatory framework for natural products is different from that for conventional pharmaceuticals. The FDA has no authority to approve herbal products before marketing. Preclinical and clinical toxicologic testing, as well as early phase clinical trials to establish safety, tolerability, and efficacy, is not required for herbals.

The current regulatory framework for marketed HDS was put into place in 1994, through the Dietary Supplement Health and Education Act (DSHEA).[22] Through this act, dietary supplements were defined as products intended to supplement the diet, but not constitute a complete meal. A dietary supplement, by definition, contains one or more ingredients; these include vitamins, minerals, herbs or other botanicals, amino acids, or extracts thereof. According to this law, the product label must identify the contents through a complete listing of ingredients. In addition, a supplement label may not claim to diagnose, treat, cure, or prevent disease. The DSHEA prohibits regulation of herbal products by the FDA, leaving policing of efficacy and safety of these products to the manufacturers.

The next significant piece of legislation following the DSHEA of 1994 was the Final Rule for Dietary Supplement Current Good Manufacturing Practices, 2007.[23] This gives guidance to the industry on production standards, and compels manufacturers to provide assurance that their product is free from adulteration and contamination. Even with these two laws, adherence by manufacturers has been inconsistent.[24] The key responsibilities that these laws impart to the manufacturer and the FDA are listed in **Table 1**.

## DIAGNOSIS OF HDS-INDUCED LIVER INJURY

The possibility that signs and symptoms of liver injury might be the consequences of HDSs requires thorough but diplomatic inquiry of the affected person as to whether an herbal or dietary supplement had been taken in the preceding months. However, patients often do not spontaneously divulge use of nonprescribed products to their providers, for a variety of reasons, including the concern that the questioning health care professional might disparage them for their use.[2,25]

Diagnosing HDS-induced liver injury (HILI) requires a systematic analytical approach, as is done for liver injury from conventional drugs. A first step is to determine the latency of the injury, namely the time interval between the start of an agent and the onset of liver dysfunction, which is helpful in recognizing injury patterns characteristic of specific classes of drugs or HDS. However, this feature may have less

**Table 1**
**Regulatory environment for HDSs in the United States**

| Regulation | Responsibilities | |
| --- | --- | --- |
| | Manufacturer | FDA |
| DSHEA (1994) | Identify product ingredients and manufacturer on the label<br>Provide disclaimer noting that product was not evaluated by the FDA for safety and efficacy, and is not intended to diagnose, treat, cure, or prevent disease | Defines supplements as vitamins, minerals, herbs, amino acids (and any concentrate, metabolite, extract thereof)<br>Investigate allegations of attributable toxicity after marketing<br>Conducts premarket review of safety data for new ingredients |
| cGMP (2007) | Must adhere to standards in identification, purity, strength, composition, and purity of the final dietary supplement<br>Must evaluate the identity, purity, strength, and composition of dietary supplements | Supplements containing contaminants or not containing labeled ingredients are considered adulterated or misbranded |

Abbreviation: cGMP, current good manufacturing practice.

value for implicating herbal products because their latency periods may be highly variable even in well-established instances of herbal hepatotoxicity. The quality or concentration of single-ingredient herbals may differ in the same product taken at different times depending on the geographic location, the growing conditions, or the extraction procedures used during its manufacture, as shown through several recently published examples.[26–28] Multiingredient products may also have problems of inconsistency from batch to batch because of poor quality control during production. Therefore, HDSs marketed under the same label but purchased on different occasions and consumed over long periods of time may have to be regarded as potentially separate agents. Individuals under consideration for HILI should therefore always be questioned about their patterns of purchase of the implicated herbal product and especially whether there had been purchase of a new batch of the product in close proximity to the onset of injury.

The next helpful step to assess the possibility of HILI is to define the injury characteristics, namely whether it presents as hepatocellular, cholestatic, or a mixed pattern of injury. The injury pattern has been a useful diagnostic clue for hepatotoxicity from conventional drugs, as for example the typical hepatocellular presentation of injury caused by isoniazid.[29,30] However, characteristic patterns of injury from HDS have been recognized for only a few products. Most notable is the presentation of liver injury from anabolic steroids, the core of bodybuilding supplements but sometimes unknowingly tainting other commercial products. Another instance is that of the pyrrolizidine alkaloids, present for example in Comfrey tea, which can lead to the development of the sinusoidal obstruction syndrome (previously, venoocclusive disease). These two examples are referred to again later in this article.

A third important step is to exclude all other causes of hepatic injury that can mimic hepatotoxicity, such as viral hepatitis, types A, B, C, and E; autoimmune and metabolic diseases; injury from coadministered conventional medications; alcohol injury; and hemodynamic insults. The approach is the same whether assessing possible liver injury from conventional drugs or HDSs. However, identifying the specific noxious ingredient in HDSs may be difficult or even impossible when the affected person is using a single herbal product that contains multiple ingredients, not all of which are identifiable, or is taking several different herbals concomitantly.

A fourth item that helps support a diagnosis of drug-induced or HDS-induced liver injury is that the biochemical abnormalities begin to subside after withdrawing the implicated agent; however, recovery from injury may be more prolonged than usually happens in recovery from acute viral hepatitis. Referred to as dechallenge, deceleration of injury can occur with variable rapidity. In some cases, the injury may progress to chronic liver disease and/or liver failure, an example being the evolution of pyrrolizidine alkaloid hepatotoxicity to the sinusoidal obstruction syndrome, as noted earlier.

In addition, the definitive indicator of DILI, whether from a conventional drug or herbal product, is that the injury subsides after discontinuing the drug but reappears when the implicated product is readministered. Even though an effective diagnostic maneuver, rechallenge is generally avoided because the recurrent liver injury may be more severe or even culminate in liver failure. The key steps in establishing an accurate diagnosis of HILI are listed in **Table 2**.

## CAUSALITY ASSESSMENT IN HILI

Once clinical, biochemical, and serologic data have been gathered, methodical causality assessment must then be performed. Because there is presently no specific

| Table 2 |
| Steps in the diagnosis of liver injury induced by HDSs |
| --- |
| Step 1 | Ascertain a history of HDS as well as all medication use that preceded liver injury, and the duration of time from starting treatment to onset of liver injury (latency) |
| Step 2 | Assign the pattern of injury as hepatocellular, cholestatic, or mixed |
| Step 3 | Exclude other causes of liver injury |
| Step 4 | Stop the implicated product and observe for improvement, or worsening on inadvertent readministration |

biomarker for hepatotoxicity, linking a drug or herbal to identified liver disease has had to be based on one of several imperfect assessment approaches: the use of scoring systems, reliance on expert opinion assessment, or using probabilistic methods of analysis. Because of its limited applicability, probabilistic methods of analysis are not discussed in this article.

### Scoring Systems

The Naranjo Adverse Drug Reaction Scale has been proposed for use in clinical trials,[31] although not specifically for assessment of DILI. This system scores a reaction from −4 to +13 and is easy to use, but several elements limit its applicability outside the research trial setting. Its primary limitation is that the scoring is based on a placebo response. Also, information is required about drug concentration and dose relationship that is difficult to obtain in liver injury from HDS. Although it has been applied to assess causality for natural products,[32] its value in this setting has been strongly questioned.[33,34]

The most widely used scoring system is termed the Roussel Uclaf Causality Assessment Method (RUCAM).[35] Created in 1989, RUCAM permits scores ranging from 1 (unlikely to be drug toxicity) to 8 (highly likely to be drug toxicity). Although commonly used by industry, it is limited in its applicability to assessing causality in the setting of clinical trials. Moreover, its applicability in clinical practice, even though problematic regarding its value, is greater for injury caused by conventional drugs than for hepatotoxicity caused by HDS products. For example, one of the multiple items to be scored in the RUCAM system requires information on whether the label on the implicated product warns about potential liver injury, whereas another item that requires a score asks for past published experience of hepatotoxicity. Information on both these items is generally unavailable for most HDS products.

The Maria and Victorino Scale is a modification of the RUCAM scale and adds drug injury features that suggest an immune or immunoallergic response, namely fever, rash, arthralgia, eosinophilia, and cytopenias.[36] This scoring system has not been evaluated as a diagnostic tool for HDS-related hepatotoxicity.

Both of these causality assessment approaches have limited value with respect to HILI, largely because of the complexity of the involved products. As already noted, the components and their concentrations may vary in natural products that are harvested at different times of the year and in different locations; commercial products generally contain multiple ingredients and may have been unknowingly contaminated or deliberately adulterated. The Maria and Victorino and Naranjo scales ask for drug concentrations, but characterizing the chemical composition of HDS is a complex and costly task. Moreover, it may be difficult or even impossible to determine which of the many constituents is responsible for causing the liver injury, let alone identifying and implicating possible contaminants.

## Assessment by Expert Opinion

Most published reports of hepatotoxicity are based on the evaluation of clinical, biochemical, and occasionally histologic features of the case but without using a uniformly established assessment process. The NIH DILIN Study Group therefore devised a graded scoring system to assess both the diagnostic likelihood of DILI and liver disease severity taking into account all the items described earlier that are required for complete causality assessment.[20] When first created, the scoring system was relevant only for liver injury caused by conventional drugs and not by HDSs. The DILIN scoring system brought uniformity to the process of causality assessment and has seemed to be more efficient in diagnosing DILI than the RUCAM method.[37] Its limitations for general application are that it used 3 independent expert reviewers, not generally available in clinical practice, and that the analytical approach remains subjective.

The DILIN Study Group recently worked to develop an expert opinion approach directed more specifically at HILI by incorporating elements that, a priori, have an impact on establishing a causal association between a liver injury event and a dietary supplement. These elements take into account the number of dietary supplements and the multiplicity of ingredients in a single product, the strength of the existing literature on the potential for hepatotoxicity of an implicated supplement, and the possibility that a concomitantly administered drug might have accounted for the presenting pattern of injury. In a small test-retest validation exercise, the developed procedure produced moderate agreement when assessed by 3 independent reviewers.[38] However, more work is needed to further improve this approach to causality assessment for potential HILI.

## CONTAMINATION AND ADULTERATION

Because of the manner in which herbals are grown, they are at risk of contamination with potentially toxic chemicals. The original plant may be acquired from the wild or specifically cultivated for eventual medicinal use. In the latter situation, they are likely to have been sprayed with pesticides. They are then harvested, dried naturally or artificially, after which constituents are extracted using organic solvents or subjected to countercurrent extraction with supercritical gases, irradiation, or cold compression. Thereafter, they are stored and eventually packaged for distribution. In view of this protracted process, there is opportunity for contamination, which has been reported to involve microbials,[39,40] mycotoxins,[41] or heavy metals[42–48] which may account for the liver injury.

More disconcerting is that some manufacturers have deliberately adulterated the herbal mixture with pharmaceutical drugs without informing the consumer or listing them in the label. There are thus reports of the identification of the following drugs found in some herbal products: corticosteroids, sildenafil citrate, diclofenac, chlordiazepoxide, chlorpheniramine, diphenhydramine, hydrochlorothiazide, promethazine, triamterene, benzodiazepines, and antiinflammatory drugs.[49] Other drugs identified in the herbal product PC-SPES used to treat prostatic cancer included indomethacin, diethylstilbestrol, and warfarin,[50–52] whereas a phosphodiesterase 5 inhibitor has been identified in a herbal product used to treat erectile dysfunction.[53] In addition to deluding the consumer into believing that the herbal product had a specific effect, whereas it was the added pharmaceutical drug of which they were unaware, it is conceivably one or other of these added products that might account for subsequent identified liver injury.

## HDSS COMMONLY ASSOCIATED WITH LIVER DISEASE

Through its experience in accruing cases of hepatotoxicity associated with drug and dietary supplements, the US DILIN offers a contemporary view of HILI. In particular, the DILIN's preliminary findings indicate that supplements used for bodybuilding and weight loss purposes, categorized as such by a review of their marketing materials, constituted the most common of the HDS products accounting for HILI (**Table 3**).[21] Furthermore, most of the implicated HDS products identified through the DILIN study consisted of multiingredient commercial mixtures. The discussion that follows regarding specific HDS products identified to have caused hepatotoxicity is therefore framed in the context of these findings. The reader is also referred to a recent comprehensive review of all published literature on HDSs implicated in liver injury.[54]

## SUPPLEMENTS USED FOR BODY AND MUSCLE BUILDING

Many products to promote building muscle mass are offered on the Internet, and most such products contain ingredients reminiscent of steroids. Whether these ingredients are true anabolic steroids or their derivatives or precursors is unclear. Regardless, the liver injury that results from them presents in a characteristic way.[55] The involved patient is typically a young man seeking to increase his muscle mass who has obtained information on the product by searching the Web; after a variable period of use, the patient develops prolonged jaundice and intense pruritus. The biochemical pattern of injury is generally a modest increase in aminotransferase levels and, early in the course, a variable increase of alkaline phosphatase levels, followed by a prolonged period, often lasting weeks to months, of hyperbilirubinemia. Complete recovery can be expected.

That anabolic steroids may cause several adverse effects including cholestasis, peliosis, or hepatic neoplasms, has long been known.[56] Despite declaring anabolic steroids as controlled substances in sporting circles because of their tendency to

**Table 3**
**DILIN patients (n = 109) by type of HDS product**

| Type of HDS Products: Main Marketed Indications for Use | DILIN Patients with Suspected HILI; n (%) |
| --- | --- |
| Bodybuilding | 36 (33) |
| Weight loss | 28 (26) |
| Immune support | 13 (12) |
| Cough/cold | 12 (11) |
| Depression/anxiety/cognition | 9 (8) |
| Multiple vitamins | 8 (7) |
| Chinese herbs | 7 (6) |
| Antiinflammatory/analgesic | 6 (6) |
| Insomnia | 4 (4) |
| Energy booster | 4 (4) |
| Joint support | 3 (3) |
| Gastrointestinal upset/diarrhea | 3 (3) |
| Sexual performance | 2 (2) |
| Chelation | 2 (2) |
| Colon cleanser | 2 (2) |
| Menopause | 2 (2) |
| Miscellaneous | 4 (4) |

cause liver injury, liver disease continues to be reported among persons who use bodybuilding supplements[57–61] and is seemingly attributable to such steroids or their derivatives.

Examples of bodybuilding supplements identified to have caused liver disease include the products T Bomb II and Superdrol.[57,58] Noteworthy, the clinical presentations in those who used these bodybuilding supplements were not always purely cholestatic because some presented with features of hepatocellular injury.

## SUPPLEMENTS COMMONLY USED FOR WEIGHT LOSS
### Conjugated Linoleic Acid

Used as a weight loss supplement, conjugated linoleic acid has been reported to cause hepatotoxicity.[62] A recent report has described fulminant liver failure leading to transplantation.[63] Injury is suspected to be a result of lipid peroxidation.

### Ephedra

Also known by its Chinese herbal name, ma huang, ephedra has been a common ingredient in weight loss supplements, exploited for its stimulant properties. However, removal of this ingredient from Hydroxycut products did not mitigate hepatotoxicity. Injury thought to be caused by ephedra presents as a hepatocellular pattern. Several reports of hepatotoxicity have been attributed to this product, with some instances leading to liver transplantation.[64–68]

### Germander

Used as an antiinflammatory agent for many ailments, as well as for weight loss, this herbal product has been linked to hepatotoxicity and has even been removed from many European markets, stemming from multiple reports of attributable hepatotoxicity, mostly from France in the early 1990s. A hepatocellular pattern of injury has been reported, as well as a few fatalities.[69–78]

### Green Tea (Camellia sinensis)

Consumed by many people around the world as a beverage, an extract of green tea (green tea extract [GTE]) is a common ingredient in many HDS products, especially those used for weight reduction. Catechins are polyphenolic compounds comprising approximately 10% GTE. These polyphenols are likely responsible for the antioxidant activity and other health benefits that have been attributed to GTE. However, GTE and at least one component, catechin (epigallocatechin-3-gallate), have been implicated through in vitro and in vivo studies as dose-dependent hepatotoxins.[79,80]

There are numerous reports of hepatotoxicity from GTE and the US Pharmacopeia has undertaken a detailed review of the issue.[32] The liver injury generally presents with a hepatocellular pattern and fatality caused by this product has been reported.[81] Particularly convincing are reports indicating recurrence of the injury on reexposure.[82,83]

### Herbalife (Herbalife International Inc)

Another compilation of agents under a single label are the Herbalife products. Weight reduction is among the marketed purposes for use. Other uses include nutritional supplementation and promotion of overall well-being. Initial reports of liver injury from these products emerged from Israel and Switzerland.[84,85] Since these initial reports, others have been published.[40,86,87] Injury is predominantly hepatocellular in nature, with highly variable latencies.

### Hydroxycut (Iovate Health Sciences Inc)

There are many products under the brand name Hydroxycut, most of which seem to be used for weight loss. The first case reports of liver injury resulting from Hydroxycut products occurred in 2005[88]; there have subsequently been others, including one describing a fatal outcome.[89–92] With this information, the FDA issued a warning and the manufacturer withdrew some of its products from the market.[93] The pattern of injury is predominantly hepatocellular, although some reports also described a protracted cholestatic course.

### Usnic Acid

In vitro and in vivo evidence has shown the potential for usnic acid to cause cell injury and necrosis.[94,95] As a weight loss supplement, it has been incorporated into other products recognized for their injurious potential, even leading to acute liver failure.[65,96–98]

## SUPPLEMENTS USED FOR JOINT HEALTH
### Flavocoxid

Flavocoxid is a medical food with the unique feature of being a dietary supplement that is administered under the supervision of a physician, as with a conventional drug, but is not required to undergo the same rigorous premarket safety and efficacy testing.[99] Flavocoxid (Limbrel) seems to have antiinflammatory properties and is therefore used for relief of osteoarthritis symptoms.[100] In a recent case series report, the type of injury noted was of a mixed hepatocellular/cholestatic pattern, with some patients experiencing severe injury.[101]

Another product implicated in causing liver injury is Move Free Advanced (Schiff Nutrition Group Inc), a complex mixture of ingredients that includes Chinese skullcap and glucosamine.[102]

## SUPPLEMENTS COMMONLY USED TO TREAT GASTROINTESTINAL COMPLAINTS
### Aloe Vera

Aside from its use as a topical emollient, aloe vera has been used to treat gastrointestinal symptoms. There are several reports of hepatocellular injury from the use of aloe vera but none that have culminated in death or liver transplantation.[103–107]

### Chaparral

Taken orally, chaparral has been used for digestive disorders such as cramps and bloating, but for other system complaints as well, such as pulmonary and respiratory disease, cancer, and infections. Most reports of chaparral-induced liver injury describe a predominantly hepatocellular pattern of injury occurring with a wide variation in latency, up to nearly a year after exposure.[108,109] Although most cases resolved with cessation, the injury has been reported to require liver transplantation.[66,110]

### Greater Celandine (Chelidonium majus)

Greater celandine has been used in the past for various gastrointestinal ailments, and greater celandine hepatotoxicity has been reported to lead to a hepatocellular pattern of injury, although cholestasis has also been described.[111–113] Injury usually appears within 3 months of use. No fatal cases have been reported.

## SUPPLEMENTS COMMONLY USED FOR PAIN RELIEF
### Black Cohosh

Black cohosh is used to relieve menopausal symptoms. Several reports of hepatotoxicity attributed to this product have appeared in the literature, prompting a comprehensive review of the subject by the US Pharmacopeia,[114] a review that has drawn criticism.[33] Affected patients are reported to develop liver disease ranging from asymptomatic increases in the aminotransferase levels to acute liver failure,[115–122] and some patients have shown autoimmune features.[123,124] Most commonly, the liver injury presents with a hepatocellular pattern.

### Comfrey

Comfrey is most commonly used as an ingredient in oral supplements and topical applications for pain relief. Often brewed as a tea, liver injury has been reported to occur after several months of use, most commonly with the features of the sinusoidal obstruction syndrome.[125–130] Patients typically develop severe liver injury characterized by right upper quadrant pain, hepatomegaly, and ascites. Increased levels of alkaline phosphatase are common and, over time, advancement to the development of posthepatic portal hypertension with ascites and, eventually, liver failure occurs. This presentation has been attributed to its component pyrrolizidine alkaloids, which create toxic intermediates that are injurious to sinusoidal endothelium, thus leading to the obstructive process.[131] Comfrey has been banned in most countries.

## SUPPLEMENTS COMMONLY USED FOR PSYCHOTROPIC EFFECTS
### Kava Kava

The active ingredients in kava preparations, thought to be responsible for its psychotropic properties, are the kavapyrones (kava lactones). Kava has traditionally been consumed as a ceremonial drink in the South Pacific, following simple aqueous extraction. Cases of liver injury in Western countries had been thought to be caused by the alcoholic and acetonic extraction process, which yields a higher concentration of kava lactones.[132–134] However, closer examination of cases suggests that the extraction process has little if any bearing on hepatotoxicity.[135]

Following a series of reports of liver injury, some severe and leading to liver transplantation and death, kava products were banned from the market in several European countries,[136–139] beginning in 2001 in the United Kingdom.[140] Some have challenged the literature on kava hepatotoxicity, suggesting inadequate causality assessment[141] or the possibility that nonkava compounds taken simultaneously are the cause for injury.[142] The case reports indicate a predominantly hepatocellular pattern of injury, with variable latency periods, suggesting an idiosyncratic mechanism of injury. Other mechanisms of injury have been considered but none have been proved.[143] Acute liver failure and transplantation have been reported as a result of kava toxicity.[139]

### Skullcap

The flavonoids that are contained in skullcap are thought to be responsible for its sedative effect. Injury tends to be hepatocellular. Attribution to skullcap has been questioned because most reported cases of hepatotoxicity seem to have been confounded by the use of other HDSs.[102,115,144]

### Valerian

Used to treat insomnia as well as other conditions, such as anxiety and digestive disorders, valerian has been implicated in cases of HILI.[145,146] However, causality in most cases was confounded by other HDSs taken concurrently. The pattern of injury is usually hepatocellular.

## SUPPLEMENTS COMMONLY USED FOR MISCELLANEOUS PURPOSES
### Noni

The fruit of the *Morinda citrifolia* plant yields noni juice, long used for a multitude of medical applications. Liver injury has been reported, occurring predominantly in a hepatocellular pattern, with resolution on cessation; confounding factors were present in some cases.[147–152] Animal and human pharmacology studies have failed to provide supporting evidence of its hepatotoxicity.[153,154]

### Pennyroyal

Pennyroyal has been used as an insect repellant, abortifacient, and to induce menses. It is derived from the plant *Mentha pulegium*, and has long been known to be toxic, inducing seizures, circulatory collapse, and multiorgan failure, with symptom onset occurring within a few hours after exposure.[155–158] The pattern of liver injury tends to be that of acute necrosis. The main constituents of pennyroyal, pulegone and menthofuran, are thought to induce hepatotoxicity in a manner similar to acetaminophen.[159]

### Traditional Remedies

Traditional remedies comprise Asian, Chinese, or ayurvedic products. The literature contains reports of liver injury attributed to various ingredients contained in traditional remedies.[160] These include ma huang, as previously described, *Atractylis gummifera*,[161,162] Ba jiao lian,[163] dai-saiko-to,[164–166] and jin bu huan.[167–170] It is common for traditional remedies to be adulterated with conventional medications[171] or heavy metals.[42]

## SUMMARY AND FUTURE DIRECTIONS

The evidence is convincing that there is extensive and even growing use of HDS products in Western countries, almost rivaling that of the use of conventional pharmaceutical drugs. Convincing also is that, contrary to popular belief, these products are no safer than prescription drugs and some may be more likely to cause harm. Past reports describing herbal hepatotoxicity focused largely on single herbal products, many used in their traditional settings, mostly but not exclusively in third world countries. What was not readily apparent was that, in westernized countries, especially the United States, the focus seems to have shifted to the use of herbals containing complex mixtures, many taken for specific reasons, mostly for bodybuilding or weight reduction purposes. This trend has become apparent from data collected In the NIH DILIN study, which enrolls all subjects identified with apparent drug-related liver injury, regardless of whether a conventional medication or a herbal product is involved. Among the enrolled cases of DILI in the DILIN database, only a few involve the single products that have been the focus of previous attention.

This finding raises the problem of needing to conduct causality assessment of products that include multiple ingredients, not all of which can be easily identified, making it difficult or even impossible to identify the component responsible for causing the liver injury. Added to this problem is the uncertainty of whether the toxic compound might be an unrecognized contaminant.

Future research must include expanding data collection of instances of HILI in real time in order to confirm and broaden knowledge of the potentially harmful effects of herbal products. These data would allow better categorization of the injury patterns according to class or use, augment the ability to chemically isolate the individual known and unknown constituents, and provide the opportunity to improve the HDS-related causality assessment process.

## REFERENCES

1. WHO. Traditional medicine. Fact sheet no. 134. December 2008. Available at: http://www.who.int/mediacentre/factsheets/fs134/en/.
2. Blendon RJ, DesRoches CM, Benson JM, et al. Americans' views on the use and regulation of dietary supplements. Arch Intern Med 2001;161:805–10.
3. Robinson A, Cooper S. Trusted information sources: the preferred option for complementary and alternative medicine users. Complement Health Pract Rev 2007;12:120.
4. Decker C, Huddleston J, Kosiborod M, et al. Self-reported use of complementary and alternative medicine in patients with previous acute coronary syndrome. Am J Cardiol 2007;99:930–3.
5. Ostrow MJ, Cornelisse PG, Heath KV, et al. Determinants of complementary therapy use in HIV-infected individuals receiving antiretroviral or anti-opportunistic agents. J Acquir Immune Defic Syndr Hum Retrovirol 1997;15:115–20.
6. Seeff LB, Curto TM, Szabo G, et al. Herbal product use by persons enrolled in the Hepatitis C Antiviral Long-Term Treatment against Cirrhosis (HALT-C) Trial. Hepatology 2008;47:605–12.
7. Izzo AA, Ernst E. Interactions between herbal medicines and prescribed drugs: an updated systematic review. Drugs 2009;69:1777–98.
8. Zeller T, Muenstedt K, Stoll C, et al. Potential interactions of complementary and alternative medicine with cancer therapy in outpatients with gynecological cancer in a comprehensive cancer center. J Cancer Res Clin Oncol 2013;139:357–65.
9. Eisenberg DM, Kessler RC, Foster C, et al. Unconventional medicine in the United States: prevalence, costs, and patterns of use. N Engl J Med 1993; 328:246–52.
10. Eisenberg DM, Davis RB, Ettner SL, et al. Trends in alternative medicine use in the United States, 1990-1997: results of a follow-up national study. JAMA 1998; 280:1569–75.
11. Block G, Cox D, Madans J, et al. Vitamin supplement use, by demographic characteristics. Am J Epidemiol 1988;127:297–309.
12. Koplan JP, Annest JL, Layde PM, et al. Nutrient intake and supplementation in the United States (NHANES II). Am J Public Health 1986;76:287–9.
13. Ervin RB, Wright JD, Kennedy-Stephenson J. Use of dietary supplements in the United States, 1988-1994. Vital Health Stat 11 1999;(244):i–iii, 1–14.
14. Radimer K, Bindewald B, Hughes J, et al. Dietary supplement use by US adults: data from the National Health and Nutrition Examination Survey, 1999-2000. Am J Epidemiol 2004;160:339–49.
15. Ni H, Simile C, Hardy AM. Utilization of complementary and alternative medicine by United States adults: results from the 1999 national health interview survey. Med Care 2002;40:353–8.
16. Kennedy J. Herb and supplement use in the US adult population. Clin Ther 2005;27:1847–58.
17. Timbo BB, Ross MO, McCarthy PV, et al. Dietary supplements in a national survey: prevalence of use and reports of adverse events. J Am Diet Assoc 2006; 106:1966–74.

18. Nahin RL, Barnes PM, Stussman BJ, et al. Costs of complementary and alternative medicine (CAM) and frequency of visits to CAM practitioners: United States, 2007. National Health Statistics Reports; no 18. Hyattsville (MD): National Center for Health Statistics; 2009.

19. Cavaliere C, Rea P, Lynch ME, et al. Herbal supplement sales rise in all channels in 2009. HerbalGram 2010;86:62–5.

20. Fontana RJ, Watkins PB, Bonkovsky HL, et al. Rationale, design and conduct of the Drug Induced Liver Injury Network prospective study. Drug Saf 2009;32: 55–68.

21. Navarro VJ, Barnhart HX, Bonkovsky HL, et al. Herbal and dietary supplement induced hepatotoxicity in the U.S. Gastroenterology 2012;142(5):S1 S-41. [Abstract #167].

22. Food and Drug Administration. Dietary supplements. Available at: http://www.fda.gov/Food/DietarySupplements/default.htm. Accessed March 25, 2013.

23. Food and Drug Administration. Food guidance documents. Available at: http://www.fda.gov/Food/GuidanceRegulation/GuidanceDocumentsRegulatory Information/default.htm. Accessed March 25, 2013.

24. Council for Responsible Nutrition (CRN). Available at: http://www.crnusa.org/FDAunity/FDAManufacturerDietarySupplements121510.pdf. Accessed March 25, 2013.

25. Robinson A, McGrail MR. Disclosure of CAM use to medical practitioners: a review of qualitative and quantitative studies. Complement Ther Med 2004; 12(2–3):90–8.

26. Komes D, Belscak-Cvitanovic A, Horzic D, et al. Phenolic composition and antioxidant properties of some traditionally used medicinal plants affected by the extraction time and hydrolysis. Phytochem Anal 2011;22:172–80, 2011.

27. Harkey MR, Henderson GL, Gershwin ME, et al. Variability in commercial ginseng products: an analysis of 25 preparations. Am J Clin Nutr 2001;73: 1101–6.

28. Ye F, Wang H, Jiang S, et al. Quality evaluation of commercial extracts of *Scutellaria baicalensis*. Nutr Cancer 2004;49:217–22.

29. Centers for Disease Control and Prevention. Severe isoniazid-associated liver injuries among persons being treated for latent tuberculosis infection-United States, 2004-2008. MMWR Morb Mortal Wkly Rep 2010;59:224–9.

30. Black M, Mitchell JE, Zimmerman HJ, et al. Isoniazid associated hepatitis in 114 patients. Gastroenterology 1975;69:289–302.

31. Naranjo CA, Busto U, Sellers EM, et al. A method for estimating the probability of adverse drug reactions. Clin Pharmacol Ther 1981;30:239–45.

32. Sarma DN, Barrett ML, Chavez ML, et al. Safety of green tea extracts: a systematic review by the US Pharmacopeia. Drug Saf 2008;6:469–84.

33. Teschke R, Schmidt-Taenzer W, Wolff A. Spontaneous reports of assumed herbal hepatotoxicity by black cohosh: is the liver-unspecific Naranjo scale precise enough to ascertain causality? Pharmacoepidemiol Drug Saf 2011; 20:567–82.

34. Teschke R, Schulze J. Suspected herbal hepatotoxicity. Requirements for appropriate causality assessment by the US Pharmacopeia. Drug Saf 2012; 35:1091–7.

35. Danan G, Benichou C. Causality assessment of adverse reactions to drugs-I. A novel methods based on the conclusions of international consensus meetings; application to drug-induced liver injuries. J Clin Epidemiol 1993;46: 1323–30.

36. Maria VA, Victorino RM. Development and validation of a clinical scale for the diagnosis of drug induced hepatitis. Hepatology 1997;26:664–9.
37. Rockey DC, Seeff LB, Rochon J, et al. US Drug-Induced Liver Injury Network. Causality assessment in drug-induced liver injury using a structured expert opinion process: comparison to the Roussel-Uclaf causality assessment method. Hepatology 2010;51:2117–26.
38. Navarro VJ, Barnhart HX, Bonkovsky HL, et al. Diagnosing hepatotoxicity attributable to herbal & dietary supplements (HDS): test-retest reliability of a novel causality assessment tool. J of Hepatol 2012;56(S2):S536 [Abstract 1364].
39. Kneifel W, Czech E, Kopp B. Microbial contamination of medicinal plants. Planta Med 2000;68:5–15.
40. Stickel F, Droz S, Patsenker E, et al. Severe hepatotoxicity following ingestion of Herbalife nutritional supplements contaminated with *Bacillus subtilis*. J Hepatol 2009;50:111–7.
41. Gray SL, Lackey BR, Tate PL, et al. Mycotoxins in root extracts of American and Asian ginseng bind estrogen receptors alpha and beta. Exp Biol Med 2004;229:560–8.
42. Saper RB, Phillips RS, Sehgal A, et al. Lead, mercury, and arsenic in US- and Indian-manufactured Ayurvedic medicines sold via the internet. JAMA 2008;300:915–23.
43. Wong MK, Tan P, Wee YC. Heavy metals in some Chinese herbal plants. Biol Trace Elem 1993;36:135–42.
44. Koh HL, Woo SO. Chinese propriety medicine in Singapore: regulatory control of toxic heavy metals and undeclared drugs. Drug Saf 2000;23:351–62.
45. Au AM, Ko R, Boo FO, et al. Screening methods for drugs and heavy metals in Chinese patent medicines. Bull Environ Contam Toxicol 2000;65:112–9.
46. Ernst E. Heavy metals in traditional Indian remedies. Eur J Clin Pharmacol 2002;57:891–6.
47. Chan K. Some aspects of toxic contaminants in herbal medicines. Chemosphere 2003;52:1361–71.
48. Centers for Disease Control and Prevention. Lead poisoning associated with use of Ayurvedic medication – five states. 2000-2003. MMWR Morb Mortal Wkly Rep 2004;53:582–4.
49. Miller GM, Streipp R. A study of western pharmaceuticals contained within samples of Chinese herbal/patent medicines collected from New York City's Chinatown. Leg Med (Tokyo) 2007;9:258–64.
50. Guns ES, Goldenberg SL, Brown PN. Mass spectral analysis of PC-SPES confirms the presence of diethylstilbestrol. Can J Urol 2002;9:1684–8.
51. Oh WK, Small EJ. Complementary and alternative therapies in prostate cancer. Semin Oncol 2002;29:575–84.
52. Sovak M, Seligson AL, Konas M, et al. Herbal composition of PC-SPES for management of prostate cancer: identification of active principles. J Natl Cancer Inst 2002;94:1275–81.
53. Fleshler N, Harvey M, Adomat H, et al. Evidence for contamination of herbal erectile dysfunction products with phosphodiesterase type 5 inhibitors. J Urol 2005;174:636–41.
54. Teschke R, Wolff A, Frenzel C, et al. Herbal hepatotoxicity: a tabular compilation of reported cases. Liver Int 2012;32:1543–56.
55. Haupt HA, Rovere GD. Anabolic steroids: a review of the literature. Am J Sports Med 1984;12:469–84.

56. Ishak KG. Hepatic lesions caused by anabolic and contraceptive steroids. Semin Liver Dis 1981;1:116–28.

57. Timchec-Hariri A, Balali-Mood M, Aryan E, et al. Toxic hepatitis in a group of 20 male body-builders taking dietary supplements. Food Chem Toxicol 2012;50: 3826–32.

58. Singh V, Rudraraju M, Carey E, et al. Severe hepatotoxicity caused by a methasteron-containing performance-enhancing supplement. J Clin Gastroenterol 2009;43:287200.

59. DesJardins M. Supplement use in the adolescent athlete. Curr Sports Med Rep 2002;1:369–73.

60. Dodge TL, Jaccard JJ. The effect of high school sports participation on the use of performance-enhancing substances in young adulthood. J Adolesc Health 2006;39:367–73.

61. Avelar-Escobar G, Mendez-Navarro J, Ortiz-Olvera N, et al. Hepatotoxicity associated with dietary energy supplements: use and abuse by young athletes. Ann Hepatol 2012;11:564–9.

62. Ramos R, Mascarenhas J, Duarte P, et al. Conjugated linoleic acid-induced toxic hepatitis: first case report. Dig Dis Sci 2009;54:1141–3.

63. Nortadas R, Barata J. Fulminant hepatitis during self-medication with conjugated linoleic acid. Ann Hepatol 2012;11:265–7.

64. Skoulidis F, Alexander GJ, Davies SE. Ma huang associated acute liver failure requiring liver transplantation. Eur J Gastroenterol Hepatol 2005;17:581–4.

65. Neff GW, Reddy R, Durazo FA, et al. Severe hepatotoxicity associated with the use of weight loss diet supplements containing ma huang or usnic acid. J Hepatol 2004;41:162–4.

66. Estes JD, Stolpman D, Olyaei A, et al. High prevalence of potentially hepatotoxic herbal supplement use in patients with fulminant hepatic failure. Arch Surg 2003;138:852–8.

67. Borum ML. Fulminant exacerbation of autoimmune hepatitis after the use of ma huang. Am J Gastroenterol 2001;96:1654–5.

68. Nadir A, Agrawal S, King PD, et al. Acute hepatitis associated with the use of a Chinese herbal product, ma-huang. Am J Gastroenterol 1996;91:1436–8.

69. Mimidis KP, Papadopoulos VP, Baltatzidis G, et al. Severe acute cholestasis caused by *Teucrium polium*. J Gastrointestin Liver Dis 2009;18:387–8.

70. Poon WT, Chau TL, Lai CK, et al. Hepatitis induced by *Teucrium viscidum*. Clin Toxicol (Phila) 2008;46:819–22.

71. Savvidou S, Goulis J, Giavazis I, et al. Herb-induced hepatitis by *Teucrium polium* L.: report of two cases and review of the literature. Eur J Gastroenterol Hepatol 2007;19:507–11.

72. Starakis I, Siagris D, Leonidou L, et al. Hepatitis caused by the herbal remedy *Teucrium polium* L. Eur J Gastroenterol Hepatol 2006;18:681–3.

73. Mazokopakis E, Lazaridou S, Tzardi M, et al. Acute cholestatic hepatitis caused by *Teucrium polium* L. Phytomedicine 2004;11:83–4.

74. Polymeros D, Kamberoglou D, Tzias V. Acute cholestatic hepatitis caused by *Teucrium polium* (golden germander) with transient appearance of antimitochondrial antibody. J Clin Gastroenterol 2002;34:100–1.

75. Laliberté L, Villeneuve JP. Hepatitis after the use of germander, a herbal remedy. CMAJ 1996;154:1689–92.

76. Mattei A, Rucay P, Samuel D, et al. Liver transplantation for severe acute liver failure after herbal medicine (*Teucrium polium*) administration. J Hepatol 1995; 22:597.

77. Mostefa-Kara N, Pauwels A, Pines E, et al. Fatal hepatitis after herbal tea. Lancet 1992;340(8820):674.
78. Larrey D, Vial T, Pauwels A, et al. Hepatitis after germander (*Teucrium chamaedrys*) administration: another instance of herbal medicine hepatotoxicity. Ann Intern Med 1992;117:129–32.
79. Lambert JD, Kennett MJ, Sang S, et al. Hepatotoxicity of high oral dose(-)-epigallocatechin-3-gallate in mice. Food Chem Toxicol 2010;48:409–16.
80. Galati G, Lin A, Sultan AM, et al. Cellular and in vivo hepatotoxicity caused by green tea phenolic acids and catechins. Free Radic Biol Med 2006;40:570–80.
81. Molinari M, Watt KD, Kruszyna T, et al. Acute liver failure induced by green tea extracts: case report and review of the literature. Liver Transpl 2006;12: 1892–5.
82. Martinez-Sierra C, Rendón Unceta P, Martin Herrera L. Acute hepatitis after ingestion of green tea. Med Clin (Barc) 2006;27:119 [in Spanish].
83. Bonkovsky HL. Hepatotoxicity associated with supplements containing Chinese green tea (*Camellia sinensis*). Ann Intern Med 2006;144:68–71.
84. Elinav E, Pinsker G, Safadi R, et al. Association between consumption of Herbalife nutritional supplements and acute hepatotoxicity. J Hepatol 2007;47: 514–20.
85. Schoepfer AM, Engel A, Fattinger K, et al. Herbal does not mean innocuous: ten cases of severe hepatotoxicity associated with dietary supplements from Herbalife products. J Hepatol 2007;47:521–6.
86. Chao S, Anders M, Turbay M, et al. Toxic hepatitis by consumption Herbalife products a case report. Acta Gastroenterol Latinoam 2008;38:274–7.
87. Manso G, Lopez-Rivas L, Salgueiro ME, et al. Continuous reporting of new cases in Spain supports the relationship between Herbalife products and liver injury. Pharmacoepidemiol Drug Saf 2011;20:1080–7.
88. Stevens T, Qadri A, Zein NN. Two patients with acute liver injury associated with use of the herbal weight-loss supplement Hydroxycut. Ann Intern Med 2005; 1426:477–8.
89. Jones FJ, Andrews AH. Acute liver injury associated with the herbal supplement Hydroxycut in a soldier deployed to Iraq. Am J Gastroenterol 2007;102:2357–8.
90. Shim M, Saab S. Severe hepatotoxicity due to Hydroxycut: a case report. Dig Dis Sci 2009;54:406–8.
91. Dara L, Hewett J, Kim JK. Hydroxycut hepatotoxicity: a case series and review of the liver toxicity from herbal weight loss supplements. World J Gastroenterol 2008;14:6999–7004.
92. Fong TL, Klontz KC, Canas-Coto A, et al. Hepatotoxicity due to Hydroxycut: a case series. Am J Gastroenterol 2010;105:1561–6.
93. Food and Drug Administration. Available at: http://www.fda.gov/oc/opacom/hottopics/hydroxycut/consumeradvisory.html. Accessed February 25, 2013.
94. Han D, Matsumaru K, Rettori D, et al. Usnic acid-induced necrosis of cultured mouse hepatocytes: inhibition of mitochondrial function and oxidative stress. Biochem Pharmacol 2004;67:439–45.
95. Pramyothin P, Janthasoot W, Pongnimitprasert N, et al. Hepatotoxic effect of (+) usnic acid from *Usnea siamensis* Wainio in rats, isolated rat hepatocytes and isolated rat liver mitochondria. J Ethnopharmacol 2004;90:381–7.
96. Favreau JT, Ryu ML, Braunstein G, et al. Severe hepatotoxicity associated with the dietary supplement LipoKinetrix. Ann Intern Med 2002;136:590–5.
97. Durazo FA, Lassman C, Han SB, et al. Fulminant liver failure due to usnic acid for weight loss. Am J Gastroenterol 2004;99:950.

98. Sanchez W, Maple JT, Burgart LJ, et al. Severe hepatotoxicity associated with the use of a dietary supplement containing usnic acid. Mayo Clin Proc 2006; 81:541–4.

99. Food and Drug Administration. Medical foods. Available at: http://www.fda.gov/food/foodsafety/product-specificinformation/medicalfoods/default.htm. Accessed March 26, 2013.

100. Altavilla D, Squadrito F, Bitto A, et al. Flavocoxid, a dual inhibitor of cyclooxygenase and 5-lipoxygenase, blunts pro-inflammatory phenotype activation in endotoxin-stimulated macrophages. Br J Pharmacol 2009;157:1410–8.

101. Chalasani N, Vuppalanchi R, Navarro VJ, et al. Acute liver injury due to Flavocoxid (Limbrel), a medical food for osteoarthritis. A case series. Ann Intern Med 2013;156:857–60.

102. Linnebur SA, Rapacchietta OC, Vejar M, et al. Hepatotoxicity associated with Chinese skullcap contained in move free advanced dietary supplement: two case reports and review of the literature. Pharmacotherapy 2010;30:750, 258e–62e.

103. Yang HN, Kim DJ, Kim YM, et al. Aloe-induced toxic hepatitis. J Korean Med Sci 2010;25:492–5.

104. Jacobsson I, Jönsson AK, Gerdén B, et al. Spontaneously reported adverse reactions in association with complementary and alternative medicine substances in Sweden. Pharmacoepidemiol Drug Saf 2009;18:1039–47.

105. Bottenberg MM, Wall GC, Harvey RL, et al. Oral aloe vera-induced hepatitis. Ann Pharmacother 2007;41:1740–3.

106. Kanat O, Ozet A, Ataergin S. Aloe vera-induced acute toxic hepatitis in a healthy young man. Eur J Intern Med 2006;17:589.

107. Rabe C, Musch A, Schirmacher P, et al. Acute hepatitis induced by an aloe vera preparation: a case report. World J Gastroenterol 2005;11:303–4.

108. Kauma H, Koskela R, Mäkisalo H, et al. Toxic acute hepatitis and hepatic fibrosis after consumption of chaparral tablets. Scand J Gastroenterol 2004;39: 1168–71.

109. Pittler MH, Ernest E. Systematic review: hepatotoxic events associated with herbal medicinal products. Aliment Pharmacol Ther 2003;18:451–71.

110. Sheikh NM, Philen RM, Love LA. Chaparral-associated hepatotoxicity. Arch Intern Med 1997;157:913–9.

111. Moro PA, Cassetti F, Giugliano G, et al. Hepatitis from greater celandine(Chelidonium majus L.): review of literature and report of a new case. J Ethnopharmacol 2009;124:328–32.

112. Hardeman E, Van Overbeke L, Ilegems S, et al. Acute hepatitis induced by greater celandine(Chelidonium majus). Acta Gastroenterol Belg 2008;71:281–2.

113. Stickel F, Pöschl G, Seitz HK, et al. Acute hepatitis induced by greater celandine(Chelidonium majus). Scand J Gastroenterol 2003;38:565–8.

114. Mahady GB, Low Dog T, Barrett ML, et al. United States Pharmacopeia review of the black cohosh case reports of hepatotoxicity. Menopause 2008;15:628–38.

115. Whiting PW, Clouston A, Kerlin P. Black cohosh and other herbal remedies associated with acute hepatitis. Med J Aust 2002;177:440–3.

116. Lontos S, Jones RM, Angus PW, et al. Acute liver failure associated with the use of herbal preparations containing black cohosh. Med J Aust 2003;179:390–1.

117. Levitsky J, Alli TA, Wisecarver J, et al. Fulminant liver failure associated with the use of black cohosh. Dig Dis Sci 2005;50:538–9.

118. Lynch CR, Folkers ME, Hutson WR. Fulminant hepatic failure associated with the use of black cohosh: a case report. Liver Transpl 2006;12:989–92.

119. Pierard S, Coche JC, Lanthier P, et al. Severe hepatitis associated with the use of black cohosh: a report of two cases and an advice for caution. Eur J Gastro-enterol Hepatol 2009;21:941–5.

120. Joy D, Joy J, Duane P. Black cohosh: a cause of abnormal postmenopausal liver function tests. Climacteric 2008;11:84–8.

121. Vannacci A, Lapi F, Gallo E, et al. A case of hepatitis associated with long-term use of *Cimicifuga racemosa*. Altern Ther Health Med 2009;15:62–3.

122. Naser B, Liske E, Teschke R. Liver failure associated with the use of black cohosh for menopausal symptoms. Med J Aust 2009;190:99–100.

123. Cohen SM, O'Connor AM, Hart J, et al. Autoimmune hepatitis associated with the use of black cohosh: a case study. Menopause 2004;11:575–7.

124. Guzman G, Kallwitz ER, Wojewoda C, et al. Liver injury with features mimicking autoimmune hepatitis following the use of black cohosh. Case Rep Med 2009; 2009:918156.

125. Sperl W, Stuppner H, Gassner J, et al. Reversible hepatic veno-occlusive dis-ease in an infant after consumption of pyrrolizidine-containing herbal tea. Eur J Pediatr 1995;154:112–6.

126. Yeong ML, Swinburn B, Kennedy M, et al. Hepatic veno-occlusive disease asso-ciated with comfrey ingestion. J Gastroenterol Hepatol 1990;5:211–4.

127. Bach N, Thung SN, Schaffner F. Comfrey herb tea-induced hepatic veno-occlusive disease. Am J Med 1989;87:97–9.

128. Weston CF, Cooper BT, Davies JD. Veno-occlusive disease of the liver second-ary to ingestion of comfrey. Br Med J 1987;295:183.

129. Huxtable RJ, Luethy J, Zweifel U. Toxicity of comfrey-pepsin preparations. N Engl J Med 1986;315:1095.

130. Ridker PM, Ohkuma S, McDermott WV, et al. Hepatic venocclusive disease associated with the consumption of pyrrolizidine-containing dietary supple-ments. Gastroenterology 1985;88:1050–4.

131. Chojkier M. Hepatic sinusoidal-obstruction syndrome: toxicity of pyrrolizidine alkaloids. J Hepatol 2003;3:437–46.

132. Currie BJ, Clough AR. Kava hepatotoxicity with Western herbal products: does it occur with traditional kava use? Med J Aust 2003;178:421–2.

133. Moulds RF, Malani J. Kava: herbal panacea or liver poison? Med J Aust 2003; 178:451–3.

134. Teschke R, Gaus W, Loew D. Kava extracts: safety and risks including rare hep-atotoxicity. Phytomedicine 2003;10:440–6.

135. Teschke R, Sarris J, Schweitzer I. Kava hepatotoxicity in traditional and modern use: the presumed Pacific kava paradox hypothesis revisited. Br J Clin Pharma-col 2011;73:170–4.

136. Kraft M, Spahn TW, Menzel J, et al. Fulminant liver failure after administration of the herbal antidepressant kavakava. Dtsch Med Wochenschr 2001;126:970–2.

137. Strahl S, Ehret V, Dahm HH, et al. Necrotizing hepatitis after taking herbal rem-edies. Dtsch Med Wochenschr 1998;123:1410–4.

138. Stevinson C, Huntley A, Ernst E. A systematic review of the safety of kava extract in the treatment of anxiety. Drug Saf 2002;25:251–61.

139. Stickel F, Baumuller HM, Seitz K, et al. Hepatitis induced by kava (*Piper methys-ticum rhizoma*). J Hepatol 2003;39:62–7.

140. Richardson WN, Henderson L. The safety of kava – a regulatory perspective. Br J Clin Pharmacol 2007;64:418–20.

141. Teschke R, Wolff A. Regulatory causality evaluation methods applied in kava hepatotoxicity: are they appropriate? Regul Toxicol Pharmacol 2011;59:1–7.

142. Teschke R, Qiu SX, Lebot V. Herbal hepatotoxicity by kava: update on piperme-thystine, flavokavain B, and mould hepatotoxins as primarily assumed culprits. Dig Liver Dis 2011;43:676–81.

143. Olsen LR, Grillo MP, Skonberg C. Constituents in kava extracts potentially involved in hepatotoxicity: a review. Chem Res Toxicol 2011;24:992–1002.

144. Yang L, Aronsohn A, Hart J, et al. Herbal hepatoxicity from Chinese skullcap: a case report. World J Hepatol 2012;4:231–3.

145. Vassiliadis T, Anagnostis P, Patsiaoura K, et al. *Valeriana* hepatotoxicity. Sleep Med 2009;10:935.

146. Cohen DL, Del Toro Y. A case of valerian-associated hepatotoxicity. J Clin Gas-troenterol 2008;42:961–2.

147. Stadlbauer V, Weiss S, Payer F, et al. Herbal does not all mean innocuous: the sixth case of hepatotoxicity associated with *Morinda citrifolia* (noni). Am J Gas-troenterol 2008;103:2406–7.

148. Millonig G, Stadlmann S, Vogel W. Herbal hepatotoxicity: acute hepatitis caused by a Noni preparation (*Morinda citrifolia*). Eur J Gastroenterol Hepatol 2005;17: 445–7.

149. Yuce B, Gulberg V, Diebold J, et al. Hepatitis induced by Noni juice from *Mor-inda citrifolia*: a rare cause of hepatotoxicity or the tip of the iceberg? Digestion 2006;73:167–70.

150. Stadlbauer V, Fickert P, Lackner C, et al. Hepatotoxicity of NONI juice: report of two cases. World J Gastroenterol 2005;11:4758–60.

151. Lopez-Cepero Andrada JM, Lerma Castilla S, Fernandez Olvera MD, et al. Hep-atotoxicity caused by a Noni (*Morinda citrifolia*) preparation. Rev Esp Enferm Dig 2007;99:179–81.

152. Yu EL, Sivagnanam M, Ellis L, et al. Acute hepatotoxicity after ingestion of *Mor-inda citrifolia* (noni berry) juice in a 14-year-old boy. J Pediatr Gastroenterol Nutr 2011;52:222–4.

153. West BJ, Su CX, Jensen CJ. Hepatotoxicity and subchronic toxicity tests of *Mor-inda citrifolia* (noni) fruit. J Toxicol Sci 2009;34:581–5.

154. West BJ, Jensen CJ, White LD, et al. A double-blind clinical safety study of noni fruit juice. Pac Health Dialog 2009;15:21–32.

155. Vallance WB. Pennyroyal poisoning: a fatal case. Lancet 1955;269(6895): 850.

156. Sullivan JB Jr, Rumack BH, Thomas H Jr, et al. Pennyroyal oil poisoning and hepatotoxicity. JAMA 1979;242:2873–4.

157. Fatality and illness associated with consumption of pennyroyal oil—Colorado. MMWR Morb Mortal Wkly Rep 1978;27:511–3.

158. Bakerink JA, Gospe SM, Dimand RJ, et al. Multiple organ failure after ingestion of pennyroyal oil from herbal tea in two infants. Pediatrics 1996;98:944–7.

159. Thomassen D, Slattery JT, Nelson SD. Menthofuran-dependent and indepen-dent aspects of pulegone hepatotoxicity: roles of glutathione. J Pharmacol Exp Ther 1990;253:567–72.

160. Seeff LB. Herbal hepatotoxicity. Clin Liver Dis 2007;11:577–96.

161. Strader DB, Navarro VJ, Seeff LB. Hepatotoxicity of herbal preparations. In: Boyer TD, Manns MP, Sanyal AJ, editors. Zakim and Boyer's hepatology: a text-book of liver disease. 6th edition. Philadelphia: Saunders; 2012. p. 462–75.

162. Ahid S, Ait El Cadi M, Meddah B, et al. *Atractylis gummifera*: from poisoning to the analytic methods. Ann Biol Clin (Paris) 2012;70:263–8.

163. Chou SL, Chou MY, Kao WF, et al. Bajiaolian poisoning-a poisoning with high misdiagnostic rate. Am J Emerg Med 2010;28:85–9.

164. Hsu LM, Huang YS, Tsay SH, et al. Acute hepatitis induced by Chinese hepato-protective herb, xiao-chai-hu-tang. J Chin Med Assoc 2006;69:86–8.

165. Itoh S, Marutani K, Nishijima T, et al. Liver injuries induced by herbal medicine, syo-saikoto (xiao-chai-hu-tang). Dig Dis Sci 1995;40:1845–8.

166. Kamiyama T, Nouchi T, Kojima S, et al. Autoimmune hepatitis triggered by administration of an herbal medicine. Am J Gastroenterol 1997;92:703–4.

167. Horowitz RS, Feldhaus K, Dart RC, et al. The clinical spectrum of Jin Bu Huan toxicity. Arch Intern Med 1996;156:899–903.

168. McRae CA, Agarwal K, Mutimer D, et al. Hepatitis associated with Chinese herbs. Eur J Gastroenterol Hepatol 2002;14:559–62.

169. Picciotto A, Campo N, Brizzolara R, et al. Chronic hepatitis induced by Jin Bu Huan. J Hepatol 1998;28:165–7.

170. Woolf GM, Petrovic LM, Rojter SE, et al. Acute hepatitis associated with the Chinese herbal product jin bu huan. Ann Intern Med 1994;121:729–35.

171. Wai CT, Tan BH, Chan CL, et al. Drug-induced liver injury at an Asian center: a prospective study. Liver Int 2007;27:465–74.

# Hepatotoxicity and Drug Interactions in Liver Transplant Candidates and Recipients

Neehar D. Parikh, MD, MS, Josh Levitsky, MD, MS*

## KEYWORDS

- DILI • Medication • Calcineurin • Immunosuppressives

## KEY POINTS

- As the US population ages, the exposure of patients to medications to treat acute and chronic conditions is also increasing.
- Health care providers must be cognizant of the risks associated with medication use and the patient characteristics, which increase risk.
- There are few medications that have been proven to increase the risk of drug-induced liver injury in patients with cirrhosis when compared with the general population.
- In posttransplant patients, drug interactions are of utmost importance because of the need to keep immunosuppressive regimens within a therapeutic range and thus mitigate the risk of drug toxicity if levels are too high or acute cellular rejection if levels are too low.
- In the new era of hepatitis C therapy with the recent advent of protease inhibitors, transplant patients with severe recurrent hepatitis C have potential treatment options, however immunosuppressive medication levels must be monitored vigilantly due to significant drug interactions.

## INTRODUCTION

It is generally accepted that the risk of drug-induced liver injury (DILI) is similar in patients with or without cirrhosis.[1] There are, however, a small number of medications that predispose patients with cirrhosis to higher risks of hepatotoxicity. DILI has a range of clinical and histopathological manifestations, from minor elevations in liver enzymes to acute or chronic hepatic failure.[2] The diagnosis is often somewhat difficult to make due to a historical lack of clear definitions and specific markers of drug injury. If DILI does occur, a cirrhotic liver is more susceptible to decompensation because of a lack of physiologic reserve.[1]

The authors have nothing to disclose.
Division of Gastroenterology and Hepatology, Department of Medicine, Northwestern University Feinberg School of Medicine, NMH/Arkes Family Pavilion 19th Floor, 676 North Saint Clair Street, Suite 1900, Chicago IL 60611, USA
* Corresponding author.
*E-mail address:* j-levitsky@northwestern.edu

Pharmacokinetic studies have found significant differences in drug metabolism and clearance in cirrhotic patients compared with healthy controls.[3,4] There is a theoretical risk of increased hepatotoxicity in patients with cirrhosis because there are numerous physiologic changes that may affect drug metabolism and the potential for DILI, including changes in drug volume of distribution,[5] renal function,[6] hepatocyte mass,[7] P450 activity,[8] and biliary excretion.[9] As these changes have variable effects on drug metabolism and excretion, the risk of hepatotoxicity remains uncertain for most medications, in addition to the fact that patients with cirrhosis are not widely tested. This often leads to uncertainty on the part of the clinician when prescribing medications in patients with advanced liver disease. However, sufficient data exist on the risk of hepatotoxicity of a small number of medications in patients with cirrhosis to guide dose adjustments and additional monitoring.

There are also important considerations with regard to the risk of drug interactions between medications after liver transplantation. The calcineurin inhibitors are largely metabolized by the P-450 enzyme system and P glycoprotein in the gastrointestinal tract and liver. Specifically the CYP3A4 and CYP3A5 enzymes are responsible for most calcineurin inhibitor clearance.[10] Similarly, the mammalian target of rapamycin (mTOR) inhibitors (sirolimus, everolimus) undergo first-pass metabolism by the CYP3A4 and CYP3A5 systems.[11] The CYP3A4/5 systems are responsible for metabolism of up to 50% of known medications; therefore, modification to activity by either up-regulation or saturation is common.[12] As a result, there are many significant drug-drug interactions to consider in postliver transplant patients that significantly affect the therapeutic levels of the immunosuppressive drugs.

In this article, the medications that increase the risk of development of DILI in patients with cirrhosis are identified. In addition, for the liver transplant recipient, drug hepatotoxicity is briefly discussed but the focus is primarily on the salient drug-drug interactions with the most commonly used immunosuppressive regimens.

## Medications that Have Increased Risk of DILI in Patients with Cirrhosis

Although the development of DILI in cirrhosis is generally similar to patients without underlying liver disease, a few notable exceptions do exist (**Table 1**).

| Table 1 Medications associated with increased risk of drug-induced liver injury in patients with cirrhosis | | |
| --- | --- | --- |
| **Medication** | **Population at Increased Risk** | **Reference** |
| Isoniazid | HBV | 27,29 |
| | HCV | 30 |
| | HCV and HIV coinfected | 30 |
| Didanosine | HCV and HIV coinfected | 38 |
| Raltegravir | HCV and HIV coinfected | 39 |
| Nevirapine | HCV and HIV coinfected | 41 |
| | HBV and HIV coinfected | 44 |
| Ritonavir | HCV and HIV coinfected | 45 |
| | HBV and HIV coinfected | 45 |
| Nelfinavir | HCV and HIV coinfected | 43 |
| Saquinavir | HCV and HIV coinfected | 34,47 |
| Indinavir | HCV and HIV coinfected | 34,47 |

### Tuberculosis medications

Isoniazid is a first-line medication used for the treatment of *Mycobacterium tuberculosis* and acts to prevent mycolic acid synthesis and tuberculosis cell wall formation.[13] It is primarily metabolized by the hepatic enzyme N-acetyltransferase-2. The hepatotoxicity associated with isoniazid use is most likely related to one of the byproducts of metabolism, hydrazine.[14] The mechanism seems to be related to hydrazine oxidative metabolism, which in rat studies, has been shown to precipitate nitrogen-free radicals.[15,16] The risk of hepatotoxicity with isoniazid ranges widely and is reported in the literature to be anywhere from 0.15% to 28%.[17–22] Demographic risk factors include advanced age (greater than 60 years old), female sex, low body mass index, and active alcohol use.[23–28] There is also evidence of increased risk of DILI in patients with chronic viral hepatitis. Wong and colleagues[27] conducted a retrospective study in patients with chronic hepatitis B (HBV) and found they had an increased risk of isoniazid-associated DILI when compared with controls (26.8% vs 8.3%). Another study by de Castro and colleagues[29] showed similar risk of liver injury in a prospective cohort of patients with HBV undergoing therapy with anti-tuberculosis medication. Hepatitis C (HCV) and human immunodeficiency virus (HIV) infection also seem to increase the risk of isoniazid-induced DILI. Based on a study by Ungo and colleagues,[30] HCV alone conferred a 5-fold increased risk of isoniazid-induced DILI, whereas coinfection with HCV and HIV increased the risk 14-fold. These studies showed these associations in small numbers of patients and a confirmatory trial is needed to corroborate the results. Nevertheless, until further evidence is available, patients with chronic liver disease needing isoniazid therapy may require more frequent monitoring of liver enzymes. In addition, although it seems that there is an increased risk of DILI with the combination of rifampin and isoniazid in normal subjects, there is no direct evidence of an increased risk in patients with cirrhosis.[31]

### HIV medications

DILI has been associated with the use of anti-retroviral therapy for HIV and all classes of medications have been shown to have some risk of hepatotoxicity.[32–34] In addition, it does seem that the risk of DILI is increased for those patients with chronic HCV and HCV infection.[35,36]

Of the nucleoside reverse transcriptase inhibitors, didanosine, zidovudine, and stavudine have been associated with mitochondrial dysfunction and development of hepatic steatosis.[37] For patients on didanosine coinfected with HCV/HIV, ribavirin has been shown to increase the potential for didanosine-related mitchondrial toxicity.[38] There is limited other evidence of increased toxicity in patients with chronic liver disease in this class of medications.

The safety of raltegravir, an integrase inhibitor, was evaluated by Vispo and colleagues[39] in a prospective study of 218 HIV-infected patients. The authors found a significantly higher incidence of liver enzyme elevation in HCV-coinfected patients than non-coinfected patients (25% vs 7.9%; relative risk: 3.1; 95% confidence interval 2.9–3.4). In addition, all of the severe DILI occurred in the coinfected patients (1.4%).

Of the nonnucleoside reverse transcriptase inhibitors, nevirapine seems to have the most significant risk of liver toxicity, estimated anywhere from 4% to 18%.[40] In one trial by Macias and colleagues[41] the rate of DILI in HIV/HCV-coinfected patients was 11%, with severe events occurring in 3.7% of patients. Liver toxicity caused therapy discontinuation in 13% of patients on nevirapine.[41] In a study of HIV/HCV-coinfected patients by Pineda and colleagues,[42] the authors found a significantly higher incidence of liver toxicity in patients with advanced fibrosis receiving efavirenz-based anti-retroviral therapy compared with those without significant fibrosis (8.9% vs 0.8%; $P<.001$).

This liver toxicity rarely led to treatment discontinuation or treatment modification (10.7% vs 3%; $P = .031$). The risk of these toxicities seems to be increased with concomitant use of a protease inhibitor. In one trial of 82 HIV/HCV-coinfected patients, the addition of nelfinavir to nevirapine significantly increased the risk of liver toxicity (adjusted odds ratio: 8.9; 95% confidence interval 1.4–54.1).[43] The use of nevirapine in patients with HBV and HCV coinfection is generally not recommended due to the risk of hepatotoxicity.[44]

The protease inhibitors alone have also been associated with an increased risk of hepatotoxicity in patients with chronic HCV and HBV infections. In a trial by Sulkowski and colleagues,[45] patients with HIV and with chronic HCV or HBV infection receiving anti-retroviral therapy had a slightly higher incidence of hepatotoxicity (12.2% vs 6.6%.) There were no differences between the coinfected and non-coinfected patients in the incidence of severe hepatotoxicity. In the trial ritonavir seemed to be the most hepatotoxic medication, and it seems that the hepatotoxic effects are accentuated in patients with concomitant viral hepatitis.[34,45,46] The incidence of hepatotoxicity with the other protease inhibitors, including nelfinavir, saquinavir, and indinavir, is also significantly elevated in patients with chronic HCV infection, although the overall risk of severe hepatotoxicity is low in this population.[34,47]

Generally the DILI seen in patients receiving anti-retroviral therapy is reversible with drug cessation and has few long-term negative consequences for the patient.[37] The impact of other forms of chronic liver disease, such as alcoholic cirrhosis, on the development of liver toxicity in patients has largely been unexplored, so it is unclear if there is something intrinsic to viral hepatitis or if the presence of chronic liver disease/cirrhosis predisposes patients to DILI. Potential mechanisms for the observed toxicity could be related to hypersensitivity reactions, intrinsic drug cytopathic effects, or immune reconstitution in patients with HIV who are coinfected.[37]

### Other classes of medications

Of the most commonly prescribed medications, there is little evidence of increased rates of DILI in patients with chronic liver disease or cirrhosis. Narcotics (+/− acetaminophen),[48–50] statins,[51,52] nonsteroidal anti-inflammatory drugs,[53] antimicrobials,[54] and cardiovascular,[55] psychiatric, and diabetes medications[56] have not been shown to cause increased rates of DILI consistently in patients with chronic liver disease or cirrhosis. Although numerous reports of medications causing hepatotoxicity exist, there are few that have increased frequency of DILI in patients with cirrhosis.

There are limited data on the risk of hepatotoxicity in patients after liver transplantation. In the largest study published by Sembera and colleagues,[57] the authors retrospectively evaluated all biopsies conducted at a single transplant center. The overall incidence of hepatotoxicity was low (1.7%; n = 29) and the most common offending agents were antibiotics, with trimethoprim-sulfamethoxazole being the most frequently implicated. The other categories of medications that were associated with hepatotoxicity included immunosuppressive agents and anti-hyperlipidemics. Resolution of liver enzyme abnormalities occurred with removal of the offending agents a median of 34 days after removal of the agents and there were no episodes of retransplantation or death due to hepatotoxicity.

### Drug Interaction in Patients After Liver Transplantation

The most commonly used immunosuppressive regimens in liver transplantation include use of a calcineurin inhibitor (tacrolimus or cyclosporine A), anti-metabolites (mycophenolate mofetil, azathioprine), and initial use of corticosteroids.[58] Alternative regimens include use of mTOR inhibitors (sirolimus or everolimus) in place of the calcineurin inhibitors. In addition, a minority of transplant centers use initial induction therapy with biologic T-cell-depleting agents (anti-CD52, OKT3, antithymocyte globulin) or non-T-cell-depleting agents (IL-2 receptor agonists, basiliximab).[59] There are numerous important drug interactions to consider that affect the serum levels of immunosuppressive medications used in liver transplantation. Reduced levels of medications predispose patients to rejection and graft loss, whereas elevated levels can lead to severe drug toxicity. An elevated serum level of calcineurin inhibitor is associated with nausea, headache, somnolence, altered mentation, hypertension, tremor, seizure, and acute kidney injury.[60,61] Increased levels of mycophenolate mofetil or azathioprine are generally well tolerated, but have been reported to result in leukopenia or pancytopenia.[62–64] Clinically significant interactions typically occur with the calcineurin inhibitors and mTOR inhibitors and are the focus of this section (**Table 2**).[65,66]

Inducers of metabolism of calcineurin inhibitors and mTOR inhibitors, which may result in decreased levels of drug, include rifampin, caspofungin, nondihydropyridine calcium channel blockers (diltiazem, verapamil), anti-epileptic medications (phenytoin, carbamazepine, and phenobarbital), and St. Johns Wort.[67–70] Increased doses of the immunosuppressive and frequent monitoring are typically required when treating a patient with these medications.

The most potent inhibitors of metabolism include the azole antifungals (ketoconazole, fluconazole, itraconazole, voriconazole), certain macrolide antibiotics (erythromycin, clarithromycin), dihydropyridine calcium channel blockers (nifedipine, nicardipine), and grapefruit juice.[71] Reduction in doses of medications and frequent monitoring of levels are required with initiation of these medications. There are many other medications that exhibit a minor inhibitory effect on the CYP3A4/5 system and may affect drug levels, although significant dose adjustment is typically not required.

The most significant recent drug-drug interactions seen with the transplant immunosuppressive agents have been with the new therapies for HCV. Patients with clinically significant recurrent genotype 1 HCV posttransplant can be treated with 2 recently approved protease inhibitors, boceprevir or telaprevir, with the addition of interferon

**Table 2**
**Clinically significant medication interactions with calcineurin inhibitor and mTOR inhibitor metabolism**

| Inducers of Metabolism | Reference |
| --- | --- |
| Rifampin | 68 |
| Caspofungin | 71 |
| Nondihydropyridine calcium channel blockers | 70 |
| Anti-epileptic medications | 69 |
| St. Johns Wort | 67 |
| **Inhibitors of Metabolism** | **Reference** |
| Azole antifungals | 71 |
| Macrolide antibiotics | 71 |
| Dihydropyridine calcium channel blockers | 71 |
| Grapefruit juice | 71 |
| Direct-acting protease inhibitors for HCV therapy | 76,77 |

and ribavirin. These medications have increased treatment success rates to near 70% for naïve patients and approach 60% for previously treated patients.[72–75] In the post-transplant population, however, there are significant concerns about drug-drug inter-actions with tacrolimus, cyclosporine, and rapamycin. In a phase I open-label study by Garg and colleagues,[76] the authors tested the effect of telaprevir on tacrolimus and cyclosporine pharmacokinetics in healthy subjects. The authors found that the levels of cyclosporine increased 4.6 times and tacrolimus increased 70 times. In a study by Hulskotte and colleagues,[77] the authors tested the pharmacokinetic effects of boce-previr on tacrolimus and cyclosporine levels. The authors found that the maximum concentration of cyclosporine increased 2.0 times and the maximum concentration of tacrolimus increased 9.9 times. With these significant drug interactions, much caution must be taken with administration of direct-acting protease inhibitors in HCV therapy. Werner and colleagues[78] published a pilot study in 9 patients with recur-rent HCV after liver transplantation that underwent therapy with a telaprevir-based regimen. Four patients were on cyclosporine, 4 on tacrolimus, and one on rapamycin. The authors found that significant dose adjustments (cyclosporine 2.5-fold, sirolimus 7-fold, and tacrolimus 22.5-fold) were necessary; however, the authors monitored immunosuppressive levels frequently and appropriately adjusted medication doses. The patients all completed 12 weeks of therapy and the main side effect was anemia, requiring erythropoietin and transfusions in two-thirds of the patients. There are limited available data on the optimal regimen for patients after transplant on triple therapy so no specific recommendations can be made on dosing or monitoring regimens. Extreme care should be taken, however, as centers have reported rare patient deaths while on triple therapy.[79]

## DISCUSSION

As the US population ages, the exposure of patients to medications to treat acute and chronic conditions is also increasing.[80] Health care providers must be cognizant of the risks associated with medication use and the patient characteristics, which increase risk. In this review the medication, which seems to have an increased risk of DILI in patients with cirrhosis and after liver transplantation, is discussed. In addition, also discussed is the important drug-drug interaction to consider in a liver transplant recipient.

There are few medications that have been proven to increase the risk of DILI in pa-tients with cirrhosis when compared with the general population. It seems that some anti-tuberculosis medications and HIV medication confer an increased risk, although the risk of severe decompensation remains very low and most patients recover with drug withdrawal. However, little drug testing occurs directly in patients with cirrhosis, so the current list of medication is by no means definitive. Efforts to collect more centralized data on drug toxicity in a standardized fashion are underway. The DILI Expert Working group recently standardized the phenotypic case definition of DILI, which will be helpful for reporting purposes and future research.[81] In addition, entities such as the DILI network, which pools multicenter data on DILI and its associated risk factors, will be instrumental in further defining the risk of hepatotoxicity in patients with chronic liver disease and cirrhosis.[82]

In the posttransplant patient, drug interactions are of utmost importance due to the need to keep immunosuppressive regimens within a therapeutic range and thus miti-gate the risk of drug toxicity if levels are too high or acute cellular rejection if levels are too low. Remaining cognizant of the most significant interaction is necessary for any transplant hepatologists coordinating the care of these patients. Untoward affects can be avoided with more frequent monitoring and prophylactic dose adjustments if drug interactions are anticipated.

In the new era of HCV therapy with the recent advent of protease inhibitors, transplant patients with severe recurrent HCV now have a potential new treatment option. The drug interactions are significant, although several small case reports and case series have shown that the interactions can be managed with frequent monitoring and dose adjustments. Further guidelines are anticipated with the publication of future trials. There are however many patients who cannot undergo repeat interferon therapy, either due to intolerance in the past or to the risk of rejection of either the liver or the kidney if the patient underwent a simultaneous liver-kidney transplantation.[83] Fortunately, there are many new oral-only regimens in the drug development pipeline and, if approved for use, further testing on the effects on immunosuppression pharmacokinetics is needed.[84,85]

## REFERENCES

1. Zimmerman HJ. Hepatotoxicity: the adverse effects of drugs and other chemicals on the liver. 2nd edition. Philadelphia: Lippincott Williams & Wilkins; 1999.
2. Wang Y, Lin Z, Liu Z, et al. A unifying ontology to integrate histological and clinical observations for drug-induced liver injury. Am J Pathol 2013;182(4): 1180–7.
3. Finucci GF, Padrini R, Piovan D, et al. Verapamil pharmacokinetics and liver function in patients with cirrhosis. Int J Clin Pharmacol Res 1988;8(2):123–6.
4. Weiler S, Zoller H, Graziadei I, et al. Altered pharmacokinetics of voriconazole in a patient with liver cirrhosis. Antimicrob Agents Chemother 2007;51(9):3459–60.
5. Henriksen JH. Volume adaptation in chronic liver disease: on the static and dynamic location of water, salt, protein and red cells in cirrhosis. Scand J Clin Lab Invest 2004;64(6):523–33.
6. DeSanto NG, Anastasio P, Loguercio C, et al. Creatinine clearance: an inadequate marker of renal filtration in patients with early posthepatitic cirrhosis (Child A) without fluid retention and muscle wasting. Nephron 1995;70(4):421–4.
7. Zuckerman E, Slobodin G, Sabo E, et al. Quantitative liver-spleen scan using single photon emission computerized tomography (SPECT) for assessment of hepatic function in cirrhotic patients. J Hepatol 2003;39(3):326–32.
8. Villeneuve JP, Pichette V. Cytochrome P450 and liver diseases. Curr Drug Metab 2004;5(3):273–82.
9. Zollner G, Fickert P, Zenz R, et al. Hepatobiliary transporter expression in percutaneous liver biopsies of patients with cholestatic liver diseases. Hepatology 2001;33(3):633–46.
10. Hu YF, Qiu W, Liu ZQ, et al. Effects of genetic polymorphisms of CYP3A4, CYP3A5 and MDR1 on cyclosporine pharmacokinetics after renal transplantation. Clin Exp Pharmacol Physiol 2006;33(11):1093–8.
11. Zochowska D, Wyzgal J, Paczek L. Impact of CYP3A4*1B and CYP3A5*3 polymorphisms on the pharmacokinetics of cyclosporine and sirolimus in renal transplant recipients. Ann Transplant 2012;17(3):36–44.
12. Luo G, Guenthner T, Gan LS, et al. CYP3A4 induction by xenobiotics: biochemistry, experimental methods and impact on drug discovery and development. Curr Drug Metab 2004;5(6):483–505.
13. Schroeder EK, de Souza N, Santos DS, et al. Drugs that inhibit mycolic acid biosynthesis in Mycobacterium tuberculosis. Curr Pharm Biotechnol 2002;3(3): 197–225.

14. Sotsuka T, Sasaki Y, Hirai S, et al. Association of isoniazid-metabolizing enzyme genotypes and isoniazid-induced hepatotoxicity in tuberculosis patients. In Vivo 2011;25(5):803–12.

15. Ranguelova K, Suarez J, Magliozzo RS, et al. Spin trapping investigation of peroxide- and isoniazid-induced radicals in Mycobacterium tuberculosis catalase-peroxidase. Biochemistry 2008;47(43):11377–85.

16. Noda A, Noda H, Ohno K, et al. Spin trapping of a free radical intermediate formed during microsomal metabolism of hydrazine. Biochem Biophys Res Commun 1985;133(3):1086–91.

17. Fountain FF, Tolley E, Chrisman CR, et al. Isoniazid hepatotoxicity associated with treatment of latent tuberculosis infection: a 7-year evaluation from a public health tuberculosis clinic. Chest 2005;128(1):116–23.

18. LoBue PA, Moser KS. Use of isoniazid for latent tuberculosis infection in a public health clinic. Am J Respir Crit Care Med 2003;168(4):443–7.

19. Fernandez-Villar A, Sopena B, Vazquez R, et al. Isoniazid hepatotoxicity among drug users: the role of hepatitis C. Clin Infect Dis 2003;36(3):293–8.

20. McNeill L, Allen M, Estrada C, et al. Pyrazinamide and rifampin vs isoniazid for the treatment of latent tuberculosis: improved completion rates but more hepatotoxicity. Chest 2003;123(1):102–6.

21. Nolan CM, Goldberg SV, Buskin SE. Hepatotoxicity associated with isoniazid preventive therapy: a 7-year survey from a public health tuberculosis clinic. JAMA 1999;281(11):1014–8.

22. Sharifzadeh M, Rasoulinejad M, Valipour F, et al. Evaluation of patient-related factors associated with causality, preventability, predictability and severity of hepatotoxicity during antituberculosis [correction of antituberculosis] treatment. Pharmacol Res 2005;51(4):353–8.

23. Ormerod LP, Horsfield N. Frequency and type of reactions to antituberculosis drugs: observations in routine treatment. Tuber Lung Dis 1996;77(1):37–42.

24. Yee D, Valiquette C, Pelletier M, et al. Incidence of serious side effects from first-line antituberculosis drugs among patients treated for active tuberculosis. Am J Respir Crit Care Med 2003;167(11):1472–7.

25. Fernandez-Villar A, Sopena B, Fernandez-Villar J, et al. The influence of risk factors on the severity of anti-tuberculosis drug-induced hepatotoxicity. Int J Tuberc Lung Dis 2004;8(12):1499–505.

26. Schaberg T, Rebhan K, Lode H. Risk factors for side-effects of isoniazid, rifampin and pyrazinamide in patients hospitalized for pulmonary tuberculosis. Eur Respir J 1996;9(10):2026–30.

27. Wong WM, Wu PC, Yuen MF, et al. Antituberculosis drug-related liver dysfunction in chronic hepatitis B infection. Hepatology 2000;31(1):201–6.

28. Saukkonen JJ, Cohn DL, Jasmer RM, et al. An official ATS statement: hepatotoxicity of antituberculosis therapy. Am J Respir Crit Care Med 2006;174(8):935–52.

29. de Castro L, do Brasil PE, Monteiro TP, et al. Can hepatitis B virus infection predict tuberculosis treatment liver toxicity? Development of a preliminary prediction rule. Int J Tuberc Lung Dis 2010;14(3):332–40.

30. Ungo JR, Jones D, Ashkin D, et al. Antituberculosis drug-induced hepatotoxicity. The role of hepatitis C virus and the human immunodeficiency virus. Am J Respir Crit Care Med 1998;157(6 Pt 1):1871–6.

31. Sarma GR, Immanuel C, Kailasam S, et al. Rifampin-induced release of hydrazine from isoniazid. A possible cause of hepatitis during treatment of tuberculosis with regimens containing isoniazid and rifampin. Am Rev Respir Dis 1986;133(6):1072–5.

32. Jones M, Nunez M. Liver toxicity of antiretroviral drugs. Semin Liver Dis 2012; 32(2):167–76.
33. Lamar ZS, Nunez M. Higher risk of severe drug-induced liver injury among Hispanic HIV-infected patients after initiation of highly active antiretroviral therapy. J Int Assoc Physicians AIDS Care (Chic) 2011;10(3):183–6.
34. Sulkowski MS. Drug-induced liver injury associated with antiretroviral therapy that includes HIV-1 protease inhibitors. Clin Infect Dis 2004;38(Suppl 2): S90–7.
35. Bonacini M. Liver injury during highly active antiretroviral therapy: the effect of hepatitis C coinfection. Clin Infect Dis 2004;38(Suppl 2):S104–8.
36. den Brinker M, Wit FW, Wertheim-van Dillen PM, et al. Hepatitis B and C virus co-infection and the risk for hepatotoxicity of highly active antiretroviral therapy in HIV-1 infection. AIDS 2000;14(18):2895–902.
37. Gupta NK, Lewis JH. Review article: the use of potentially hepatotoxic drugs in patients with liver disease. Aliment Pharmacol Ther 2008;28(9):1021–41.
38. Balzarini J, Lee CK, Herdewijn P, et al. Mechanism of the potentiating effect of ribavirin on the activity of 2',3'-dideoxyinosine against human immunodeficiency virus. J Biol Chem 1991;266(32):21509–14.
39. Vispo E, Mena A, Maida I, et al. Hepatic safety profile of raltegravir in HIV-infected patients with chronic hepatitis C. J Antimicrob Chemother 2010;65(3): 543–7.
40. Rivero A, Mira JA, Pineda JA. Liver toxicity induced by non-nucleoside reverse transcriptase inhibitors. J Antimicrob Chemother 2007;59(3):342–6.
41. Macias J, Neukam K, Mallolas J, et al. Liver toxicity of initial antiretroviral drug regimens including two nucleoside analogs plus one non-nucleoside analog or one ritonavir-boosted protease inhibitor in HIV/HCV-coinfected patients. HIV Clin Trials 2012;13(2):61–9.
42. Pineda JA, Neukam K, Mallolas J, et al. Hepatic safety of efavirenz in HIV/hepatitis C virus-coinfected patients with advanced liver fibrosis. J Infect 2012; 64(2):204–11.
43. Mira JA, Macias J, Giron-Gonzalez JA, et al. Incidence of and risk factors for severe hepatotoxicity of nelfinavir-containing regimens among HIV-infected patients with chronic hepatitis C. J Antimicrob Chemother 2006;58(1):140–6.
44. Dieterich DT, Robinson PA, Love J, et al. Drug-induced liver injury associated with the use of nonnucleoside reverse-transcriptase inhibitors. Clin Infect Dis 2004;38(Suppl 2):S80–9.
45. Sulkowski MS, Thomas DL, Chaisson RE, et al. Hepatotoxicity associated with antiretroviral therapy in adults infected with human immunodeficiency virus and the role of hepatitis C or B virus infection. JAMA 2000;283(1):74–80.
46. Aceti A, Pasquazzi C, Zechini B, et al. Hepatotoxicity development during antiretroviral therapy containing protease inhibitors in patients with HIV: the role of hepatitis B and C virus infection. J Acquir Immune Defic Syndr 2002; 29(1):41–8.
47. Monforte Ade A, Bugarini R, Pezzotti P, et al. Low frequency of severe hepatotoxicity and association with HCV coinfection in HIV-positive patients treated with HAART. J Acquir Immune Defic Syndr 2001;28(2):114–23.
48. Duh MS, Vekeman F, Korves C, et al. Risk of hepatotoxicity-related hospitalizations among patients treated with opioid/acetaminophen combination prescription pain medications. Pain Med 2010;11(11):1718–25.
49. Tegeder I, Lotsch J, Geisslinger G. Pharmacokinetics of opioids in liver disease. Clin Pharmacokinet 1999;37(1):17–40.

50. Kuffner EK, Green JL, Bogdan GM, et al. The effect of acetaminophen (four grams a day for three consecutive days) on hepatic tests in alcoholic patients–a multicenter randomized study. BMC Med 2007;5:13.

51. Avins AL, Manos MM, Ackerson L, et al. Hepatic effects of lovastatin exposure in patients with liver disease: a retrospective cohort study. Drug Saf 2008;31(4): 325–34.

52. Bhardwaj SS, Chalasani N. Lipid-lowering agents that cause drug-induced hepatotoxicity. Clin Liver Dis 2007;11(3):597–613, vii.

53. Chavez E, Castro-Sanchez L, Shibayama M, et al. Effects of acetyl salycilic acid and ibuprofen in chronic liver damage induced by CCl4. J Appl Toxicol 2012; 32(1):51–9.

54. Brown SJ, Desmond PV. Hepatotoxicity of antimicrobial agents. Semin Liver Dis 2002;22(2):157–67.

55. Andrade RJ, Lucena MI, Kaplowitz N, et al. Outcome of acute idiosyncratic drug-induced liver injury: long-term follow-up in a hepatotoxicity registry. Hepatology 2006;44(6):1581–8.

56. Gundling F, Seidl H, Strassen I, et al. Clinical manifestations and treatment options in patients with cirrhosis and diabetes mellitus. Digestion 2013;87(2): 75–84.

57. Sembera S, Lammert C, Talwalkar JA, et al. Frequency, clinical presentation, and outcomes of drug-induced liver injury after liver transplantation. Liver Transpl 2012;18(7):803–10.

58. Wiesner RH, Fung JJ. Present state of immunosuppressive therapy in liver transplant recipients. Liver Transpl 2011;17(Suppl 3):S1–9.

59. Rostaing L, Saliba F, Calmus Y, et al. Review article: use of induction therapy in liver transplantation. Transplant Rev (Orlando) 2012;26(4):246–60.

60. Scott LJ, McKeage K, Keam SJ, et al. Tacrolimus: a further update of its use in the management of organ transplantation. Drugs 2003;63(12):1247–97.

61. Ceschi A, Rauber-Luthy C, Kupferschmidt H, et al. Acute calcineurin inhibitor overdose: analysis of cases reported to a national poison center between 1995 and 2011. Am J Transplant 2013;13(3):786–95.

62. Wu SW, Chang HR, Lai YR, et al. Non-life-threatening leukopenia in a renal transplant recipient with acute overdose of mycophenolate mofetil. Transplant Proc 2008;40(10):3770–1.

63. Bebarta VS, Heard K, Nadelson C. Lack of toxic effects following acute overdose of cellcept (mycophenolate mofetil). J Toxicol Clin Toxicol 2004;42(6): 917–9.

64. Kruger C, Jungert J, Schmitt-Grohe S, et al. Azathioprine ingestion with suicidal intent by an adolescent with chronic juvenile polyarthritis. Klin Padiatr 1998; 210(3):136–8 [in German].

65. Levitsky J. Next level of immunosuppression: drug/immune monitoring. Liver Transpl 2011;17(Suppl 3):S60–5.

66. Wallemacq P, Armstrong VW, Brunet M, et al. Opportunities to optimize tacrolimus therapy in solid organ transplantation: report of the European consensus conference. Ther Drug Monit 2009;31(2):139–52.

67. Madabushi R, Frank B, Drewelow B, et al. Hyperforin in St. John's wort drug interactions. Eur J Clin Pharmacol 2006;62(3):225–33.

68. Borcherding SM, Baciewicz AM, Self TH. Update on rifampin drug interactions. II. Arch Intern Med 1992;152(4):711–6.

69. Ruffmann C, Bogliun G, Beghi E. Epileptogenic drugs: a systematic review. Expert Rev Neurother 2006;6(4):575–89.

70. Bunnag S, Vareesangthip K, Ong-ajyooth L. Effect of diltiazem on the pharma-cokinetics of microemulsion cyclosporine A in renal transplantation. J Med Assoc Thai 2006;89(Suppl 2):S228–34.

71. Iwasaki K. Metabolism of tacrolimus (FK506) and recent topics in clinical phar-macokinetics. Drug Metab Pharmacokinet 2007;22(5):328–35.

72. McHutchison JG, Manns MP, Muir AJ, et al. Telaprevir for previously treated chronic HCV infection. N Engl J Med 2010;362(14):1292–303.

73. McHutchison JG, Everson GT, Gordon SC, et al. Telaprevir with peginterferon and ribavirin for chronic HCV genotype 1 infection. N Engl J Med 2009; 360(18):1827–38.

74. Poordad F, McCone J Jr, Bacon BR, et al. Boceprevir for untreated chronic HCV genotype 1 infection. N Engl J Med 2011;364(13):1195–206.

75. Bacon BR, Gordon SC, Lawitz E, et al. Boceprevir for previously treated chronic HCV genotype 1 infection. N Engl J Med 2011;364(13):1207–17.

76. Garg V, van Heeswijk R, Lee JE, et al. Effect of telaprevir on the pharmaco-kinetics of cyclosporine and tacrolimus. Hepatology 2011;54(1):20–7.

77. Hulskotte E, Gupta S, Xuan F, et al. Pharmacokinetic interaction between the hepatitis C virus protease inhibitor boceprevir and cyclosporine and tacrolimus in healthy volunteers. Hepatology 2012;56(5):1622–30.

78. Werner CR, Egetemeyr DP, Lauer UM, et al. Telaprevir-based triple therapy in liver transplant patients with hepatitis C virus: a 12-week pilot study providing safety and efficacy data. Liver Transpl 2012;18(12):1464–70.

79. Pungpapong S, Aqel BA, Koning L, et al. Multicenter experience using telaprevir or boceprevir with peginterferon and ribavirin to treat hepatitis C genotype 1 after liver transplantation. Liver Transpl 2013;19(7):690–700.

80. Yong TY, Lau SY, Li JY, et al. Medication prescription among elderly patients admitted through an acute assessment unit. Geriatr Gerontol Int 2012;12(1): 93–101.

81. Aithal GP, Watkins PB, Andrade RJ, et al. Case definition and phenotype stan-dardization in drug-induced liver injury. Clin Pharmacol Ther 2011;89(6):806–15.

82. Fontana RJ, Watkins PB, Bonkovsky HL, et al. Drug-Induced Liver Injury Network (DILIN) prospective study: rationale, design and conduct. Drug Saf 2009;32(1):55–68.

83. Hassan Q, Roche B, Buffet C, et al. Liver-kidney recipients with chronic viral hepatitis C treated with interferon-alpha. Transpl Int 2012;25(9):941–7.

84. Suzuki Y, Ikeda K, Suzuki F, et al. Dual oral therapy with daclatasvir and asunap-revir for patients with HCV genotype 1b infection and limited treatment options. J Hepatol 2013;58(4):655–62.

85. Fontana RJ, Hughes EA, Appelman H, et al. Case report of successful peginter-feron, ribavirin, and daclatasvir therapy for recurrent cholestatic hepatitis C after liver retransplantation. Liver Transpl 2012;18(9):1053–9.

# How to Avoid Being Surprised by Hepatotoxicity at the Final Stages of Drug Development and Approval

Arie Regev, MD

## KEYWORDS

• Drug-induced liver injury • Hy's Law • Causality assessment • Drug development

## KEY POINTS

- Despite ongoing efforts to develop preclinical approaches and biomarkers that would help in predicting the risk of idiosyncratic drug-induced live injury (DILI) in earlier phases of drug development, such approaches and biomarkers are not yet ready for prime time.
- Data pertaining to milder liver injury occurring during clinical development, when assessed correctly, may enhance our ability to predict the potential of the drug to cause severe liver injury after marketing.
- Although increase of alanine aminotransferase (ALT) levels is a sensitive marker for hepatocellular DILI, the specificity of such an increase is low, and it is generally considered a poor predictor of severe hepatotoxicity.
- The most specific indicator during a clinical trial for a drug's potential to cause severe DILI is occurrence of cases of drug induced hepatocellular injury accompanied by evidence of altered liver function (elevated direct bilirubin level or prolonged PT-INR).
- High increases in ALT level and increases accompanied by signs of hypersensitivity or symptoms of liver injury may also have some predictive value, and should be taken seriously.
- Meticulous causality assessment of individual hepatic cases and adherence to predetermined discontinuation rules are critical to a timely and thorough understanding of the hepatic safety profile of the drug.

## INTRODUCTION

Drug-induced live injury (DILI) has been a major cause of drug withdrawal, nonapproval, and regulatory action in the last 50 years. In most cases, drugs that caused severe DILI did so infrequently and unexpectedly, in a manner consistent with idiosyncratic DILI. Most of the drugs withdrawn from the market for hepatotoxicity have caused liver failure

Global Patient Safety, Eli Lilly and Company, Lilly Corporate Center, Indiana University School of Medicine, Drop Code 2121, Indianapolis, IN 46285, USA
E-mail address: regev_arie@lilly.com

Clin Liver Dis 17 (2013) 749–767
http://dx.doi.org/10.1016/j.cld.2013.07.014
1089-3261/13/$ – see front matter © 2013 Elsevier Inc. All rights reserved.

liver.theclinics.com

leading to death or transplantation at frequencies lower than 1 per 10,000. Consequently, most drug development databases, which typically include up to a few thousand subjects, have not shown any cases of severe liver injury, even when the drug was later found to have a high potential of causing DILI. Despite intensive research and development efforts, there are no specific biomarkers that can accurately predict idiosyncratic DILI in preclinical or clinical phases of drug development.[1] In addition, most drugs that were later found to cause severe DILI, did not show any clear unequivocal signals in preclinical studies.[2] In most cases, drugs that caused severe DILI in humans have not shown hepatotoxicity in animals and have not shown clear predictive signals in cell cultures. Preclinical studies have been more useful in detecting overtly hepatotoxic agents that cause dose-related DILI (eg, carbon tetrachloride, chloroform, methylene chloride). As a result, drugs that cause such predictable and dose-related injury generally are discovered and rejected in preclinical testing.[2] In contrast, identifying drugs that cause idiosyncratic DILI during drug development remains a major challenge, because this type of DILI seems to depend not only on the administered drug but on individual susceptibility of affected patients, which has not yet been well characterized. Nevertheless, in the last 3 decades, it has become increasingly clear that meticulous collection and evaluation of clinical trial data during drug development may uncover evidence and signals of the potential of a drug to cause severe DILI, even in the absence of cases of severe DILI.

DILI may mimic almost any known liver disease.[3,4] Of the many clinicopathologic types of DILI, acute hepatocellular injury has been associated with most of the significant hepatotoxic drugs.[2] Although there are a few exceptions, hepatocellular DILI typically tends to progress more rapidly and has a higher tendency to lead to liver failure and death compared with other types. Furthermore, most (although not all) of the cases of drug withdrawal and nonapproval in the last 50 years have been related to hepatocellular DILI. As a result, efforts to identify and predict DILI have largely been directed at this type of injury. This review focuses on the recommended approaches to data collection and assessment during clinical phases of drug development, which are aimed at predicting the potential of a drug to cause severe idiosyncratic DILI.

## HISTORICAL PERSPECTIVE

In several well-documented cases of drugs associated with DILI, hepatotoxic drugs were identified after being approved by regulators and marketed for several months or years. For example: ticrynafen (tienilic acid), a loop diuretic, was approved by the US Food and Drug Administration (FDA) on May 2, 1979 for the treatment of hypertension. During the months after its approval, several hundreds of cases of liver injury were reported to the manufacturer.[5,6] A retrospective analysis of 340 of these cases showed that most of them presented with hepatocellular injury and jaundice. Jaundice was recorded in 246 of 287 patients with sufficient clinical information, and about 10% of the patients who had jaundice died.[6] Ticrynafen was withdrawn from the US market in 1980.

Bromfenac is a nonsteroidal antiinflammatory drug, which was approved by the FDA in July, 1997 for short-term use. During the months after its approval, the drug maker and the FDA received numerous reports of liver injury and hepatic failure, including fatal cases and cases requiring liver transplantation. In most cases, patients who suffered hepatotoxicity had taken the medication for longer than the recommended 10-day period. A few of these cases were reported in the medical literature.[7–10] Bromfenac was withdrawn from the market in June, 1998, 11 months after its approval.

Troglitazone was approved by the FDA in January, 1997 for the treatment of type 2 diabetes mellitus. After marketing, the drug maker and the FDA received numerous reports of severe liver injury associated with troglitazone use, and several reports of acute liver failure caused by troglitazone were published in the medical literature.[11–13] Troglitazone was withdrawn from the US market in March, 2000. A retrospective analysis of the combined North American clinical trials of troglitazone, revealed that increases in serum alanine aminotransferase (ALT) concentrations to more than 3 times the upper limit of normal (ULN) were detected in 1.9% of the troglitazone-treated patients and in 0.6% of the patients given placebo (**Table 1**).[14] Treatment was discontinued because of abnormal liver chemistry in 20 troglitazone-treated patients (0.8%) and in no placebo-treated patients. Twelve of these 20 patients had peak serum ALT levels of more than 10 times the ULN, and 5 had levels of more than 20 times the ULN. In all 20 patients in whom therapy was discontinued, serum ALT levels returned to baseline. None of the placebo-treated patients had reached ALT levels of 10 or 20 times the ULN. The onset of the increases in serum ALT level was typically delayed; in most patients, the peak values occurred between the third and seventh months. Two troglitazone-treated patients (and no placebo-treated patients) had ALT levels increase to more than 3 times the ULN and concomitant increase in total bilirubin (TBL) level to more than 2 times the ULN, which was believed to be drug-related, consistent with the definition of Hy's Law cases (see **Table 1**).[14]

In other cases of hepatotoxic drugs, DILI has led to nonapproval or abandonment of drug development during the last phases of drug development or final stages of new-drug application (NDA). Delevalol is a nonselective β adrenoreceptor antagonist, which was developed for treatment of hypertension. Clinical trials showed 2 Hy's Law cases[2] in about 1000 exposures. The NDA was filed in 1986, but the manufacturer subsequently withdrew the application and discontinued the registration and marketing program worldwide because of these cases, as well as other clinical trial DILI cases, and cases discovered after approval in Portugal and Japan.[15]

In 2006, the manufacturer of ximalagatran, an oral anticoagulant (antithrombin), withdrew a pending application to the FDA for marketing approval because of reports of abnormal liver tests and DILI occurring during clinical trials.[16,17] Review of the clinical trial data showed that 7.9% of patients receiving ximelagatran had ALT level increase to more than 3 times ULN, compared with 1.2% of the comparator group. Combined increases of ALT level of more than 3 times ULN and TBL level of more than 2 times ULN, regardless of cause, were observed in 37 patients (0.5%) treated with ximelagatran. Eleven of these patients were found to have no alternative cause for liver injury. One of these patients sustained severe liver damage with liver failure and died.[17] At the time of withdrawal of pending application to the FDA, the drug had already been approved in several European and South American countries,

| Table 1 Combined results of North American clinical studies with troglitazone | | |
|---|---|---|
| | **Troglitazone** | **Placebo** |
| Total number of subjects | 2510 | 475 |
| Any ALT increase | ↑↑ | ↑↑↑ |
| ALT >3 × ULN | 48 (1.9%) | 3 (0.6%) |
| ALT >15 × ULN | 10 | 0 |
| ALT >20 × ULN | 5 | 0 |
| Hy's law levels | 2 | 0 |

*Data from* Watkins PB, Whitcomb RW. Hepatic dysfunction associated with troglitazone. N Engl J Med 1998;338:916–7.

including Germany, Portugal, Sweden, Finland, Norway, Iceland, Austria, Denmark, France, Switzerland, Argentina, and Brazil.

## SIGNALS OF DILI DURING DRUG DEVELOPMENT
### Hepatic Injury Versus Adaptation

Individuals who are exposed to a new drug or chemical may generally be divided into 3 main groups based on the pattern of their hepatic response.[18]

### Tolerators

In most cases of drug ingestion, there are no significant changes in hepatic biochemical tests. ALT and aspartate aminotransferase (AST) remain within the patient's baseline levels or close to them and the patient remains asymptomatic. This group, which typically includes the vast majority of the patients, has been dubbed tolerators. Typically, these patients tolerate the drug well throughout the treatment and do not develop DILI related to this specific drug.

### Adapters

Another group may show transient increases in ALT and AST levels, which eventually return to baseline levels despite continuation of the drug (**Fig. 1**). During the last 3 decades, it has become increasingly apparent that intransient increase in ALT and AST levels occurs commonly during the first few months of exposure to a new drug and, in most cases, constitutes a poor predictor of the potential of the drug to cause DILI. This phenomenon has been called adaptation, and patients showing these changes have been dubbed adapters.[18] Although adaptation has been described with some drugs (eg, isoniazid) even after significant liver injury had developed,[18–20] in its clean form, it typically involves transient increases in ALT and AST levels, which are usually asymptomatic and not accompanied by signs of decreased liver function (eg, jaundice, increased direct bilirubin level, prolonged prothrombin time [PT] or increased international normalized ratio [INR]). The mechanism behind adaptation remains unclear. It may represent true mild liver injury with spontaneous resolution[21] or may have another underlying mechanism, but it does not represent clinically important liver injury. Changes in aminotransferases (ATs) consistent with adaptation occur with numerous drugs, many of which are rarely if ever associated with clinically significant DILI, such as hydroxyl-methylglutaryl coenzyme A-reductase inhibitors (statins), aspirin,

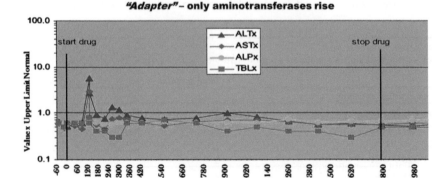

**Fig. 1.** Time course of liver tests in an adapter exposed to a new drug.

heparin,[22–24] tacrine,[25] and others.[2] In some individuals exposed to heparin, increased ALT and AST levels have been shown to be accompanied by changes in other biomarkers, such as sorbitol dehydrogenase, glutamate dehydrogenase, and micro RNA-122, indicating high likelihood of true liver injury[21]; however, these patients invariably adapted to the drug and did not develop any signs or symptoms of clinically significant hepatic injury. Based on growing experience with adapters, it looks like they typically do not experience DILI related to the specific drug to which they adapted.

The frequency and magnitude of ALT and AST changes occurring during adaptation vary between individual drugs. Higher frequency of increase in AT level, although deserving of full attention during drug development, does not point against the possibility of adaptation. Of the patients receiving heparin, about 15% would develop increases in ALT level to more than 3 times ULN; however, there have been no reliable reports of serious DILI in association with this drug. In patients receiving tacrine, about 25% showed increase in ALT level to more than 3 times the ULN, whereas about 2% showed increase to more than 20 times ULN. Nevertheless, no patient had increase of TBL level to more than 2 times ULN, and no one experienced liver dysfunction.[24,25]

### Susceptibles

The third group of patients experience, after receiving a new drug, a progressive increase in AT level, which continues increasing while they are on the drug and evolves into clinically significant liver injury. This injury is often accompanied by symptoms such as fatigue, nausea, vomiting, right upper quadrant pain or tenderness, and in some cases, fever, rash, or eosinophilia. Occasionally, these patients may show signs of decreased liver function, such as jaundice, increased direct bilirubin levels, or prolonged PT, and some progress to overt liver failure. This group has been dubbed susceptibles, and is the main focus of endeavors to identify and predict idiosyncratic DILI during drug development.

Although for some drugs, only 1 or 2 of the 3 groups may exist (for example, only tolerators and adapters have been well described for heparin and tacrine[23–25]). For many drugs, all 3 groups may be found, and the difference between safe drugs and those that are considered less safe to the liver may depend on the relative frequency of tolerators, adapters, and susceptibles. For example, statins are considered safe to the liver, although rare cases of susceptible patients with severe DILI have been described. On the other hand, isoniazid is considered hepatotoxic, because it causes clinically significant DILI, in about 0.5% to 1% of patients and severe DILI, with acute liver failure, in about 1 in 1000.[26] In many cases, drugs that are considered safe to the liver and hepatotoxic drugs are on a continuum, in which the former are associated with rare cases of susceptibles who develop severe DILI (generally, safer drugs are associated with DILI in <1 per million cases) and the latter are associated with higher frequency of susceptibles who develop severe DILI (typically >1 per 10,000).

Because benign reversible increase in ALT and AST levels occurs frequently during the first months of exposure, it is critical to differentiate between self-limiting increases in AT level, which represent adaptation, and significant hepatic injury, which may indicate a potential of the drug to cause severe liver injury. The following are considered warning signs that may suggest that the abnormality in AT is associated with clinically significant hepatic injury:

1. Symptoms suggestive of clinically significant liver injury such as:
   a. Right upper abdominal pain, right upper abdominal discomfort or tenderness
   b. Worsening fatigue or malaise
   c. Jaundice
   d. Nausea or vomiting

2. Symptoms or laboratory changes suggestive of hypersensitivity-type reaction such as:
   a. Rash
   b. Fever
   c. Lymphadenopathy
   d. Eosinophilia
3. Signs or laboratory changes suggestive of decreased liver function or liver failure, such as:
   a. A significant increase in serum bilirubin level, not accompanied by cholestasis (ie, increased alkaline phosphatase [ALP] levels)
   b. Ascites
   c. Hepatic encephalopathy
   d. Increased PT or INR

The appearance of any one of these signs or symptoms should be taken seriously, and should prompt a thorough discussion on whether or not the study drug should be discontinued. An important part of this discussion should focus on the likelihood that the study drug is the cause of the observed manifestations (see later discussion). This discussion should optimally take place before the decision on discontinuation has been finalized.

### ALT Increase Versus Hy's Law During Drug Development

ALT is a sensitive marker for hepatocellular DILI; however, as discussed earlier, the finding of a higher rate of ALT increases in drug-treated individuals than in a control group is a nonspecific signal of a potential to cause severe DILI. ALT increase is therefore a necessary, but not sufficient, signal of the potential of the drug to cause severe hepatocellular DILI. For other types of DILI, such as drug-induced cholestasis (as seen with drugs such as amoxicillin clavulanate),[27] mitochondrial toxicity (eg, fialuridine),[28] or hepatic steatosis/fibrosis (eg, methotrexate),[29] ALT is a less sensitive marker than it is for hepatocellular DILI.

As mentioned earlier, high frequency of increases in serum AT level during a clinical trial also is not a good indicator of a potential for severe DILI.[25] High levels of ALT (eg, >10 × ULN or >15 × ULN) may be a better indicator, but still carry less than optimal specificity for prediction of severe DILI.[2]

The most specific indicator during a clinical trial for a potential of the drug to cause severe DILI is occurrence of cases of drug-induced hepatocellular injury (increased AT level) accompanied by evidence of altered liver function, such as increased serum TBL level, prolonged PT, or increased INR.

The combination of increased AT level equal to or higher than 3 times the ULN and increased serum TBL equal to higher than 2 times the ULN, not explained by any other cause, in the absence of evidence of cholestasis, has been dubbed Hy's Law after Hymann Zimmerman.[30] The significance of this combination was based on Zimmerman's observation that drug-induced hepatocellular injury (ie, increased ALT level) accompanied by jaundice had a poor prognosis, with more than 10% mortality from acute liver failure without liver transplantation.[31] The explanation for this outcome has been that hepatocellular injury that is sufficient to cause jaundice or even mild hyperbilirubinemia (ie, a bilirubin level >2 × ULN) represents an extent of liver injury so great that recovery may not be possible in some cases. Concomitant increase of ALT to more than 3 × ULN and TBL to more than 2 × ULN during a clinical trial has been used by the FDA to identify drugs likely to be capable of causing severe liver injury.[2] Drugs that cause such injury during drug development raise serious concerns about liver safety in the postmarketing phase, when more patients are exposed to the drug.[32] Furthermore, Hy's Law allows for a rough estimation of the rate of severe DILI likely to occur after marketing, which is roughly one-tenth the rate of Hy's Law cases observed during clinical development.[2] In the last decade, Hy's Law has gained support from 2 population-based studies. In 1 study, Bjornsson and Olsson[33] found a mortality or transplantation rate of 9.2% in patients with hepatocellular DILI who had concomitant TBL level greater than or equal to 2 times the ULN. Similarly, Andrade and colleagues[34] found a mortality of 11.7% among patients with suspected DILI and concomitant jaundice.[34] Both studies offer support to the notion that hepatocellular DILI with jaundice or hyperbilirubinemia is a serious entity, with a potentially severe outcome.

To define a clinical trial subject as a Hy's Law case, the following 4 components need to be present.[2,30]

1. ALT increase to a level equal to or higher than 3 times ULN
2. TBL increase to a level equal to or higher than 2 times ULN
3. No significant increase of ALP (initial ALP value does not reach 2 times ULN)
4. No other cause is found to explain the liver injury, such as viral hepatitis A, B, C, or E; autoimmune hepatitis; acute gallstone disease, alcoholic liver disease; congestive heart failure or another drug that is known to cause the observed injury

The following considerations are important in the assessment of suspected cases of Hy's Law:

The Hy's Law criteria outlined above pertain to patients who had normal or near normal liver tests at baseline. Because one of the criteria for Hy's Law is absence of a coexisting liver disease, there are no universally accepted criteria equivalent to Hy's Law for patients who had abnormal liver tests at baseline.

Hy's Law cases typically appear on a background of several cases of increases in ALT level to more than 3 times ULN (see later discussion on evaluation of drug-induced serious hepatotoxicity). Generally, a drug that causes hepatocellular DILI is likely to show a higher incidence of 3-fold or greater increases in ALT level above the ULN than placebo or a comparator, assuming that the comparator does not itself cause increases in ALT level. A case that meets the 4 Hy's Law criteria but is not accompanied by increased incidence of increased ALT level should be viewed with suspicion, because it is unlikely to be drug induced.

Based on the FDA guidance from 2009: "Finding one Hy's Law case in the clinical trial database is worrisome; finding two is considered highly predictive that the drug has the potential to cause severe DILI when given to a larger population."[2]

Hy's Law cases were observed in clinical trials with delevalol, tasosartan, ximelagatran, and troglitazone, which were either abandoned or withdrawn from the market because of DILI.[2,14,17]

## ORGANIZATION AND ANALYSIS OF HEPATIC SAFETY DATA
### Evaluation of Drug-induced Serious Hepatotoxicity

Because the most reliable and specific biomarker for DILI prediction is the concomitant increase of serum ALT and serum TBL levels, there is a great advantage to an efficient and comprehensive approach to monitoring and assessment of concomitant changes in ALT and TBL levels during a clinical trial. Modern phase 3 clinical trials may have many thousands of data points related to liver tests. Such data are often difficult to visualize and assess. The potential difficulty is increased by the need for an in-depth case-by-case analysis of patients with treatment-emergent hepatic abnormalities.

An efficient method to visualize, assess, and summarize ALT and TBL levels in a clinical trial is the recently introduced evaluation of drug-induced serious hepatotoxicity (eDISH), which was developed by Guo and Senior at the FDA to allow medical reviewers to display the peak serum ALT and TBL values for every individual in a clinical trial (**Fig. 2**).[35] eDISH allows each point in the display to be directly linked to each individual's clinical and laboratory data for a full evaluation of the clinical picture and history related to the hepatic abnormality. It is being used by FDA medical reviewers when evaluating liver safety databases from phase 3 clinical trials, and is gradually being adopted by drug makers in the United States and Europe. It may be useful in presenting liver safety data to FDA-appointed Advisory Committees.[36]

On the eDISH plot, the peak serum ALT level is shown along the x-axis, and the peak serum TBL level is shown along the y-axis as multiples of the ULN on log scales (see **Fig. 2**). Four quadrants are defined by a line corresponding to 3 times the ULN for serum ALT and a line corresponding to twice the ULN for TBL.

The right upper quadrant includes all individuals with serum ALT level greater than 3 × ULN and serum TBL greater than 2 × ULN. This quadrant is referred to as "Hy's Law range." ALT level >3 × ULN and TBL level >2 × ULN are only 2 of the 4 criteria for the definition of a Hy's Law case. The ability to use the specific point on the eDISH plot as a link to the rest of the individual's clinical data is helpful in allowing assessment of the other 2 criteria (initial ALP level <2 × ULN, and no other cause explaining the hepatic injury). Furthermore, when true Hy's Law cases are present, there should be a higher incidence of ALT increases greater than 3 × ULN in the drug-treated individuals relative to individuals treated with the comparator, assuming that the comparator does not itself cause increased ALT levels.

The right lower quadrant shows individuals who had increases in ALT level to more than 3 × ULN without increases of TBL to >2 × ULN. This quadrant has been labeled Temple's Corollary, reflecting an observation first made by Dr Robert Temple of the FDA that an imbalance in this quadrant between those subjects treated with study drug and those treated with placebo (or a nonhepatotoxic comparator) has been reliably present with drugs capable of causing serious liver injury.[2] As discussed earlier, an imbalance of increase in ALT level between treatment and comparator does not in

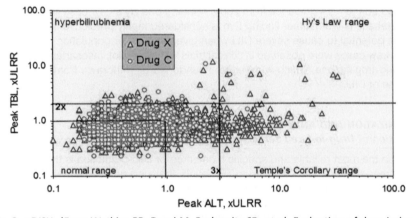

**Fig. 2.** eDISH. (*From* Watkins PB, Desai M, Berkowitz SD, et al. Evaluation of drug-induced serious hepatotoxicity (eDISH) application of this data organization approach to phase III clinical trials of rivaroxaban after total hip or knee replacement surgery. Drug Saf 2011;34(3):247; with permission.)

itself constitute a clear liver safety signal, because ALT level is often increased in drugs that rarely if ever cause severe liver injury.

The left upper quadrant has been labeled hyperbilirubinemia or cholestasis quadrant. It represents individuals with TBL levels greater than 2 × ULN along with ALT levels less than 3 × ULN. An overrepresentation of points on study drug would be expected in this quadrant for drugs that are associated with cholestatic liver injury.

The left lower quadrant represents individuals who never showed ALT levels greater than 3 times the ULN or TBL levels greater than twice the ULN.

eDISH seems to be an effective method to visualize, summarize, and assess hepatic safety data during randomized controlled clinical trials. It may be instrumental in identifying drugs with a potential to cause severe DILI after marketing.

## HEPATIC DISCONTINUATION RULES AND THEIR IMPORTANCE FOR ASSESSMENT OF HEPATIC SAFETY PROFILE DURING DRUG DEVELOPMENT

In most DILI cases, the only effective treatment is discontinuation of the causal agent. Delayed discontinuation may occasionally lead to worsening of the liver injury, which may result in liver failure and death. On the other hand, automatic discontinuation of a trial drug on finding of a mild abnormality in liver enzymes (eg, increase of ALT or AST levels to >3 × ULN) is not only unnecessary but may render it impossible to differentiate between drugs that cause benign self-limiting increases in AT level and those that may cause a clinically significant liver injury.[2] The correct timing of discontinuation of an investigational drug when faced with abnormal liver tests has been a matter of debate, and in the absence of systematic and prospective studies addressing this question, drug makers and regulators have suggested arbitrary hepatic stopping rules. In general, although early discontinuation of the drug may better protect individuals in a study from a rare DILI event, it may lead to failure to identify the potential of the drug to cause severe DILI, and consequently may lead to an increased risk of DILI after marketing.

As discussed earlier, most patients who show mild increases of AT level are likely to adapt to the drug despite continued exposure. Stopping a drug at the first hint of increased ALT or AST levels precludes the drug maker from learning whether adaptation occurs. Furthermore, regulators may justifiably be reluctant to approve marketing of a drug that was repeatedly discontinued at low increases in ALT level during clinical development. Under these circumstances, regulators may prefer to prevent exposure of a larger population, which is typically less closely monitored and less likely to be identified as DILI.

Based on these considerations, the FDA has suggested the following discontinuation rules for drugs in clinical phases of development.[2]

- ALT or AST level greater than 8 × ULN
- ALT or AST level greater than 5 × ULN for more than 2 weeks
- ALT or AST level greater than 3 × ULN and (TBL >2 × ULN or INR >1.5)
- ALT or AST level greater than 3 × ULN with the appearance of fatigue, nausea, vomiting, right upper quadrant pain or tenderness, fever, rash, or eosinophilia (>5%)

The decision on whether or not a study drug should be discontinued, when hepatic abnormalities reach these levels, may be influenced by several considerations. First, when applying these discontinuation rules, it is assumed that the study drug is the cause of abnormal hepatic tests. Discontinuation of the study drug may not be necessary if the abnormality is caused by an intercurrent viral hepatitis, a concomitantly administered drug, or gallstones. Consequently, a timely and comprehensive causality assessment (discussed later) may help prevent an unnecessary early discontinuation of the study drug. Second, when recommending these specific discontinuation rules, the FDA assumed that the patient's baseline hepatic tests levels were either within or close to normal levels. For study patients who are enrolled with abnormal tests because of an underlying hepatic or systemic disorder, discontinuation rules may need to be adjusted. Third, the decision on whether to discontinue the drug or not may be influenced by our knowledge of the probability of effect of the drug, and the potential importance of that effect to the patient's health. An investigator may be less inclined to discontinue a drug that has a high likelihood of saving the patient's life (eg, an anticancer drug) than a drug that has no proven benefit.

Clinical trial investigators who are not experienced with hepatic disorders or DILI may tend to discontinue the drug long before the hepatic abnormalities meet the FDA's recommended discontinuation rules. Drug makers often need to use intensive guidance and training, and maintain close communication with their clinical trial investigators, to prevent unnecessary early discontinuation. The importance of such training and close communication cannot be overemphasized.

## CAUSALITY ASSESSMENT FOR SUSPECTED DILI DURING DRUG DEVELOPMENT

Causality assessment is a critical component in the process of understanding the hepatic safety profile of a drug and predicting its potential to cause severe DILI. Causality assessment for suspected DILI is still a major challenge in clinical practice and even more so during drug development. In contrast to many other liver disorders, there is no specific biomarker or a combination of tests that can establish the diagnosis of DILI and differentiate it from other causes of liver injury. Furthermore, DILI may resemble almost any type of liver disease.[37] The diagnosis of DILI is therefore almost always presumptive, because it is based on clinical assessment and exclusion of other possible causes rather than on absolute criteria and specific diagnostic tests. Abnormal hepatic biochemical tests may be caused by many liver diseases as well as extrahepatic disorders (**Box 1**), most of which (eg, viral hepatitis, alcoholic liver

---

**Box 1**
**Alternative causes of abnormal hepatic biochemical tests**

Hepatitis viruses A,B,C,D,E

Other infectious agents (cytomegalovirus, Epstein-Barr virus, herpes simplex virus)

Alcoholic liver disease

Nonalcoholic fatty liver disease and nonalcoholic steatohepatitis

Autoimmune hepatitis

Ischemic hepatopathy

Congestive heart failure

Systemic infection/sepsis

Wilson disease

Primary or secondary hepatic tumors

Gallstone disease

Vascular disorder (Budd-Chiari, portal vein thrombosis)

disease, gallstone disease) are considerably more common than is typical DILI. It is therefore critical to exclude other liver diseases before attributing a liver injury to a drug. Exclusion of other causes requires detailed information pertaining to the patient's clinical course and laboratory data. Failure to evaluate the patient for other causes may result in omission of critical information, and may lead to erroneously attributing a liver injury to a study drug.

### Causality Assessment Methods

There are 2 types of approaches to causality assessment for suspected DILI: approaches that rely on expert opinion and those that rely on scoring instruments such as the Roussel Uclaf Causality Assessment Method (RUCAM),[38] and the Maria and Victorino method (M&V),[39] which attempt to standardize the process of causality assessment and increase its objectivity.

#### Causality assessment based on expert opinion

Causality assessment by expert opinion is considered more reliable than the standardized instruments[40]; however, it requires specific expertise in the fields of liver disease and DILI, which is not always readily available. It is based largely on detailed clinical evaluation and is focused on 4 major components: (1) compatible clinical course, including typical time to onset and time to resolution, typical changes in hepatic biochemical tests, and compatible extrahepatic manifestations; (2) exclusion of all other reasonable causes, including but not limited to viral hepatitis, alcoholic liver disease, gallstone-related disorders, autoimmune hepatitis, metabolic and inherited liver diseases, and DILI related to a concomitant drug; (3) resemblance of clinical and pathologic features to known features of liver injury related to the drug in question (also called the drug signature); and (4) increased DILI incidence in patients treated with the drug compared with control or nonhepatotoxic comparators. A new drug candidate in clinical development often lacks data pertaining to the last 2 components, which renders causality assessment more complicated. Nevertheless, some data pertaining to the drug signature may be gleaned during a clinical trial from careful review of hepatic biochemical changes in milder cases of liver injury.

Despite its many advantages, causality assessment based on expert opinion is largely subjective, and suffers from interobserver variance.[40] Furthermore, the use of this approach requires the availability of hepatology experts, which is not always feasible. Under optimal circumstances during drug development, this type of assessment should be performed by hepatology experts. At a minimum, it is advisable to use hepatology experts for causality assessment in more severe cases of liver injury, such as cases with increased ALT levels to more than 3 × ULN with increased TBL levels to more than 2 × ULN, or cases with liver failure. When using expert opinion to assess hepatic cases, it is probably advantageous to use at least 3 experts to increase the chances of a majority opinion, especially in cases of serious liver injury. In general, each expert should perform causality assessment independently, and each expert should be blinded to treatment assignment when feasible. Discrepant scores between reviewers can be resolved through subsequent communications to achieve consensus, or at least a majority opinion.

#### Causality assessment based on standardized instruments

In an attempt to standardize the process of causality assessment for liver injury and achieve an objective assessment, 2 causality assessment instruments were developed. Despite some advantages, these instruments have several shortcomings, which limit their accuracy and restrict their routine use during drug development. Of the

2 instruments, the RUCAM is the most well recognized and is considered superior to the M&V method.[27] RUCAM was developed in 1989 by a group of experts at the request of the Council for International Organizations of Medical Sciences. It is based on 7 criteria, which may receive scores ranging from −3 to +3. The total score for acute liver injury can range between −7 and +14. The final score is classified into 5 categories of relatedness: when the score is equal to or less than 0, the relationship is classified as excluded; 1–2, unlikely; 3–5, possible; 6–8, probable; more than 8, highly probable.[38]

In a study by the Drug Induced Liver Injury Network (DILIN),[40] which assessed the reliability of RUCAM in well-defined cases of hepatotoxicity, RUCAM was found to have low test-retest reliability (0.54), and low interrater reliability (0.45). The investigators concluded that RUCAM had mediocre reliability, which was problematic for future DILI studies. They suggested that alternative methods, including modification of the RUCAM, developing drug-specific instruments, or causality assessment based on expert opinion, may be more appropriate.[40]

When used in the setting of clinical trials for new drugs, RUCAM has additional limitations:

1. RUCAM relies heavily on response to readministration (rechallenge) of the drug after resolution of liver injury. Although this may be justified in specific circumstances in clinical practice (eg, when a clear benefit of the drug is established, and the risk-benefit is favorable), rechallenge is not recommended under most circumstances pertaining to clinical trials.[41]
2. RUCAM requires previous information on the typical features of liver injury related to the drug (drug signature), which is often lacking in clinical trials, especially in early phases.
3. RUCAM includes pregnancy and excessive alcohol consumption as potential risk factors for DILI, but both pregnancy and excessive alcohol drinking are considered exclusion criteria for most clinical trials. Furthermore, the role of these conditions as general risk factors for DILI has not been clearly established.

Consequently, RUCAM, in its present form, may not be suitable for causality assessment in clinical trials. There is a great need for a systematic revision of RUCAM that renders it more suitable for the setting of clinical trials and drug development.

### Causality assessment scales

The use of an appropriate causality assessment scale is critical for complete assessment of treatment-emergent cases of liver injury, and full understanding of the hepatic safety profile of the drug in development. The DILIN has defined categories based on percent likelihood (**Table 2**),[10] which may be helpful in further defining the association, particularly by nonhepatologists. These categories range from definite to unlikely.

The definite category requires a typical temporal relationship with no competing diagnosis. The event should fit a pattern (signature) of liver hepatic biochemistry abnormality observed in other patients treated with the study drug but not the comparator.

The highly likely category requires a convincing temporal relationship and no competing diagnosis.

The probable category requires a temporal relationship considered to be compatible with drug-related injury, with no competing causes or, if competing causes are present, they should be considered less likely than is injury from the study drug.

In the possible category, there is at least 1 other reasonable diagnosis that is more likely than the drug to be the cause of liver injury.

| Table 2 | | |
| --- | --- | --- |
| Causality assessment scoring based on the DILIN prospective study | | |
| Causality Score | Likelihood (%) | Description |
| 1 = definite | >95 | Liver injury is typical for the drug or herbal product (signature or pattern of injury, timing of onset, recovery). The evidence for causality is beyond a reasonable doubt |
| 2 = highly likely | 75–95 | The evidence for causality is clear and convincing but not definite |
| 3 = probable | 50–74 | The causality is supported by the preponderance of evidence as implicating the drug but the evidence cannot be considered definite or highly likely |
| 4 = possible | 25–49 | The causality is not supported by the preponderance of evidence; however, the possibility cannot be definitively excluded |
| 5 = unlikely | <25 | The evidence for causality is highly unlikely based on the available information |
| Insufficient data | Not applicable | Key elements of the drug exposure history, initial presentation, alternative diagnoses, or diagnostic evaluation prevent determination of a causality score |

*From* Fontana RJ, Watkins PB, Bonkovsky HL, et al. Drug-Induced Liver Injury Network (DILIN) prospective study: rationale, design and conduct. Drug Saf 2009;32(1):55–68; with permission.

In the unlikely category, the temporal relationship is atypical for DILI, or another cause is considered to be responsible for the reaction.

The indeterminate or unassessable category is reserved for cases that have insufficient data to arrive at a reasonable causality assessment.

The 5-category scale has been favored by DILIN and other academic investigators. However, several drug makers have preferred the use of a 3-category scale, namely unlikely, possible, and probable (**Table 3**), for the following reasons: (1) cases recorded during drug development are often not as completely evaluated as are DILIN cases and it is rarely possible to reach the same granularity in causality classification as DILIN with the data available to drug makers. Therefore, it is often impossible, to differentiate between probable, highly likely, and definite. (2) From the regulatory perspective, there is generally no significant difference in the approach toward cases that are classified as probable versus those that are classified as highly likely or definite. (3) The differentiation between probable, highly likely, and definite requires reviewers with competence in the fields of liver disease and knowledge of DILI. In many cases, the level of proficiency among assessors of causality in pharmaceutical companies may not be as high as that of DILIN investigators, and the differentiation between probable, highly likely, and definite may not be a realistic expectation for these assessors. (4) From the statistical standpoint, the 5-category classification system may be viewed as an unbalanced rating scale, because it consists of more high categories than low categories. Although this type of scale may be suitable for studies such as that of DILIN, it may introduce a potential bias when used during drug development. Scales that are balanced toward higher categories are more likely to provoke an apparently higher response level.[42,43] The unbalanced 5-category scale might therefore provoke higher causality assessment responses, which may lead to skewed assessments, especially when used by nonexperts. Although formal recommendations are lacking, it may be preferable for pharmaceutical companies to use a

**Table 3**
**A 3-category causality assessment scale for possible DILI**

| Causality Score | Likelihood (%) | Description |
|---|---|---|
| 1 = probable | 50–100 | The causality is supported by the preponderance of evidence, and the drug is more likely than not to be the causal agent. Other likely causes have been ruled out with appropriate tests |
| 2 = possible | 25–49 | The causality is not supported by the preponderance of evidence; however, the possibility cannot definitively be excluded. Another cause is more likely to be the cause of liver injury |
| 3 = unlikely | <25 | The evidence for causality is highly unlikely based on the available information. Another cause is likely to be the cause of abnormal hepatic biochemical tests |
| Insufficient data | Not applicable | Key elements of the drug exposure history, initial presentation, alternative diagnoses, or diagnostic evaluation prevent determination of a causality score |

3-category scale (probable, possible, unlikely) for causality assessment during drug development.

### Critical Data for Causality Assessment During Drug Development

The following data should be collected and assessed in every case of possible DILI during drug development:

#### Time to onset and time to resolution
These are critical components for causality assessment. Time to onset is the time from the first exposure to the drug to the first hepatic biochemical abnormality or hepatic symptoms (ie, right upper quadrant abdominal pain/discomfort, nausea, vomiting, increasing fatigue, jaundice) if they preceded the laboratory tests.[2,44] Time to resolution is the time between the discontinuation of the drug and return of hepatic biochemical test to baseline. It is critical to continue monitoring hepatic biochemical tests after drug discontinuation until they return to baseline. In the absence of accurate information on time to onset and time to resolution, assigning causality is often impossible.

#### Pattern and severity
The pattern is usually described as hepatocellular, cholestatic, or mixed based on the R value, using the first set of tests when the event meets the threshold for DILI. R is the ratio of serum activity of ALT divided by serum activity of ALP (ALT×ULN/ALP×ULN). Each activity is expressed as a multiple of ULN, and both should be measured together at the time of recognition of liver injury. Liver injury is designated hepatocellular when there is an increase greater than 3 × ULN in ALT alone or when R is 5 or greater. Liver injury is designated cholestatic when there is an increase greater than 2 × ULN in ALP alone or when R is 2 or less. Liver injury is designated mixed when there is an increase greater than 2 × ULN in ALT and an increase in ALP and R is between 2 and 5.

In addition to the pattern, it is also important to record the peak values of AT, TBL, and ALP and to define the severity of the injury based on to the existing definitions.[44]

#### Exclusion of other disorders
Exclusion of other potential causes of liver injury (see **Box 1**) is an essential part of causality assessment. The frequency of specific liver disorders varies widely

according to populations and geographies. In general, the frequency of many non–drug-related causes is often considerably higher than that of DILI. For example, although the incidence of DILI for specific drugs has typically ranged between 1:10,000 and 1:100,000, the US prevalence of hepatitis C alone is 1.8%. The prevalence of hepatitis B[45] and hepatitis E[46] in the United States is also considerably higher than that of DILI. The likelihood that abnormal hepatic biochemical tests are related to viral hepatitis is therefore relatively high, so that if specific tests for viral hepatitis have not been performed, assigning high causality to a drug is problematic at best. In 1 analysis,[47] two-thirds of cases initially reported as drug-induced chronic hepatitis were subsequently attributed to chronic hepatitis C. In the US DILIN registry,[48] 3% of the cases initially believed to be highly likely or definitely caused by DILI were later determined to be a result of acute hepatitis E infection.

In most cases of treatment-emergent liver injury, autoimmune hepatitis should be evaluated by testing for antinuclear antibody, smooth muscle antibody, immunoglobulin profile, and in certain circumstances (eg, acute hepatitis in pediatric patients), liver-kidney microsomal antibody and soluble liver/liver-pancreas antibody.[49,50] Other infectious agents such as cytomegalovirus (cytomegalovirus serology) and Epstein-Barr virus (Epstein-Barr Virus serology) should also be excluded, particularly when extrahepatic manifestations are present.

Gallstone disease is common in certain populations, and as high as 24% of cases of increased AST levels higher than 400 U/L have been shown to have an underlying pancreaticobiliary disorder on investigation.[51] Imaging to exclude biliary obstruction is therefore essential in cases of suspected DILI during clinical trials. In addition, hepatic ischemia and hypoxia caused by circulatory or cardiac failure can present with acute hepatocellular form of liver injury indistinguishable from DILI,[51] and systemic sepsis should also be considered as an alternative diagnosis in an appropriate clinical scenario.[44] In cases with increased TBL, it is imperative to consider the possibility of Gilbert syndrome, which may affect as much as 10% of the population, and may be mistakenly diagnosed as severe DILI or a Hy's Law case.

However, exclusion of all of these conditions alone does not guarantee that a drug is the causative agent underling liver injury. Acute seronegative hepatitis of unknown cause, indistinguishable from DILI, accounts for many patients developing acute liver failure even in extensively investigated cohorts.[52,53]

Other potential causes of liver injury, which need to be excluded in treatment-emergent hepatic abnormality, are herbal products and food supplements. Both are emerging as important causes of DILI, including severe liver injury and liver failure leading to liver transplantation.[54] It is important to obtain a full history regarding such products in every patient with suspected DILI.

A thorough evaluation for other causes of abnormal liver tests is critical to the process of causality assessment for suspected DILI. It is also good practice to save samples in suspected DILI cases to allow further investigations if uncertainty persists after initial evaluation.

## Risk factors

Although risk factors for DILI are often mentioned in drug labels, the role of most potential risk factors has not been clearly established and is still a matter of debate.[55,56] Furthermore, information regarding potential risk factors that may increase the susceptibility to DILI is unlikely to be known during drug development. Nevertheless, information regarding factors such as age, gender, ethnicity, body mass index, diabetes, metabolic syndrome, alcohol intake, smoking, and other comorbidity should be collected whenever possible.

## Extrahepatic features

Clinical symptoms and biochemical changes other than hepatic may be helpful in defining the phenotype or signature of a specific drug, and may be instrumental in guiding the causality assessment. For example, the presence of rash, fever, arthralgia, lymphadenopathy, or eosinophilia may be typical for certain drugs and may be helpful in differentiating liver injury caused by a particular drug from other causes. Occasionally, involvement of other organs (eg, kidney, lungs, pancreas) may point to a specific drug and assist in the causality assessment. It is therefore important to collect and document information regarding these manifestations in all cases with treatment-emergent hepatic abnormalities.

## SUMMARY

Despite ongoing efforts to develop preclinical approaches and biomarkers that would help in predicting the risk of idiosyncratic DILI in earlier phases of drug development, such approaches and biomarkers are not yet ready for prime time. Nevertheless, clinical trial databases may show evidence of the potential of a drug for severe DILI if clinical and laboratory data are properly collected, organized, and evaluated for evidence of milder liver injury. Data pertaining to milder liver injury occurring during clinical development, when assessed correctly, may enhance our ability to predict the potential of the drug to cause severe liver injury after marketing. Although increased ALT levels are a sensitive marker for hepatocellular DILI, the specificity of such increase is low, and it is generally considered a poor predictor of severe hepatotoxicity. On the other hand, the occurrence of Hy's Law cases may be a significant and specific predictor of the ability of a drug to cause severe DILI after marketing. In addition, high increases in ALT levels and increases accompanied by signs of hypersensitivity or symptoms of liver injury may also have some predictive value and should be taken seriously. To maximize the success of this approach, drug developers must use meticulous causality assessment in patients in clinical trials with treatment-emergent abnormal hepatic biochemical tests and strict hepatic discontinuation rules to prevent unnecessary early discontinuation of the study drug. Adherence to predetermined discontinuation rules is critical to a timely and thorough understanding of the hepatic safety profile of the drug.

## REFERENCES

1. Navarro VJ, Senior JR. Drug-related hepatotoxicity. N Engl J Med 2006;354(7): 731–9.
2. FDA, Guidance for industry. Drug-induced livery injury: premarketing clinical evaluation. July 2009 [online]. Available at: http://www.fda.gov/downloads/Drugs/GuidanceComplianceRegulatoryInformation/Guidances/UCM174090.pdf. Accessed December 17, 2009.
3. Goodman Z. Drug hepatotoxicity. Clin Liver Dis 2002;6(2):381–9.
4. Lewis JH, Ahmed M, Shobassy A, et al. Drug-induced liver disease. Curr Opin Gastroenterol 2006;22(3):223–33.
5. Manier JW, Chang WW, Kirchner JP, et al. Hepatotoxicity associated with ticrynafen–a uricosuric diuretic. Am J Gastroenterol 1982;77(6):401–4.
6. Zimmerman HJ, Lewis JH, Ishak KG, et al. Ticrynafen-associated hepatic injury: analysis of 340 cases. Hepatology 1984;4(2):315–23.
7. Moses PL, Schroeder B, Alkhatib ON, et al. Severe hepatotoxicity associated with bromfenac sodium. Am J Gastroenterol 1999;94(5):1393–6.

8. Hunter EB, Johnston PE, Tanner G, et al. Bromfenac (Duract)-associated hepatic failure requiring liver transplant. Am J Gastroenterol 1999;94(8):2299–301.

9. Rabkin JM, Smith MJ, Orloff SL, et al. Fatal fulminant hepatitis associated with bromfenac use. Ann Pharmacother 1999;33(9):945–7.

10. Fontana RJ, McCashland TM, Benner KG, et al. Acute liver failure associated with prolonged use of bromfenac leading to liver transplantation. Liver Transpl Surg 1999;5(6):480–4.

11. Gitlin N, Julie NL, Spurr CL, et al. Two cases of severe clinical and histologic hepatotoxicity associated with troglitazone. Ann Intern Med 1998;129(1):36–8.

12. Vella A, deGroen PC, Dinneen SF. Fatal hepatotoxicity associated with troglitazone. Ann Intern Med 1998;129(12):1080.

13. Herrine SK, Choudary C. Severe hepatotoxicity associated with troglitazone. Ann Intern Med 1999;130(2):163–4.

14. Watkins PB, Whitcomb RW. Hepatic dysfunction associated with troglitazone. N Engl J Med 1998;338:916–7.

15. Maria VA, Victorino RM. Hypersensitivity immune reaction as a mechanism for dilevalol-associated hepatitis. Ann Pharmacother 1992;26(7):924–6.

16. He R. Clinical review of exanta (ximelagatran) tablets, FDA Cardiovascular and Renal Drugs Advisory Committee Briefing Information. 2004. Available at: http://www.fda.gov/ohrms/dockets/ac/04/briefing/2004-4069B1_04_FDA-Backgrounder-MOR-180.pdf. Accessed January 20, 2013.

17. Lee WM, Larrey D, Olsson R, et al. Hepatic findings in long-term clinical trials of ximelagatran. Drug Saf 2005;28(4):351–70.

18. Senior John. Lessons from isoniazid. Would it be approved today? March, 2008. Available at: www.fda.gov/downloads/Drugs/ScienceResearch/.../ucm076755.pdf. Accessed December 12, 2012.

19. Mitchell JR, Long MW, Thorgeirsson UP, et al. Acetylation rates and monthly liver function tests during one year of isoniazid preventative therapy. Chest 1975;68(2):181–90.

20. Nolan CM, Goldberg SV, Buskin SE. Hepatotoxicity associated with isoniazid preventative therapy: a 7-year survey from a public health tuberculosis clinic. JAMA 1999;281(11):1014–8.

21. Harrill AH, Roach J, Fier I, et al. The effects of heparins on the liver: application of mechanistic serum biomarkers in a randomized study in healthy volunteers. Clin Pharmacol Ther 2012;92(2):214–20.

22. Olsson R, Korsan-Bengtsen BM, Korsan-Bengtsen K, et al. Serum aminotransferases after low-dose heparin treatment. Acta Med Scand 1978;204(3):229–30.

23. Dukes GE Jr, Sanders SW, Russo J Jr, et al. Transaminase elevations in patients receiving bovine or porcine heparin. Ann Intern Med 1984;100(5):646–50.

24. Carlson MK, Gleason PP, Sen S. Elevation of hepatic transaminases after enoxaparin use: case report and review of unfractionated and low-molecular weight heparin induced hepatotoxicity. Pharmacotherapy 2001;21(1):108–13.

25. Watkins PB, Zimmerman HJ, Knapp MJ, et al. Hepatotoxic effects of tacrine administration in patients with Alzheimer's disease. JAMA 1994;271:992–8.

26. NIDDK, LiverTox, Clinical and research information on drug-induced liver injury. Available at: http://livertox.nlm.nih.gov/Isoniazid.htm. Accessed December 20, 2012.

27. Lucena MI, Molokhia M, Shen Y, et al. Susceptibility to amoxicillin-clavulanate-induced liver injury is influenced by multiple HLA class I and II alleles. Gastroenterology 2011;141(1):338–47.

28. Kleiner DE, Gaffey MJ, Sallie R, et al. Histopathologic changes associated with fialuridine hepatotoxicity. Mod Pathol 1997;10(3):192–9.

29. Berends MA, Snoek J, De Jong J, et al. Liver injury in long-term methotrexate treatment in psoriasis is relatively infrequent. Aliment Pharmacol Ther 2006;24: 805–11.

30. Temple R. Hy's law: predicting serious hepatotoxicity. Pharmacoepidemiol Drug Saf 2006;15:241–3.

31. Zimmerman HJ. Drug-induced liver disease. In: Hepatotoxicity, the adverse effects of drugs and other chemicals on the liver. 2nd edition. Philadelphia: Lippincott Williams & Wilkins; 1999. p. 428–33.

32. Senior JR. Regulatory perspectives. In: Kaplowitz N, DeLeve LD, editors. Drug-induced liver disease. New York: Marcel Dekker; 2003. p. 739–54.

33. Björnsson E, Olsson R. Outcome and prognostic markers in severe drug-induced liver disease. Hepatology 2005;42:481–9.

34. Andrade RJ, Lucena MI, Fernandez MC, et al. Drug-induced liver injury: an analysis of 461 incidences submitted to the Spanish registry over a 10-year period. Gastroenterology 2005;129:512–21.

35. Guo T, Gelperin K, Senior J. A tool to help you decide (detect potentially serious liver injury). March 2008 [online]. Available at: http://www.fda.gov/downloads/Drugs/ScienceResearch/ResearchAreas/ucm076777.pdf. Accessed December 17, 2009.

36. Watkins PB, Desai M, Berkowitz SD, et al. Evaluation of drug-induced serious hepatotoxicity (eDISH) application of this data organization approach to phase III clinical trials of rivaroxaban after total hip or knee replacement surgery. Drug Saf 2011;34(3):243–52.

37. Chitturi S, Farrell GC. Drug induced liver disease. In: Schiff ER, Maddrey WC, Sorrell MF, editors. Schiff's diseases of the liver. 11th edition. Oxford, UK: Wiley-Blackwell; 2012. p. 703–82.

38. Danan G, Benichou C. Causality assessment of adverse reactions to drugs: I. A novel method based on the conclusions of international consensus meetings: applications to drug induced liver injury. J Clin Epidemiol 1993;46:1323–30.

39. Maria VA, Victorino AJ. Development and validation of a clinical scale for the diagnosis of drug-induced hepatitis. Hepatology 1997;26:664–9.

40. Rochon J, Protiva P, Seef LB, et al. Reliability of the Roussel Uclaf causality assessment method for assessing causality in drug-induced liver injury. Hepatology 2008;48:1175–83.

41. Papay JI, Clines D, Rafi R, et al. Drug-induced liver injury following positive drug rechallenge. Regul Toxicol Pharmacol 2009;54(1):84–90.

42. Brown G, Copeland T, Willward M, et al. Monadic testing of new products–an old problem and some partial solutions. J Mark Res Soc 1973;15:112–31.

43. Friedman HH, Amoo T. Rating the rating scales. J Market Manag 1999;9:114–23.

44. Aithal GP, Watkins PB, Andrade RJ, et al. Case definition and phenotype standardization in drug-induced liver injury. Clin Pharmacol Ther 2011;89(6):806–15.

45. Kowdley KV, Wang CC, Welch S, et al. Prevalence of chronic hepatitis B among foreign-born persons living in the United States by country of origin. Hepatology 2012;56(2):422–33.

46. Kunihom MH, Purcell RH, McQuillan GM, et al. Epidemiology of hepatitis E virus in the United States: results from the third National Health and National Health and Nutritional Examination survey, 1988-1994. J Infect Dis 2009;200:48–56.

47. Laurent-Puig P, Dussaix E, de Paillette L, et al. Prevalence of hepatitis C RNA in suspected drug induced liver injury [letter]. J Hepatol 1993;19:487–9.

48. Davern TJ, Chalasani N, Fontana RJ, et al. Acute hepatitis E infection accounts for some cases of suspected drug-induced liver injury. Gastroenterology 2011; 141:1665–72.
49. Desmet VJ, Gerber M, Hoofnagle JH, et al. Classification of chronic hepatitis: diagnosis, grading and staging. Hepatology 1994;19:1513–20.
50. Czaja AJ. Acute and acute severe (fulminant) autoimmune hepatitis. Dig Dis Sci 2013;58(4):897–914.
51. Whitehead MW, Hawkes ND, Hainsworth I, et al. A prospective study of the causes of notably raised aspartate aminotransferase of liver origin. Gut 1999; 45(1):129.
52. Bernal W, Ma Y, Smith HM, et al. The significance of autoantibodies and immunoglobulins in acute liver failure: a cohort study. J Hepatol 2007;47(5):664–70.
53. Marudanayagam R, Shanmugam V, Gunson B, et al. Aetiology and outcome of acute liver failure. HPB (Oxford) 2009;11(5):429–34.
54. Mindikoglu AL, Regev A, Schiff ER. Hepatitis B virus reactivation after cytotoxic chemotherapy: the disease and its prevention. Clin Gastroenterol Hepatol 2006; 4:1076–81.
55. Rosenberg P, Urwitz H, Johannesson A, et al. Psoriasis patients with diabetes type 2 are at high risk of developing liver fibrosis during methotrexate treatment. J Hepatol 2007;46:1111–8.
56. Chalasani N, Bjornsson E. Risk factors for idiosyncratic drug-induced liver injury. Gastroenterology 2010;138:2246–59.

# Index

*Note:* Page numbers of article titles are in **boldface** type.

Clin Liver Dis 17 (2013) 769–786
http://dx.doi.org/10.1016/S1089-3261(13)00083-4
1089-3261/13/$ – see front matter © 2013 Elsevier Inc. All rights reserved.

# United States Postal Service

## Statement of Ownership, Management, and Circulation
### (All Periodicals Publications Except Requestor Publications)

| 1. Publication Title | 2. Publication Number | 3. Filing Date |
|---|---|---|
| Clinics in Liver Disease | 0 1 6 - 7 5 7 4 | 9/14/13 |

| 4. Issue Frequency | 5. Number of Issues Published Annually | 6. Annual Subscription Price |
|---|---|---|
| Feb, May, Aug, Nov | 4 | $282.00 |

7. Complete Mailing Address of Known Office of Publication (Not printer) (Street, city, county, state, and ZIP+4®)

Elsevier Inc.
360 Park Avenue South
New York, NY 10010-1710

Contact Person
Stephen R. Bushing
Telephone (Include area code)
215-239-3688

8. Complete Mailing Address of Headquarters or General Business Office of Publisher (Not printer)

Elsevier Inc., 360 Park Avenue South, New York, NY 10010-1710

9. Full Names and Complete Mailing Addresses of Publisher, Editor, and Managing Editor (Do not leave blank)
Publisher (Name and complete mailing address)

Linda Belfus, Elsevier, Inc., 1600 John F. Kennedy Blvd. Suite 1800, Philadelphia, PA 19103-2899
Editor (Name and complete mailing address)

Kerry Holland, Elsevier, Inc., 1600 John F. Kennedy Blvd. Suite 1800, Philadelphia, PA 19103-2899
Managing Editor (Name and complete mailing address)

Adrianne Brigido, Elsevier, Inc., 1600 John F. Kennedy Blvd. Suite 1800, Philadelphia, PA 19103-2899

10. Owner (Do not leave blank. If the publication is owned by a corporation, give the name and address of the corporation immediately followed by the names and addresses of all stockholders owning or holding 1 percent or more of the total amount of stock. If not owned by a corporation, give the names and addresses of the individual owners. If owned by a partnership or other unincorporated firm, give its name and address as well as those of each individual owner. If the publication is published by a nonprofit organization, give its name and address.)

| Full Name | Complete Mailing Address |
|---|---|
| Wholly owned subsidiary of | 1600 John F. Kennedy Blvd., Ste. 1800 |
| Reed/Elsevier, US holdings | Philadelphia, PA 19103-2899 |

11. Known Bondholders, Mortgagees, and Other Security Holders Owning or Holding 1 Percent or More of Total Amount of Bonds, Mortgages, or Other Securities. If none, check box ☐ None

| Full Name | Complete Mailing Address |
|---|---|
| N/A | |

12. Tax Status (For completion by nonprofit organizations authorized to mail at nonprofit rates) (Check one)
The purpose, function, and nonprofit status of this organization and the exempt status for federal income tax purposes:
☐ Has Not Changed During Preceding 12 Months
☐ Has Changed During Preceding 12 Months (Publisher must submit explanation of change with this statement)

PS Form **3526**, September 2007 (Page 1 of 3 (Instructions Page 3)) PSN 7530-01-000-9931 PRIVACY NOTICE: See our Privacy policy in www.usps.com

| 13. Publication Title | | 14. Issue Date for Circulation Data Below |
|---|---|---|
| Clinics in Liver Disease | | August 2013 |

| 15. Extent and Nature of Circulation | | Average No. Copies Each Issue During Preceding 12 Months | No. Copies of Single Issue Published Nearest to Filing Date |
|---|---|---|---|
| a. Total Number of Copies (Net press run) | | 400 | 390 |
| b. Paid Circulation (By Mail and Outside the Mail) | (1) Mailed Outside-County Paid Subscriptions Stated on PS Form 3541. (Include paid distribution above nominal rate, advertiser's proof copies, and exchange copies) | 150 | 140 |
| | (2) Mailed In-County Paid Subscriptions Stated on PS Form 3541 (Include paid distribution above nominal rate, advertiser's proof copies, and exchange copies) | | |
| | (3) Paid Distribution Outside the Mails Including Sales Through Dealers and Carriers, Street Vendors, Counter Sales, and Other Paid Distribution Outside USPS® | 83 | 82 |
| | (4) Paid Distribution by Other Classes Mailed Through the USPS (e.g. First-Class Mail®) | | |
| c. Total Paid Distribution (Sum of 15b (1), (2), (3), and (4)) | ▶ | 233 | 222 |
| d. Free or Nominal Rate Distribution (By Mail and Outside the Mail) | (1) Free or Nominal Rate Outside-County Copies Included on PS Form 3541 | 75 | 74 |
| | (2) Free or Nominal Rate In-County Copies Included on PS Form 3541 | | |
| | (3) Free or Nominal Rate Copies Mailed at Other Classes Through the USPS (e.g. First-Class Mail) | | |
| | (4) Free or Nominal Rate Distribution Outside the Mail (Carriers or other means) | | |
| e. Total Free or Nominal Rate Distribution (Sum of 15d (1), (2), (3) and (4)) | ▶ | 75 | 74 |
| f. Total Distribution (Sum of 15c and 15e) | ▶ | 308 | 296 |
| g. Copies not Distributed (See instructions to publishers #4 (page #3)) | ▶ | 92 | 94 |
| h. Total (Sum of 15f and g) | ▶ | 400 | 390 |
| i. Percent Paid (15c divided by 15f times 100) | ▶ | 75.65% | 75.00% |

16. Publication of Statement of Ownership

☐ If the publication is a general publication, publication of this statement is required. Will be printed in the **November 2013** issue of this publication. ☐ Publication not required

17. Signature and Title of Editor, Publisher, Business Manager, or Owner

*Stephen R. Bushing*

Stephen R. Bushing – Inventory Distribution Coordinator

Date
September 14, 2013

I certify that all information furnished on this form is true and complete. I understand that anyone who furnishes false or misleading information on this form or who omits material or information requested on the form may be subject to criminal sanctions (including fines and imprisonment) and/or civil sanctions (including civil penalties).

PS Form **3526**, September 2007 (Page 2 of 3)

Printed and bound by CPI Group (UK) Ltd, Croydon, CR0 4YY

03/10/2024

01040409-0010